Bottom Line's
HEALTH 2024
BREAKTHROUGHS

Belvoir

Bottom Line's Health Breakthroughs 2024

Bottom Line Books® is an imprint of Belvoir Media Group, LLC.

Belvoir

© 2023 Belvoir Media Group, LLC.

10 9 8 7 6 5 4 3 2 1

ISBN 978-0-88723-024-0

Bottom Line Books® publishes the advice of expert authorities in many fields. These opinions may at times conflict as there are often different approaches to solving problems. The use of this material is no substitute for health, legal, accounting or other professional services. Consult competent professionals for answers to your specific questions.

Telephone numbers, addresses, prices, offers and websites listed in this book are accurate at the time of publication, but they are subject to frequent change.

Bottom Line Books® is a registered trademark of Belvoir Media Group, LLC.
535 Connecticut Avenue, Norwalk, CT 06854-1713

Belvoir.com || BottomLineInc.com

Bottom Line Books® is an imprint of Belvoir Media Group, LLC, publisher of print and digital periodicals, books and online training programs. We are dedicated to bringing you the best information from the most knowledgeable sources in the world. Our goal is to help you gain greater wealth, better health, more wisdom, extra time and increased happiness.

Printed in the United States of America

Contents

Contents

Contents

10 • GET THE BEST MEDICARE CARE

11 • INFECTIOUS DISEASE

12 • MEDICAL NEWS ALERTS

Contents

13 • MEDICATION SMARTS

14 • MEN'S HEALTH

15 • NATURAL REMEDIES AND SUPPLEMENTS

Contents

Preface

We are proud to bring you the all-new *Bottom Line's Health Breakthroughs 2024*. This collection represents a year's worth of the latest health news and scientific discoveries in a broad spectrum of fields.

When you choose a Bottom Line book, you are turning to a stellar group of experts in a wide range of specialties—medical doctors, alternative practitioners, renowned nutrition experts, research scientists, and consumer-health advocates, to name a few.

We go to great lengths to interview the foremost health experts. Whether it's cancer prevention, breakthrough arthritis treatments, or cutting-edge nutritional advice, our editors talk to the true innovators in health care.

How do we find all these top-notch professionals? Over the past 40 years, we have built a network of leading physicians in both alternative and conventional medicine. They are affiliated with the world's premier medical institutions. We follow the medical research and bring the latest information to our readers. We also regularly talk with our advisers in teaching hospitals, private practices, and government health agencies.

Bottom Line's Health Breakthroughs 2024 is a result of our ongoing research and contact with these experts, and is a distillation of their latest findings and advice. We hope that you will enjoy the presentation and glean helpful information about the health topics that concern you and your family.

As a reader of a Bottom Line book, please be assured that you are receiving reliable and well-researched information from a trusted source. But, please use prudence in health matters. Always speak to your physician before taking vitamins, supplements or over-the-counter medication…changing your diet…or beginning an exercise program. If you experience side effects from any regimen, contact your doctor immediately.

The Editors, Bottom Line Books, Norwalk, Connecticut.

CHAPTER 1

Aging Gracefully

What Happens as You Get Older

As a geriatrician who has spent 40 years treating older patients, Rosanne M. Leipzig, M.D., Ph.D, hears the same question day in and day out—"Is [XYZ symptom] a normal part of aging?" *Here's what Dr. Leipzig tells them…*

Many changes in your physical, mental, and emotional health can be chalked up to "normal" aging…and some physical and cognitive changes are inevitable. Needing assistive devices such as eyeglasses or hearing aids and occasionally losing your train of thought are to be expected as you age.

But: That doesn't mean a 75-year-old can't be full of energy and free from symptoms of most chronic diseases.

Many of these changes, such as having the occasional "senior moment"…not being able to

handle alcohol as well as decades earlier…and needing to use the bathroom several times a night may be manageable. Others, including poor vision or becoming off balance more easily, can be more concerning if they put you at risk for falls and other incidents. But only 20 percent of people age 65 and over…and 40 percent of those over 85…experience significant limitations in cognition, vision, hearing, mobility, communication, or the ability to continue caring for themselves.

Still, Dr. Leipzig does not agree with the saying, "80 is the new 60"—even though the intentions behind it are good.

Her take: Old age is a new stage of life, and it's not the same as middle age. One of the keys to healthy aging is accepting the fact that

Rosanne M. Leipzig, M.D., Ph.D., the Gerald and May Ellen Ritter Professor and Vice Chair Emerita for the Brookdale Department of Geriatrics and Palliative Medicine at Icahn School of Medicine at Mount Sinai. She is editor-in-chief of the monthly newsletter *Focus on Healthy Aging*, coeditor of the fourth edition of *Geriatric Medicine*, and author of *Honest Aging: An Insider's Guide to the Second Half of Life*. RosanneMD.com

1

humans change as the years march on—hair turns gray, weight shifts to the belly, eyesight gets weaker. You don't need to enjoy these changes, but learning your options for navigating your new normal can enhance your well-being while helping you cultivate a positive mindset.

According to researchers at Yale University School of Public Health, older adults with negative perceptions of aging performed worse on memory and hearing tests than similar older adults with positive perceptions of aging. Positive perceptions of aging also were linked with longer life span…and those extra years (7.5 to be exact) were more likely to be independent.

Ready to make peace with aging? Dr. Leipzig explains what you can expect and how to manage these changes…

CHANGE #1: Medications will affect you differently.

What's happening: The kidneys and liver play a role in processing medications. These organs change with age. Not only do they receive less blood flow, but the number of cells within the organs begin to dwindle. Both changes decrease the speed with which medications are eliminated from the body. This causes increased blood levels of medications, possibly leading to adverse drug events (ADEs) such as confusion (with common acid reducers like Tagamet and Pepcid) or hypoglycemia and fainting (with insulin). This can happen with new drugs or with drugs you've been taking for decades.

Higher-than-usual drug levels also can be caused by drug-drug interactions. Older adults often take multiple medications, some of which may no longer be needed and others that are prescribed to treat side effects from a preexisting drug. This *polypharmacy* often leads to ADEs. The more drugs you take, the greater the chance for side effects.

Lastly, aging brains often grow more sensitive to common medications, including antihistamines like *diphenhydramine* (Benadryl)… sleeping pills such as *zolpidem* (Ambien)…and muscle relaxants like *cyclobenzaprine* (Flexeril). This can lead to greater sedation than usual, confusion, and falls.

Alcohol hits harder, too. Body composition changes with age—muscle mass decreases, as does the amount of water stored in your body. Because alcohol is absorbed into the bloodstream—and blood is mostly water—this decrease in water results in an increased concentration of alcohol, so you feel every sip more than you used to. A 70-year-old liver also takes more time to metabolize wine, beer, and liquor than a 30-year-old liver.

What to do: Practice Goldilocks's motto, and take what's just right for you. Tell each of your physicians and health-care providers that you'd like to be thoughtful with your prescription regimen, and confirm that you need every medication you're prescribed and that you are taking the proper doses for your age and body composition. That includes medications that treat chronic conditions such as high blood pressure and diabetes—you may have taken them for years, but the dose you need may have changed with age. Or perhaps you've made a major lifestyle change such as losing weight or quitting smoking and no longer need a particular medication at all.

Reminder: Part of ensuring the appropriate dose also involves checking for *underdosing.*

Important: Never stop taking a drug without talking to your provider first. That may cause uncomfortable—even life-threatening—withdrawal symptoms.

CHANGE #2: You'll need to urinate more frequently.

What's happening: With age, the urge to empty the bladder often grows stronger—even with smaller volumes of urine. This can be chalked up to spasms known as *uninhibited bladder contractions* that signal the brain to void the bladder. Nighttime urination, called *nocturia,* also becomes more frequent thanks to a natural decline in production of antidiuretic hormone (ADH). Production of ADH is robust in younger adults and helps ensure that the majority of urination occurs during the daytime.

Your bladder also may not fully empty each time you urinate due to age-weakened bladder muscles…enlarged prostate in men, also called benign prostatic hyperplasia (BPH), which narrows the urethra…pelvic organ prolapse in women, in which age-weakened support structures allow the bladder or uterus to drop down into the vagina…or severe constipation, common in older years.

What to do: Use the bathroom regularly during the day. Avoid "holding it" for long periods—doing so can stretch and weaken the bladder over time. Ask your doctor for help resolving any problems with constipation. Starting around 4 p.m. each day, decrease your fluid intake, especially of alcohol and caffeinated and carbonated beverages, all of which are diuretics or bladder irritants.

Caution: Don't stop drinking altogether—that can lead to unintentional dehydration. Ask your doctor to evaluate you for pelvic organ prolapse or BPH—both conditions are treatable. If nocturia keeps you up at night, ask your doctor if any medications you are taking increase fluid retention. These include nonsteroidal anti-inflammatory drugs (NSAIDs) such as *ibuprofen* (Motrin, Advil)…neurogenic pain medications including *gabapentin* (Neurontin) and *pregabalin* (Lyrica)…and calcium channel blockers such as *amlodipine* (Norvasc) and *nifedipine* (Procardia).

What is not normal: *Consult your doctor if you experience…*

•**Urine loss without warning** (and not triggered by coughing, sneezing, laughing or movement)

  •**Inability to urinate**
  •**Blood in the urine**
  •**Sudden incontinence in a man**
  •**Pelvic pain or pain when urinating.**

CHANGE #3: Your mood may shift…but in surprising, enjoyable ways. A patient once said to me, "It seems like old people have plenty of reasons to feel down. Their lives are filled with losses, physical illnesses, problems getting around, and memory glitches. I'm only 50, but I dread getting older. How does anyone cope?"

Reality: Older adults tend to be quite content. In fact, older people tend to be better emotionally adjusted than their younger counterparts because they remember positive images and statements more than negative ones and their successes more than their mistakes… they are less likely to have strong or negative responses to major stressors and emotional events…and they are less likely to develop major depressive disorder. This isn't to say older people don't get sad or mad—they do. But thanks to what's known as the *paradox of aging*, it happens less frequently, is less intense, and fizzles out relatively quickly.

Drastic or sudden changes in personality or self-esteem usually are due to illness (stroke, Parkinson's disease, dementia)…or personal circumstances (intense grief, depression).

If you find yourself feeling sad or anxious, isolated, or like you have nothing to look forward to: It is time to talk to a professional. Ditto if you feel like your sad, mad or hopeless feelings are interfering with daily life.

One tip for boosting mood: Go outside! Force yourself to leave the house and feel the sunlight on your face. Bright light is wonderful for mood, as is exercise.

A Nutrient Found in Strawberries and Apples May Fight Aging

Matthew Yousefzadeh, Ph.D, postdoctoral fellow at the University of Minnesota. *Disclosure:* He serves as an unpaid advisor on the scientific advisory board for SRW Laboratories, which produces a supplement with fisetin.

Every cell in your body has a predetermined life span. Some cells live for a few days, while others live for decades. At the end of that life span, each cell undergoes a process called *apoptosis:* The cell breaks apart and the immune system carries the pieces away. But as we age, this system can go awry.

Enter senescent cells. These dysfunctional cells earned the nickname of *zombie cells* because they are neither alive and multiplying nor are they broken down and carted off by apoptosis. Instead, they build up and interfere with how healthy cells communicate with each other, impair the body's ability to get rid of old mitochondria (the powerhouse of the cell),

Choosing a Supplement

When choosing any supplement, including fisetin, look for a brand that has good manufacturing practice (GMP) designation. GMP is a system that ensures that products are consistently produced and controlled according to quality standards. The United States Pharmacopeia (USP), the Natural Products Association (NPA), and NSF International (NSF) are three GMP certification programs. Look for products with a seal from one of those organizations or search their databases.

USP: https://www.usp.org/reference-standards/reference-standards-catalog

NPA: https://www.npanational.org/certifications/npa-gmp-certification-program/gmp-certified-companies/

NSF: https://www.nsf.org/certified-products-systems

reduce the function of stem cells, and damage the healthy cells around them. Ultimately, they cause everything from frailty and cognitive impairment to inflammation and chronic diseases. They can even worsen viral infections like COVID-19, my colleagues and I reported in the journal *Science.*

There is research being done every day to investigate what permanently kills off these cells, and after conducting several trials and studies, we may have an answer.

SENOLYTICS AND FISETIN

Drugs and nutraceuticals called senolytics are designed to rid the body of senescent cells by inducing apoptosis. They include *dasatinib* (a cancer drug), *quercetin*, and *fisetin*. The latter two are plant flavonols. *Fisetin, the more powerful of the two, can be found in many fruits and vegetables…*

- **strawberries:** 160 microgram/gram (µg/g)
- **apples:** 26 µg/g
- **persimmons:** 10.6 µg/g
- **onions:** 4.8 µg/g
- **grapes:** 3.9 µg/g
- **kiwi fruit:** 2.0 µg/g

A healthy diet that contains fruits and vegetables that are high in fisetin is extremely beneficial and will result in positive long-term effects for your body. But it is difficult to get the amount needed to get rid of senescent cells through food alone, so a senolytic or nutraceutical supplement might be beneficial.

Supplements are available in 100- to 500-mg strengths, but there are no human studies on the most effective dosage. Animal trials suggest that range is safe, but more human trials are needed. It's important that you consult with your doctor before beginning any supplement. (See the sidebar for more safety tips.)

Key to Healthy Aging— Friendship

Marisa G. Franco, Ph.D., psychologist, speaker, and assistant clinical professor at University of Maryland, College Park. She is author of *Platonic: How the Science of Attachment Can Help You Make—and Keep—Friends.* DrMarisaGFranco.com

A good friend can be hard to find—especially in your older years. Friendships form frequently—and quite easily—in childhood, but they are relatively rare in adulthood, leaving many older adults lonely. This doesn't just detract from their social lives…it can significantly impact their health.

Researchers at BYU who examined the results of 148 published longevity studies concluded that when it comes to living a long life, having a large social network matters even more than exercising or losing weight.

Meanwhile, a study by psychologists at the University of Illinois and University of Pennsylvania found that the most pronounced difference between happy and unhappy people was not whether good or bad things happened to them—it was their level of social connection.

Fortunately, it is possible to form new friendships during adulthood—even if you aren't naturally outgoing. It just takes a little more effort than it did when you were a kid.

DON'T WAIT FOR FRIENDSHIP

School was an excellent setting for friendship formation when we were kids. Sociologist Rebecca Adams, Ph.D., has said that we're especially likely to form friendships with people with whom we have repeated unplanned interactions that include shared vulnerability. We had that with our classmates, but it's rare in the adult world.

It may be surprising to learn that vulnerability plays a critical role in forming friendship—vulnerability is widely viewed as dangerous and best avoided, especially by men. But the risks associated with showing vulnerability in social settings are greatly outweighed by the benefits that vulnerability offers in the form of strengthened social bonds. A series of studies conducted by researchers at Florida State, Yale, and Carnegie Mellon universities found that participants who shared their negative emotions, such as nervousness about an upcoming project, received more assistance and formed more friendships than those who didn't.

All of this is good news for adults—we don't lose our ability to form new friendships as we age...we just need to find new ways to display the vulnerability that was unavoidable in school and then do so with people with whom we interact regularly.

THE RIGHT KIND OF VULNERABLE

Most people respond positively to vulnerability, but some instead pull away or seek to exploit the situation. To gauge who will respond well, ask acquaintances unconventional, probing questions outside the bounds of normal small talk.

Examples: "What would constitute a perfect day?" or "Among everyone in the world, whom would you want as a dinner guest?" People who respond to questions such as these openly also tend to respond well to vulnerability...while people who become evasive or judgmental tend to be "avoidant" and respond poorly to vulnerability.

Caution: Attempts to be vulnerable also fail when people overshare, burying acquaintances under laundry lists of painful personal details. Vulnerability facilitates friendship most effectively when it's limited in scope. *How to be vulnerable...*

•**Open up about one thing you've struggled with recently.** This could be "I'm having the hardest time staying on a diet" or "I haven't been able to figure out this new client."

•**Share your joy about one positive aspect of your life.** Perhaps "I'm really proud of how well my daughter has done for herself" or "I worked hard my whole career so I could afford this car—and I love it." This is a form of vulnerability because we're opening up about something that matters to us and trusting that the people we're speaking with won't consider us braggarts. Moderation is key.

•**Voice a positive opinion about the person you're speaking to.** This could be "You always have something intelligent to say" or "I'm so blown away with your sense of style." Complimenting people who are not yet close friends shows vulnerability because we can't be certain how our praise will be received.

WHAT PREVENTS POTENTIAL FRIENDSHIPS

Have you ever stood quietly in a corner at a social gathering and wondered, Why is everyone here so unfriendly? They probably weren't unfriendly—they feared social rejection. By standing in a corner not speaking, you send a signal that you're the sort of antisocial person likely to reject anyone who approaches.

To escape this trap: Be the friend you want to meet. If you wish someone would strike up a conversation, walk up to someone else and strike up a conversation. If you wish someone would say something nice about you, say something nice about someone else.

Reassure yourself that most people probably like you more than you think—and there's science to prove it. Participants in a study conducted by Cornell University researcher Erica Boothby, Ph.D., were asked to interact with strangers. The study participants later were asked how much they liked the people they met...and to estimate how much the people they met liked them. Virtually everyone reported thinking others liked them less than others actually did. In other words, virtually everyone underestimates how much other people like them—and that probably includes you.

Socializing Is More Protective for Your Health Than Exercise

In a landmark study conducted at Brigham Young University in Utah, Julianne Holt-Lunstad, Ph.D., and her colleagues analyzed data from 148 other studies on social relationships, involving more than 300,000 people. The results proved the importance of socializing for better health and longevity. Strong social relationships were linked to a 50 percent increased likelihood of living rather than dying during the study period, which averaged 7.5 years. *To put that finding in perspective, strong social relationships may be significantly more protective of longer life than…*

- **Regular exercise**
- **Maintaining normal weight**
- **Getting a flu vaccine**
- **Taking medication for high blood pressure**
- **Cardiac rehabilitation** (exercise therapy) after a heart attack.

One lifestyle change that strong social relationships didn't beat was quitting smoking. The two factors were equally protective. Looked at another way, weak social relationships were as risky to long life as smoking 15 cigarettes a day.

Julianne Holt-Lunstad, Ph.D., professor of psychology and neuroscience and director of the social neuroscience lab at Brigham Young University in Provo, Utah. She is the founding scientific chair for the U.S. Coalition to End Social Isolation and Loneliness, and the Foundation for Social Connection.

TO IDENTIFY POTENTIAL FRIENDS

Our odds of forming successful friendships are greatest with certain sorts of people…

- **Fellow members of groups and clubs that meet regularly.** Not only do these organizations bring together people who share common interests, they're a way to take advantage of the mere exposure effect. People who see us regularly are predisposed to like us—even if we've never spoken to them. Researchers at the University of Pittsburgh put this to the test—they instructed strangers to show up in college classes but not interact with anyone else. When other students in those classes later were shown photos of these strangers, they expressed more favorable opinions about the strangers who had been in their classes most often—even though they'd never spoken with them and often couldn't recall where they'd seen them before.

- **Neighbors.** A study conducted by a University of California, San Francisco, researcher found that the higher the cost of continuing a friendship in terms of resources such as time, the greater the odds that the friendship will fail. Someone who lives five minutes from your house is thus a better friendship candidate than someone who lives a half-hour away.

- **People who display signs of social acceptance.** If a conversation partner smiles… leans slightly toward you…and nods his/her head as you speak, those are signals he's on the same page as you, greatly improving the odds he's interested in forming a friendship.

#1 Cause of Senior Falls

Brad Manor, Ph.D., associate scientist, Hinda and Arthur Marcus Institute for Aging Research, and assistant professor of medicine, Harvard Medical School, writing at Health.Harvard.edu/blog.

Dual-tasking—standing or walking while also doing a separate mental or physical task—is the most common cause of falls among older adults, according to recent research. Standing and walking require more cognitive effort as people age, leaving less cognition available for other tasks. Moving while trying to read, talk, or carry a cup of coffee increases fall risk.

Safer: Pay attention to surroundings…minimize distractions when walking on uneven pavement, in a crowded room or when in a hurry…try to avoid talking while moving…improve balance with mind-body exercises such as dancing, tai chi, or yoga.

How to Prevent a Dangerous Fall

Patricia A. Quigley, Ph.D., MPH, APRN, past president of the Association of Rehabilitation Nurses, clinical nurse specialist, and a nurse practitioner in rehabilitation based in Saint Petersburg, Florida. Dr. Quigley is a leading expert on falls and served as the principal or co-investigator in more than 35 research studies.

Take the following anti-fall precautions to prevent not only injury but also fear of falling, which can push you toward a sedentary lifestyle…

•**Be realistic about your physical abilities.** Climbing ladders to clean gutters or trim trees even though you shouldn't can lead to debilitating falls.

•**Don't multitask.** It is easy to not pay attention to your surroundings…and multitasking often means you don't have a hand free to break a fall.

•**Compensate for sensory changes.** Particularly if you have diabetes, changes in sensation in your feet can cause changes to your gait. Talk to your doctor about blood sugar control, medication, and exercises to increase circulation to the nerves in your feet. Mention any tingling you feel at night. Always wear appropriate shoes (with a closed toe and heel).

•**Have your depth perception and visual acuity checked at eye exams.** A loss of depth perception affects how you see your environment.

Also: Going down stairs poses a greater risk than going up. Be cautious for a few weeks when your eyeglass prescription changes.

•**Schedule a medication review.** Discuss with your health-care provider(s) alternatives to drugs that increase your fall risk because of dizziness, confusion, and changes in balance. When you're prescribed a new drug or a dosage, ask if it could increase your fall risk.

•**Get evaluated for causes of dizziness.** These include vertigo, and postural hypotension, which occurs when you stand after sitting or lying down. Always report these to your provider.

•**Manage urge incontinence and frequent nighttime urination.** Slow your gait to avoid falling on the way to the bathroom. Get proper lighting along the way to the toilet. Talk to your doctor about stopping liquids after 7 p.m. and trying "prompted voiding" (urinating before your bladder is full).

•**Safeguard your sleeping environment.** Switch to a nightstand with rounded corners, and place a thick nonskid floor mat along your bedside if you do not have carpet.

•**Get a strength assessment.** Do you need to push off the sofa or grab the sink to pull yourself up from the toilet? You might be compensating for muscle weakness or limitations from arthritis, chronic back, hip or knee pain, and other conditions. Physical therapy can address these mobility limitations…or you may need assistive devices such as grab bars, a cane, or a walker.

•**Consider protective clothing and devices.** There are slim styles of padded hip protectors and wearable smart belts that sense a fall and deploy an airbag to reduce impact. Smartwatches can detect when you fall and call for help. MedicAlert.org offers wearable IDs and a subscription membership service that stores your health profile and activates an emergency response in case you fall.

How to Avoid Fatal Fractures

Jacqueline Center, Ph.D, co-lead of the Skeletal Diseases Program at Garvan Institute of Medical Research, Sydney, Australia, and conjoint professor at the School of Medicine at University of New South Wales. She is coauthor of the paper "Association of Multimorbidity and Excess Mortality After Fractures Among Danish Adults," published in *JAMA Network Open*. Garvan.org.au

A broken rib or upper-arm bone might be more than a painful inconvenience. For some, it could increase the odds of dying in the months that follow. It is known that older adults' mortality rates rise following hip fractures, but new research from Australia's University of New South Wales, University of Southern Denmark, and elsewhere found that other broken bones are associated with elevated mortality risks as well—and some older adults are at far greater risk than others.

In addition to hips, broken ribs, vertebrae and upper-arm and upper-leg bones are associated with increased mortality rates. Breaks to bones located farther from the torso, including hands, feet, ankles, wrists, and forearms, were not associated with increased mortality rates.

Who is most at risk? Post-fracture fatality rates are greatest among adults who have preexisting health problems such as diabetes, cancer, cardiovascular and—for men but not women—liver/inflammatory disease. But not every patient who has one of these preexisting issues is at elevated risk following a fracture—patients who have multiple serious health issues are in the most danger.

Example: Otherwise healthy people with diabetes without any associated complications may have post-fracture fatality rates similar to those of people without diabetes…but diabetics who also suffer from associated heart or kidney disease are at far greater risk.

What to do: Adults over age 50 who have multiple serious chronic health issues should take an aggressive approach to fracture prevention—discuss balance and bone-strength concerns and treatment options with doctors ideally before breaking a bone in a fall and certainly after a break.

Problem: Doctors sometimes fail to prescribe osteoporosis medications to patients who have multiple major health issues—bone strength seems like the least of these patients' problems. But the elevated post-fracture fatality risk suggests that osteoporosis medication could be a potential lifesaver.

Even relatively healthy older adults who experience fractures to bones in or near the torso as a result of falls should discuss bone strength and balance concerns with their doctors. In fact, have these conversations even if the fracture is to an extremity. A broken hand or foot isn't directly associated with elevated risk of dying, but any break is associated with increased odds of broken bones in the years ahead—the next fracture might be more problematic.

Your Pelvic Floor

John O.L. DeLancey, M.D., eminent pelvic floor authority, Norman F. Miller professor of gynecology at University of Michigan Medical School, Ann Arbor, and director of Pelvic Floor Research in the university's department of obstetrics and gynecology. UMich.edu

A well-functioning pelvic floor is important for both men and women for a number of reasons, all of which are easier to understand once you know where it sits within the body.

The pelvic floor is a sheet of muscles known as the *levator ani* with openings that allow canals, such as the urethra and the rectum, to pass through. There are sphincter muscles that squeeze these canals closed when you aren't eliminating. The pelvic floor provides structural support to keep your organs, including the bowel and bladder—and the prostate for men and the vagina and uterus for women—in place when you jump, run, sneeze, cough, and more. It is also essential for the stability of your spine and for good posture and is involved in sexual performance.

To identify exactly where your pelvic floor is: The next time you're on the toilet—and your bladder is not overly full—deliberately stop the flow of urine just for a second (you will be using the same muscles used to prevent passing gas). Think of pulling up as opposed to pushing down.

Other ways to know if you've activating the right muscles: Sit on an arm of a couch. When you tighten the pelvic floor, you should feel your bottom lift up. Or sit on a cushion with a button and try to "pick up" the button with your butt.

When the pelvic floor doesn't function optimally, you can experience incontinence, pelvic organ prolapse (when an organ, such as the uterus or the rectum, starts to come out of the body), and/or pain during sex for women and erectile dysfunction in men.

Common causes of a weak pelvic floor include…

•**Old age.** As with other parts of the body, your pelvic floor simply may not work as well as it did when you were 30 years old.

•**Childbirth.** Part of the levator ani can be torn during vaginal delivery and, unfortunately, the tear can't be repaired, but healing, along with strengthening the other muscle sections, can help compensate.

•**Enlarged prostate or prostate surgery.** Both can create challenges that the pelvic floor must deal with and lead to a weak urine stream or incontinence.

•**Strenuous exercise.** Athletes—in particular, runners and weightlifters—who do intense exercise that puts significant demands on the pelvic floor may experience weakness and its negative effects.

Example: Many female athletes on major university basketball teams leak urine when they play because the sport's intense bouncing stresses the pelvic floor. While this isn't damaging, it puts extreme demands on the system.

•**Obesity.** Excess body fat presses down on the pelvic floor and can stress its muscle and ligaments. Studies show that losing as little as 15 pounds can reduce incontinence.

REENGAGING YOUR PELVIC FLOOR

You can train your pelvic muscles to engage when you need them, easing urine leakage and other symptoms of a weak pelvic floor. You may have heard about Kegel exercises, but there are some misconceptions about how these help...how often to do them...and how to do them correctly.

What they are: Kegel exercises involve isolating the internal pelvic muscles and contracting them to activate and strengthen them. Contracting, or engaging, the pelvic floor is different from weight training a large muscle group.

To understand the difference: You might strengthen your leg muscles to have the stamina needed to walk a golf course, but if you want to improve your putting, you aren't heading to the weight room—you're going to develop that skill so that, over time, it becomes a positive habit that takes over when needed. This is especially helpful if you have bladder leakage that's bothersome but not to the point of requiring surgery.

There are many different approaches to pelvic floor training, but two are most successful...

•**The "Knack."** Janis Miller, Ph.D., a nurse practitioner and researcher at the University of Michigan, suggests contracting the pelvic floor muscles in the moment, say when you're about to cough or sneeze, to prevent leakage, rather than doing the exercises at set times during the day when you might not have any leakage risk. This technique is referred to as "the Knack maneuver"—you get into the habit of engaging that muscle at the precise time you need it. Once you get the knack of doing it purposefully and skillfully, your body may do it instinctively.

Try it out before you need it: Pull your pelvic floor up and in, do a fake cough, and then relax your pelvic floor. Do this consistently whenever you feel an imminent leakage trigger coming on.

To determine if you are doing it right: Dr. Miller's website, MyConfidentBladder.org,

---

Pelvic Pain Syndrome

It's possible to have tightness, spasms, and pain emanating from the pelvic floor and from some of the same things that cause weakness—childbirth, aging, and obesity. Pelvic pain syndrome affects primarily women, but men may experience it as well. (It is unclear what comes first—does pain make the muscle spastic...or is a spastic muscle responsible for the pain?)

A physical therapist can help, although it may take some research to find one who is trained to work with the male pelvic floor.

The American Physical Therapy Association has a searchable database (APTA.org), but also ask any therapist you contact if he/she is familiar with and treats pelvic pain.

Also: The Australia-based PelvicPain.org has a one-minute relaxation technique for men—think of it as reverse Kegels—on its website at PelvicPain.org.au (click on For Men under the Learn drop-down menu).

—John O.L. DeLancey, M.D.

The Eight-Glass Myth

The idea that everyone needs to drink eight glasses of water a day stemmed from an old recommendation to prevent dehydration in the elderly. But the advice was co-opted by marketers pushing bottled water, and now many people are flooding themselves with fluids that can aggravate incontinence. If you're eating high-water-content fruits and vegetables, cereal with milk at breakfast, maybe a cup of soup at lunch or dinner, plus tea or coffee, you don't need eight glasses of water on top of it. If your body needs more water, your thirst will tell you so!

offers a simple way to test if you're contracting correctly and how well it's working as well as many other practical ways to reduce or eliminate incontinence. The paper towel test is done with a modestly full bladder. Place three or four stacked paper towels against the urethra, cough three times without contracting the pelvic floor, and see how much wetness is on the towel, circling the wet area with a marker. Then repeat this using fresh paper towels and tightening the muscles as you cough, again circling any wetness with the marker. Compare the circles—if the wet area is reduced, you're doing the Knack maneuver correctly.

More detailed training program: Another successful approach has been created by Kari Bø, Ph.D., exercise scientist and professor at Norwegian School of Sport Sciences in Norway. She has studied the pelvic floor extensively and works with patients who have an exercise lifestyle, are committed to keeping their body in shape, and want to improve bladder weakness and/or sexual performance. You have to be highly motivated to improve your pelvic floor with her programs, but research has found that people who do her training for 20 minutes three times a week experience noticeable results.

For a 34-minute video on pelvic floor work: Go to https://bit.ly/2xrccnt.

For specific help with pelvic prolapse: Go to https://bit.ly/3Nm3N6r.

WHEN EXERCISE ISN'T ENOUGH

If contracting the pelvic floor on your own isn't helping, work with a physical therapist who has special training in pelvic floor issues. Specialists who can help are urogynecologists, ob-gyns with three years of additional training, and, for men, urologists. You can look for one at VoicesForPFD.org/find-a-provider.

Routines Keep Older Adults Happier and Their Brains Sharper

Study of 1,800 people over age 65 by researchers at University of Pittsburgh, published in *JAMA Psychiatry*.

According to recent research, older adults who got up before 7 a.m. and stayed active for 15 hours or more daily (37.6 percent of participants) were happiest, less depressed, and scored highest for cognitive function. Participants who also had consistent activity patterns but for an average 13.4 hours per day (32.6 percent of participants) had more depression symptoms and poorer cognition than the most active group. The remaining 29.8 percent of those studied had erratic periods of activity and inconsistent daily life patterns...and scored lowest for both happiness and cognition. The research suggests that it is not just staying active that keeps us mentally and physically fit as we age, but also having consistent routines for activity.

Eat Less to Live More

Susan B. Racette, Ph.D, professor of medicine in the Department of Medicine at Washington University School of Medicine in St. Louis, Missouri. Dr. Racette is a contributing author to 18 studies on CALERIE, the first randomized, controlled trial of calorie restriction in non-obese people.

If you've ever tried to lose weight (and most of us have), you're familiar with calorie restriction (CR) or eating less than you usually do to shed extra pounds. Over the last 90 years, scientists have investigated CR for another purpose: to see if it slows aging and adds extra years to the average life span.

In fact, a scientific paper that was published in the *Journal of Nutrition* goes so far as to say that—because aging is the leading risk factor for chronic diseases and disability—CR for slower aging is "the most important health intervention that has ever been studied."

CR IN THE LAB

The first research on CR and aging was published in 1935 by Clive McCay, Ph.D., a professor at Cornell University. He found that feeding rats a calorie-restricted diet with adequate vitamins and minerals nearly doubled their life span.

Since then, there have been similar findings in fruit flies, worms, rodents, and non-human primates like rhesus monkeys—with most research showing significant increases in life span. CR doesn't just support *longer* life in animal models: It also supports *healthier* life as an organism ages.

But fruit flies and worms aren't people. Would calorie restriction have the same effects in us humans?

CR IN HUMANS

To find out, scientists conducted so-called "observational" studies on people who had chosen CR as a lifestyle (such as members of the Calorie Restriction Society). Investigators found very low levels of cholesterol and triglycerides, very low blood pressure, levels of inflammation 20 times lower than normal, and hearts that resembled those of people 17 years younger.

But there had never been a rigorous study of the effects of calorie restriction in people who weren't obese until the CALERIE Trials, the largest and most systematic examinations of prolonged CR in nonobese people. The most recent study was CALERIE 2. This two-year study involved 220 people: 145 who participated in CR and 75 who were eating a normal diet. The participants were 21 to 50 years old, healthy, and of normal weight. The study aimed to cut calories by 25 percent in the participants' diets, but participants averaged a reduction of 11.9 percent. That's a reduction of

---

See Your Doctor Before Restricting Calories

It's good to have regular physical checkups if you decide to practice daily calorie restriction. Risks include anemia and decreased bone density. However, CALERIE scientists say the loss of bone mass in CR may simply accompany weight loss and isn't a health problem. Also, if you've had an eating disorder of any kind, you shouldn't practice calorie restriction.

---

about 300 calories a day in the recommended calorie intake for an adult man (2,500 calories) and a reduction of about 240 calories in the recommended intake for an adult woman (2,000 calories).

Even with an 11.9 percent reduction, the benefits were remarkable.

MANY BENEFITS OF CR

In a recent issue of the journal *Nutrition Reviews*, a team of CALERIE 2 researchers summarized the many benefits of an 11.9 percent calorie restriction.

•**Weight loss.** Although they weren't overweight, people in the CR group lost an average of 10 percent of their body weight. They lost body fat generally and abdominal fat in particular. Reductions in abdominal fat are linked to a lower risk of heart disease and type 2 diabetes.

•**Less oxidation.** The CR group participants had lower levels of several key markers of oxidation, a kind of cell- and tissue-destroying inner rust that is linked to chronic disease.

•**Slower aging.** The researchers used two algorithms to estimate the rate of biological aging or deterioration of tissues and body systems and found that the control group was aging nearly seven times faster than the CR group.

•**Less inflammation.** Low-level, chronic inflammation is linked to many chronic diseases, and the CR group had a 40 to 50 percent average reduction in two biomarkers of inflammation.

•**Lower insulin resistance.** Insulin is the hormone that ushers glucose (blood sugar) out of the bloodstream and into the cells. Insulin resistance—where the hormone's action is blocked—is linked to increased risk for type 2 diabetes, cardiovascular disease, cancer, and a shorter life. The CR group had a 20 to 30 percent reduction in insulin resistance.

•**Better blood fats.** After 24 months, the CR group had lower "bad" LDL cholesterol and higher "good" HDL cholesterol, while the control group had no changes. The CR group also had lower levels of triglycerides, another heart-hurting blood fat.

•**Lower blood pressure.** The CR group had a significant drop of both systolic (upper reading) and diastolic (lower reading) blood pressure.

•**Healthier livers.** The CR group had improvement in several biomarkers of liver health.

•**Improved immunity.** The thymus gland generates the T-cells that help fight off infectious microbes, like viruses and bacteria. After two years, the CR group had healthier glands with less fat and more volume.

•**Improved mood.** The CR group had improvements in mood, tension, and anxiety, compared with the control group.

•**Better memory.** The CR group had greater improvements in working memory—the ability to work with information without losing track of what you're doing.

•**More regulated eating.** The CR group had a better ability to regulate food intake, particularly in social settings and during physical discomfort.

•**Higher sex drive, better relationships.** The CR group had a small improvement in sex drive and the quality of their relationships, compared with the control group.

GETTING STARTED

Implementing CR is a two-step process: 1) figuring out how many calories you eat on average; 2) cutting calories.

1. Determine daily calories. There are many apps for both Android and iPhone

---

Calorie-Cutting Strategies

Several strategies have been effective in weight-loss studies…

•**Cut out calories from beverages.** Stick with black coffee, tea, and water, and limit diet sodas to no more than two per day. (Diet sodas increase sugar cravings.)

•**Limit highly processed foods—particularly fast foods.** Processed foods are loaded with calories, increase hunger and cravings, and increase inflammation.

•**Eat more vegetables, fruits, and legumes.** Eating more whole, nutrient-dense foods will help you displace the processed foods in your diet.

•**Use time-restricted eating.** In this dietary strategy, you eat only during a limited period of the day (four to 10 hours), such as 8 a.m. to 6 p.m., or noon to 8 p.m., which helps restrict calorie intake.

•**Choose spices over sauces.** Spices can make food flavorful without the fat.

•**Use smaller plates.** Studies show that the size of your plate affects the portions that you eat.

•**Eat a salad or low-calorie soup before your meal.** You'll feel fuller faster and be less likely to overeat. Instead of pouring dressing over your salad, put it in a small bowl on the side and dip your fork before each bite.

•**Doggy bag it.** When eating out, ask for half of your meal to be placed into a take-out container to enjoy later.

•**Cook light.** Replace oil frying with air frying, steaming, grilling, and broiling.

---

that help you determine your current calorie count, such as MyFitnessPal, Lose It, FatSecret, Cronometer, and Noom. MyFitnessPal, for example, has a database that includes 5 million foods, including many restaurant foods. Track your calories for seven days to create a daily average. Now you're ready to reduce calories by around 12 percent.

2. Reduce daily calories. In CALERIE 2, the researchers found that reducing calories was very individualized, with different dietary strategies working for different people. (See the sidebar on previous page for some suggestions.) Once you've put your strategies in place, continue to track your daily calories so you're sure they're reduced by approximately 12 percent.

Save Your Sight

Jeffrey Anshel, OD, optometrist, founder, and past president of the Ocular Wellness and Nutrition Society and author or coauthor of *Smart Medicine for Your Eyes, What You Must Know About Age-Related Macular Degeneraton* and the recently published *What You Must Know About Eyestrain.*

Are you noticing changes to your vision with each passing year—nearsightedness or cloudy or blurry vision? Some of this is normal—but some changes are more serious than others. We asked Jeffrey Anshel, OD, what changes to look for...and what you can do to preserve your vision.

•**Presbyopia,** a loss of focusing ability, commonly starts around age 40 and is most noticeable among people who hadn't needed vision correction earlier. Presbyopia makes it harder to read at a distance of 16 inches—where we tend to hold reading material—and difficult to make out small print. (If you're nearsighted, you probably know that taking off your glasses and holding the print closer to your eyes makes it more legible.) Presbyopia occurs because the lens of the eye becomes less flexible over time, hampering focusing ability. *What to do...*

•Wear reading glasses—but not drugstore "readers." These cause eyestrain—both lenses are the same power, while your eyes might require different powers...they don't correct for astigmatism...and the "optical center" of each lens likely will not align properly with the distance between your eyes.

•If you already wear glasses, talk to your eye doctor about a prescription for multifocal or progressive lenses, so you won't have to switch glasses for reading and distance.

•If you wear contacts, you can wear reading glasses over your lenses. Or try multifocal contact lenses or monovision correction with one contact lens for near vision, the other for distance.

•For computer work, try occupational progressive lenses that correct intermediate- and near-vision. Typical "reading lenses" are single-vision only and so may not be the correct prescription for computer work.

To avoid eyestrain from your screens: Relieve your eyes with the 20-20-20 rule—every 20 minutes, take 20 seconds to look 20 feet away.

To make reading easier in general: Improve your lighting...choose a large-print format...use an e-reader that lets you adjust the lighting and font size...and listen to audiobooks on occasion.

•**Night driving can be challenging for people with presbyopia.**

Possible solution: If you wear monovision contact lenses, ask your doctor to place a prescription lens for distance in an eyeglass frame on only the side that matches up to your near-vision contact lens (the lens in the other side of the frame remains clear). This way, you will have both eyes corrected for distance vision. Wear these glasses over your contacts when driving.

•**Dry eye occurs when your tear glands don't work well.** It's most common in women over 40 because tear production is linked to estrogen production, so women may experience it throughout and after menopause. Symptoms vary with the type of dry eye—your eyes might produce fewer tears...or your tears may evaporate quickly, leaving you with a gritty, stinging or burning feeling and then you may make too many tears in response. *What to do...*

•Over-the-counter eyedrops such as Systane may soothe your eyes temporarily, but ask your eye doctor about specific lubricating eyedrops or ointments.

Three prescription medications for dry eyes: Restasis, Xiidra, and Cequa.

Caution: Do not use eye "whiteners," which, surprisingly, can make your eye red and uncomfortable in the long term.

•Take supplements such as MaxiTears Pro, HydroEye, and EZ Tears. There are over-the-counter versions of these, but ask your doctor which nutritional supplements he/she recommends for dry eyes—he may write a prescription.

•Switch to daily disposable lenses if you wear contacts—they will be more comfortable than monthlies.

•Use a humidifier in your bedroom and, if possible, at work to add moisture to the air…or try an air purifier to remove irritants that bother your eyes—some devices do both. If your house is very dry, a whole-house humidifier will have a big impact, though it must be installed by an HVAC professional.

•**Age-related macular degeneration (AMD).** This disorder stems from changes to the macula, the small central portion of the retina, and causes vision to become blurred or distorted. There are two types of AMD—dry and wet.

•Dry AMD is more common and occurs as the macula thins with advancing age. It progresses over years through three stages—early, intermediate, and late. There's no treatment for late stage, so catching it early is imperative.

•Wet AMD, caused by damage to the macula from abnormal blood vessel growth in the back of the eye, is always considered late stage and causes faster vision loss, but there are treatments.

What to do…

•**Take OTC supplements known as the AREDS2 formula**—named for the "Age-Related Eye Disease Study 2." The formula contains specific amounts of vitamin C, vitamin E, zinc, copper, lutein, and zeaxanthin. These supplements can slow the advance of both types of AMD (they do not prevent the condition).

•**Injections into the eye of biologic drugs,** such as *bevacizumab* and *aflibercept,* may help some cases of wet AMD. While the injections are not painful, advances may soon reduce the frequency of the injections from every six to eight weeks to just twice a year.

•**Cataracts** are cloudy areas in the lens that prevent light from passing through to the back of the eye. The result is blurry or hazy vision that worsens over time—you may not even realize it is happening at first.

Why it happens: The lens gets nutrients, including vitamin C, from a fluid in the eye called *aqueous humor.* As the lens thickens with age, it's difficult for it to get those nutrients and it starts to lose transparency. Some cataracts stay small and don't impact vison, but if yours interfere with your lifestyle, cataract surgery can replace the clouded lens with a clear plastic one.

Reminder: Even though cataract surgery is the most common surgery performed by ophthalmic surgeons in the U.S., it does have risk. Some conditions, including dry eye, may get worse after the procedure. But it usually is worth the risk because your vision will continue to decline as the cataract gets denser.

•**Glaucoma.** This threat to vision is more commonly linked to the aqueous humor—when this fluid can't drain properly, it builds up, increasing pressure in the eye and causing optic nerve damage. Types of glaucoma include "open angle" with no early symptoms and "closed angle" with symptoms that come on quickly, including eye pain, redness, and blurred vision as well as a severe headache, nausea, and vomiting. If either type of glaucoma progresses unchecked, it can lead to vision loss and, ultimately, irreversible blindness. *What to do…*

•Prescription eyedrops sometimes can control glaucoma, though laser treatment or surgery may be needed.

•The combination supplement Mitrogenol, which contains French maritime pine bark (Pycnogenol) and bilberry extract, has been found by some studies to enhance traditional treatments. Talk to your doctor.

•Control your blood sugar if you have diabetes. Some studies have pointed to a greater risk for open-angle glaucoma among people with diabetes.

•**Floaters and flashes.** Nearly everyone has floaters, pieces of cells stuck inside the eye, but they're not always noticeable or can be ignored.

Why they occur: Before you're born, blood vessels grow through the center of the eye and then dissolve to leave the area clear. Some cells remain suspended in the vitreous humor, a gel that sits between the lens and the retina. You may see floaters when you're facing a bright wall or ceiling or staring at a display screen. Because the gel softens as you get older, you're likely to see them more often.

Beware: Suddenly seeing floaters along with flashes of light in the front of an eye can signal a detached retina. See an eye-care specialist immediately. If the retina loses its connection to the brain, you may lose all vision permanently.

•**Diabetic retinopathy.** Diabetes risk tends to increase with age—about 25 percent of Americans over age 60 have this chronic disease. When diabetes is uncontrolled, one of the many complications is diabetic retinopathy, when blood vessels can't nourish the retina properly. There are no warning signs in the early stages, but as it progresses, you may experience cloudiness or blind spots in your field of vision. Ultimately, blood vessels can bleed into the eye, leading to significant vision loss or even blindness.

What to do: Controlling blood sugar is essential. If you develop swelling of the retina, caused by poor integrity of the blood vessels, treatment may involve injections and/or laser therapy.

What to Do About Dry Eye Disease

Esen Karamursel Akpek, M.D., professor of ophthalmology at the Johns Hopkins University School of Medicine. Dr. Akpek is the director of the Ocular Surface Disease and Dry Eye Clinic at the Wilmer Eye Institute at Johns Hopkins and has led numerous studies on dry eye disease.

Anyone with a television has heard of dry eye, thanks to decades of commercials for prescription dry-eye treatments.

The condition is very common: Up to 30 percent of people over age 55 have dry-eye symptoms, such as frequent stinging, burning, grittiness, blurry vision, fluctuating vision, redness, or pain. About half of those people, if thoroughly checked by an eye doctor, turn out to have clear physical signs of dry eye, meaning they don't produce enough tears or tears of good enough quality, or they have damage to the cornea, the clear, dome-shaped window on the front of the eye.

But many people with dry eye never get properly diagnosed, so they don't benefit from a growing list of effective treatments. Those treatments include not only prescription medications, but also some helpful procedures and lifestyle changes.

Some people with dry eye disease also have another serious condition that causes the dryness, such as autoimmune diseases, most common of which is Sjogren's syndrome. A delay in diagnosis can have especially serious consequences for them.

In any case, untreated dry eye can interfere with reading, driving, and any other activity that requires clear, comfortable, consistent vision.

DIAGNOSIS

Even if you get regular eye exams, dry eye can go unnoticed. That's because your eye doctor can't tell you have the condition just by looking at you or running the usual eye tests. But if you tell your doctor about your symptoms, you may get tests that check for problems with how your eyes make or use tears and for damage to your corneas and eye surface.

The doctor might test the quality of your tears with a handheld device that briefly touches your tears. In another test, paper strips might be applied to the inside of your lower lid for a few minutes to see how much moisture they collect. To check for corneal damage, a paper strip containing dye might be applied to your eye. Using a special blue light, the doctor will be able to see if the dye stains the cornea, indicating damage. The eye doctor also should ask about your medical history, medications, and other factors that might contribute to your symptoms.

OTC RELIEF

Some people without advanced dry eyes can get relief without prescription medications or medical procedures. *You can try…*

•**Artificial tears sold over the counter.** These come in different brands and formulations, so you may have to try a few. Your doctor may have some recommendations.

•**Lifestyle and environmental changes.** If the air in your home is part of the problem, you might benefit from a humidifier or air purifier. If you work long hours in front of a screen, you might need more breaks.

A good rule of thumb: Every 20 minutes, take at least a 20-second break, and blink your eyes forcefully to stimulate tear production.

•**Warm compresses.** Pressing a warm, wet, cloth to your eyes can provide soothing relief

Who Is at Risk for Dry Eye Disease?

While the exact causes of dry eye can vary from person to person, several factors can increase your risk or make symptoms worse…

- **Aging.** The prevalence of dry eye increases every five years after age 50.
- **Hormonal changes.** Postmenopausal women have a higher risk than men.
- **Medications.** Any drug that causes dryness, including antihistamines, decongestants, anti-depressants, and some blood-pressure medications, such as diuretics and beta blockers, can contribute to dry eyes. So can medications that reduce the sensitivity of the cornea, leading to less blinking. Some eye drops for glaucoma are in that category.
- **Medical conditions,** including diabetes, thyroid disease, Sjogren's syndrome, and rheumatoid arthritis, can cause dry eyes. Dry eyes, often along with a dry mouth, can be major warning signs of Sjogren's syndrome.
- **Environmental factors,** such as pollution, smoke, wind, and dry indoor or outdoor air.
- **Work** that requires long hours of visual attention.
- **Contact lens use.** One reason is that contact wearers may blink less.
- **Eye surgeries,** including LASIK procedures and cataract removal. These surgeries can lead to decreased cornea sensitivity, which leads to less blinking.

- **Prescription medications.** The mainstays of treatment are prescription drops containing the anti-inflammatory drug *cyclosporine* (brand names Restasis and Cequa) or another anti-inflammatory medicine, *lifitegrast* (Xiidra). These medications can take several months to produce results. Another medicine, a steroid eye drop called *loteprednol* (Eysuvis), can be used for two weeks at a time for flare-ups. A newer medication, *varenicline* (Tyrvaya), comes in a nasal spray and seems to boost tear production by stimulating a nerve inside the nose.

- **Procedures.** Your eye doctor may suggest several procedures, alone or in combination. One involves inserting plugs in your tear ducts to help more tears stay in your eyes. Plug procedures are covered by insurance when they are medically necessary.

People with more severe symptoms may benefit from procedures that involve scrubbing the eyelid margins to remove debris, and using heat, gentle massage, or other means to open up oil glands in the lids. These procedures need to be repeated every few months and generally are not covered by insurance.

- **Autologous serum tears.** When artificial tears are ineffective or irritating, some people have tears made from their own blood. These drops contain more nutrients than artificial tears. They do require blood draws and careful handling (they must be frozen, and then refrigerated between uses), so they aren't for everyone.

and help release oil from the eyelid glands, improving tear quality. To keep the cloth warm for a longer time, try wrapping it around a reusable heated gel pack.

- **Omega-3 fatty acids.** Diets rich in these healthy fats, found in fatty fish, walnuts, and flaxseed, may help with dry eyes. Studies of omega-3 supplements have produced mixed results. A dose of 1,000 milligrams a day may be worth trying, but you should always discuss the pros and cons of any supplement with your doctor.

WHEN HOME REMEDIES AREN'T ENOUGH

When these steps don't help, it's time to ask your doctor about next steps…

Better Vision Through Eye Drops

Michael J. Shumski, M.D., MSE, cataract and refractive surgeon with Magruder Laser Vision, in Orlando, Florida.

Reading glasses are a necessity for almost everyone over age 50, but a newly approved eye drop promises to make them obsolete. We reached out to Michael J. Shumski, M.D., MSE, a cataract and refractive surgeon at Magruder Laser Vision, to find out if Vuity (pilocarpine hydrochloride ophthalmic solution 1.25 percent) lives up to the hype. Pilocarpine has been used as a glaucoma medication for many decades, but this is a new indication.

WHAT IS VUITY?

Starting in the mid-40s the natural lens inside the eye starts to stiffen, resulting in a loss of one's range of vision. This is called presbyopia, and it's why we eventually all need reading glasses. Some people become bothered by these symptoms in their mid-40s, while others make it a little longer until closer to 50. This is a natural part of aging and eventually happens to everyone.

Vuity works by constricting the pupil, which causes a pinhole effect. (It's similar to squinting to see better.) When peripheral light rays are blocked from making their way to the retina, and central light rays don't have to be refracted as much by the cornea and lens, the depth of focus is extended. To benefit from Vuity, you must have good uncorrected *distance* vision. The drops then extend that range of vision to include intermediate and near vision without the need for reading glasses.

IMPLICATIONS FOR CATARACT SURGERY

When you have cataract-removal surgery, you are usually offered the option to replace your natural lens with one that corrects your vision. This is called an intraocular lens (IOL). Vuity does not change the prescription of the eye, so it should not be considered as an alternative to an upgraded IOL. However, if you have already had cataract surgery and are happy with your distance vision, you may be a good candidate for Vuity to replace your reading glasses.

THINGS TO WATCH OUT FOR

When using Vuity, be cautious when driving at night or working in poor illumination. Don't drive or use machinery if your vision isn't clear. If you wear contact lenses, wait 10 minutes after administering the eye drop before inserting the contacts. If you have an increased risk of retinal detachment or iritis, you may need to take additional precautions. One of the most common side effects of Vuity is a mild headache.

Fewer Injections for Macular Degeneration Patients

Nancy Holekamp, M.D., director of retina services at the Pepose Vision Institute in St. Louis, Missouri. Pepose Vision.com

Standard treatment for wet age-related macular degeneration (AMD)—which causes vision loss in the central field of vision—has been monthly injections into the eye of the drug ranibizumab.

New: The FDA has approved Susvimo, a device implanted into the white of the eye that holds a continuous-release six-month supply of ranibizumab that can be refilled twice a year. Susvimo is for people who have already responded to ranibizumab injections.

A Temporary Fix

The medication in Vuity works temporarily. U.S. Food and Drug Administration studies showed that peak improvement in near vision occurs one hour after the drops are put in the eyes and gradually wears off over 10 hours. Near vision will likely degrade over the day if the drops are placed in the morning.

Brian Boxer Wachler, M.D., *All About Vision*, AllAbout Vision.com

Warning: Eye Floaters and Flashes Can Signal a Serious Vision Problem

Jeffrey Anshel, OD, an optometrist with a consulting practice in Kapaa, Hawaii, and founder and past president of the Ocular Wellness and Nutrition Society. OcularNutritionSociety.org

Seeing a few floaters is normal. But suddenly seeing dozens, especially if accompanied by flashes of light, could mean that your retina is torn and that you should see a doctor immediately. Retinal tears are painless but left untreated can lead to a detached retina and blindness.

Clearing Up the Clouds: New Treatments for Cataracts

Marc Grossman, OD, LAc, doctor of optometry and licensed acupuncturist in New Paltz and Somers, New York, and cofounder of NaturalEyeCare, Inc. He is coauthor of *Natural Eye Care: Your Guide to Healthy Vision & Healing.* DrGrossman2020.com

Got cataracts? You're in good company. Half of all 75-year-olds have developed this vision-obscuring clouding of the lens in one or both eyes…and by age 85, that percentage jumps to 70 percent.

Conventional cataract treatment involves surgically replacing the lens of the eye. About four million cataract removals and replacements are performed annually in the U.S.. The success rate is impressive—about 90 percent of patients see their vision improve.

But not everyone is a candidate for the procedure. Some patients have to wait until other medical conditions have been treated. Co-occurring eye diseases such as macular edema or retinal detachment, heart disease, or a history of retinal bleeding may render some people poor surgical candidates. Sometimes medication, including alpha-blockers such as *tamsulosin* (Flomax) and *terazosin* (Hytrin) used to treat symptoms of an enlarged prostate, makes someone a poor surgical candidate. And in some cases, the patient just has to wait for the right insurance to come into effect.

Even though complications are rare, risks associated with cataract surgery include swelling, bleeding, light sensitivity, retinal detachment, and dry eyes.

Fortunately, there are nutritional and life-style changes to help prevent—and possibly reverse—early-stage cataracts. (Surgery is the only treatment for significantly developed cataracts.)

We asked holistic eye doctor Marc Grossman, OD, LAc, for his recommendations to improve your cataracts and your surgical outcome…

***STRATEGY #1:* Eat an antioxidant-rich diet.** After age 40, proteins in the lens begin to break down through a process called oxidation, causing the lens to get cloudy and obscuring vision. Fruits and vegetables are full of antioxidants that slow cellular damage throughout the body, including in the eyes. This, in turn, may reduce the risk for cataracts.

It's best to obtain antioxidants from food, not supplements, because produce and other antioxidant-rich items contain healthful substances that work synergistically to boost the antioxidant effect.

Caution: Studies have failed to show that antioxidant supplementation prevents cataracts…and there are health risks to overdosing on certain vitamins and minerals. *The best eye-friendly nutrients…*

•**Vitamin C.** The eyes contain more vitamin C than nearly any other organ in the body—there's 50 times more vitamin C in the fluid in the eye than in blood. A 2020 study by researchers at The University of Auckland published in *Nutrients* went so far as to compare the vitamin to sunscreen for the eyes, thanks to its ability to help absorb ultraviolet light—a known cause of cataracts.

Best sources: Citrus fruits, peppers, broccoli, Brussels sprouts, strawberries, and tomatoes.

•**Vitamin E.** Some studies show that sufficient vitamin E levels reduce cataract risk…others do not. But we know that a diet with adequate amounts of vitamin E seems to protect cells in the eyes from cellular damage, which may ultimately slow or prevent cataract development.

Best sources: Olive oil, avocados, almonds, and sunflower seeds.

•**Zinc.** This mineral aids in the production of *melanin*, a protective pigment in the eyes. (Melanin also is responsible for skin and hair color.)

Best sources: Beans, lentils, seeds, eggs, seafood, red meat, and dairy.

•**Lutein and zeaxanthin.** This dynamic duo has been well-studied for its potential to lower risk for several chronic eye diseases. Lutein and zeaxanthin are found in the retina, particularly in the macula, which is critical for vision. They protect against cellular damage and UV light. Lutein and zeaxanthin are found together in many foods.

Best sources: Leafy green vegetables (spinach, kale, swiss chard), asparagus, broccoli, raspberries, mangoes, peaches, and papaya.

STRATEGY #2: **Try a glutathione supplement.** Most cataract patients are deficient in the nutrient glutathione, a crucial-for-vision antioxidant that not only protects against oxidation but also helps prevent sugar and protein molecules from binding together in the eye—a contributing factor to cataract formation. A 2017 chemical analysis of both cataract and clear lenses done by researchers at the Post Graduate Institute of Medical Education and Research in Chandigarh, India, and published in *International Journal of Ophthalmology,* found that cataract lenses contained far less glutathione than healthy lenses. Onions, garlic, leafy greens, and cruciferous veggies such as broccoli and cauliflower can increase glutathione levels, but to reach a level necessary for protection from cataracts, a supplement usually is necessary.

Glutathione is not well-absorbed when taken in capsule or tablet form, so I recommend an oral spray such as ACG Glutathione Extra Strength by Results RNA ($39.99 for two ounces, BlueSkyVitamin.com). Try six sprays in the mouth, twice a day.

In addition, you can take two supplements that, once ingested, act as building blocks for glutathione—*N-acetyl cysteine* and *alpha lipoic acid.* Take 600 mg to 1,200 mg of N-acetyl cysteine and 300 mg to 600 mg of alpha lipoic acid a day to gradually build glutathione levels.

STRATEGY #3: **Wear sunglasses.** Sunlight's UVA and UVB rays can have damaging effects on eye health, thinning out the protective pigments and increasing risk for cataracts and other vision disorders. More than 60 percent of UVA rays and more than 90 percent of UVB rays are absorbed by the cornea, according to a 2021 *Translational Research in Anatomy* study.

UV-blocking sunglasses help immensely. Wear them whenever you're outdoors, even on gray days—UV rays still sneak through the clouds. You may think that darker sunglass lenses offer more protection, but that's not necessarily the case. Instead, make sure the lenses are labeled "UV 400," which means they provide close to 100 percent protection from harmful UV rays. (The 400 refers to the wavelengths of light included.)

Best: When trying on sunglasses, ask if you can walk outside the store to see how effective they are in sunlight. Wraparound styles are ideal, considering that about one-third of UV rays sneak in through the tops and sides of standard shades.

STRATEGY #4: **Use cataract-fighting eyedrops.** For more than a century, people in India, Europe, and South America have used a homeopathic formula incorporating a flowering plant called *cineraria* to help treat cataracts. Cineraria eyedrops, which contain compounds that help clear and heal the lens, work best in the early stages of cataract formation, though they may help in more moderate stages, too. In my practice, I've seen them reverse early cataracts about 25 percent of the time. Everybody over age 70 could consider using these drops as a preventive—one drop per day. Cineraria is considered safe, but signs of an allergic reaction include itching or hives, swelling in face or hands, swelling or tingling in the mouth or throat, and trouble breathing.

N-acetyl carnosine eyedrops are another potent cataract treatment. N-acetyl carnosine is an anti-glycation agent, meaning that it helps break up clumps of protein that collect in the lens, creating cloudy cataracts. Everybody over age 70 could consider using these drops as a preventive—one drop per day.

My protocol below uses cineraria and N-acetyl carnosine drops, plus an anti-inflammatory eyedrop pretreatment called *methylsulfonylmethane* (MSM), which softens eye tissues, making it easier for drugs and nutrients to be absorbed. These products all are available over the counter. (*Note:* If you are concerned about a sensitivity to sulfur, check with your health-care practitioner before using this protocol.) *You can try this on your own or under a doctor's supervision…*

- **One to two drops of MSM**
- **Two drops of cineraria**

• **Wait 15 minutes or longer**
• **One to two drops of MSM**
• **One to two drops of N-acetyl carnosine**

Repeat this sequence two or three times a day. You may notice your eyeglass prescription starts to feel off. If your eyesight improves, that is good—it means the cataract is breaking up and more light is coming through your lens, allowing you to see better. If your eyesight gets worse or you don't notice an improvement in three months, this protocol likely is not going to work for you. As with anything that you put into your eyes, side effects can include stinging/redness, widened pupils and blurred vision, which warrant a call to a doctor or pharmacist.

***STRATEGY #5:* Quit smoking.** Add cataracts to the long list of ways smoking damages your health. Each cigarette robs the body of 25 mg of vision-protective vitamin C. Smokers also tend to have elevated cholesterol levels and higher body fat levels, both of which increase the risk for severe cardiovascular disease. That, in turn, causes blood vessels in the eye to narrow, starving the eye of vital nutrients. Smokers are two to three times as likely to develop cataracts as nonsmokers.

Microstents Help Glaucoma

Iqbal Ike K. Ahmed, M.D., professor of ophthalmology and visual sciences at University of Utah, Salt Lake City, and leader of a study of 556 patients presented at the annual meeting of the American Academy of Ophthalmology.

Patients with glaucoma and cataracts whose eyes were fitted with microstents during cataract surgery retained more benefit from the surgery after five years than similar patients who had only cataract surgery. Microstents, roughly the size of an eyelash, are commonly inserted via open-angle glaucoma surgery to lower eye pressure. Patients who got the stents also had a nearly 50 percent lower rate of visual field loss compared with patients who just had surgery.

Your Eyes Will Thank You for Exercising!

Study of 52 adults led by researchers at University of Cape Coast, Cape Coast, Ghana, published in *Experimental Eye Research*.

Tear production and quality of tears were better for people who exercised on a treadmill at least five times a week than for those who performed the same exercise only once a week. Those who exercised five times a week produced more tears…and the tear film on the eye remained stable for longer before beginning to dry. Having a healthy tear film on the eyes keeps eyes from itching, stinging, and burning and protects the eyes against dust, dirt, and other irritants.

Are OTC Hearing Aids Right for You?

Barbara Weinstein, Ph.D., professor of audiology and founding executive officer of the Graduate Center at City University of New York (CUNY) in New York City. She is a leading hearing expert and creator of widely used screening tools for hearing loss. GC.CUNY.edu

You have undoubtedly heard that the Food and Drug Administration has approved the sale of hearing aids over the counter (OTC) and without a prescription —that's welcome news for the 54 million Americans over age 12 with self-perceived mild-to-moderate hearing difficulty.

Despite the availability of prescription hearing aids, only about 20 percent of people with hearing loss use them. Why? They may lack access to providers or don't admit to needing them…or it may be because prescription hearing aids are expensive and often not covered by insurance and Medicare.

Good news: UnitedHealthcare is partnering with AARP to offer benefits for both OTC and traditional prescription hearing aids. *What you should know before you buy OTC hearing aids…*

• **Who can benefit from them?** OTC hearing aids are meant for adults over age 18 with mild-to-moderate hearing difficulty. They are not suitable for people with severe to profound hearing loss, which needs to be managed by an audiologist—a hearing specialist who can offer strategies and adaptations to help you hear and communicate better with prescribed technology. Before buying OTC hearing aids, it can be helpful to have your hearing assessed by an audiologist or do an auditory hearing test through your smartphone using an app such as Mimi Hearing Test or SonicCloud.

Nonprescription hearing aids are particularly suited to tech-savvy people in their mid-50s who are experiencing noise-induced hearing loss, which is on the rise due to the widespread use of earbuds and the high noise levels at concerts and in restaurants. OTC hearing aids are worn discreetly behind or inside the ear, just like prescription aids.

Bonus: If the hearing aids you buy can be paired with your smartphone, you also can listen to music and answer calls through them.

•**Where should you buy them?** OTC aids are available at pharmacies…big-box stores such as Costco and BJ's…Best Buy and other electronics stores…and online from companies like Bose. Many are comparable in quality to traditional entry-level prescription hearing aids that cost much more. Since OTC hearing aids are new to the marketplace, educate yourself before making a purchase.

•**How much do they cost?** Prices for OTC hearing aids range from $200 to $1,600 per pair—versus as much as $7,000 for prescription devices.

Buyer beware: Be sure the manufacturer offers a 30-day trial period—that gives you enough time to see if you can adjust to using the aids—and allows returns.

Optimism Boosts Life Span

Journal of the American Geriatrics Society.

Higher levels of optimism were associated with longer life span in a study led by researchers at Harvard T.H. Chan School of Public Health. Among 159,255 participants in the Women's Health Initiative, the most optimistic people had a 5.4 percent longer life span and a 10 percent greater likelihood of living beyond age 90 than the least optimistic. The investigators reported in the *Journal of the American Geriatrics Society* that lifestyle factors, such as regular exercise and healthy eating, accounted for less than a quarter of the association.

"A lot of previous work has focused on deficits or risk factors that increase the risks for diseases and premature death," said lead author Hayami Koga, PhD. "Our findings suggest that there's value to focusing on positive psychological factors, like optimism, as possible new ways of promoting longevity and healthy aging across diverse groups."

Why Are Your Hands Trembling?

Charles Adler, M.D., Ph.D, Wayne and Kathryn Preisel Professor of Neuroscience Research, and professor of neurology at Mayo Clinic, Scottsdale, Arizona. MayoClinic.org

You may attribute your trembling hands to getting older or heredity…or you may fear that you have Parkinson's disease (PD). *But there are several treatable reasons for developing a tremor, including…*

•**Medications,** including cardiac medications, thyroid medicines, epilepsy drugs, and psychiatric meds.

•**Treatable health conditions,** such as hypothyroidism and hyperthyroidism. Even stress and anxiety can cause tremor.

The disorder most likely to be mistaken for PD is known as essential tremor (ET). This common condition is marked by trembling in the hands when they're in use, known as "action tremor"—when they're grasping objects or being used to perform an activity. Tremor also can appear in your head and/or your voice. ET slowly gets worse over years, but it is not life-threatening, and for many patients, it's simply a minor annoyance. But ET can be disabling when it interferes with your ability to use your hands.

Example: A surgeon with mild ET may find it impossible to work.

No one knows what causes ET (although 50 percent or more of cases are hereditary)…and there's no cure or treatment that slows its progression. *But there are treatments for its symptoms…*

•**Medications.** Most doctors treat by trial and error, prescribing a series of beta-blockers, antiseizure medications, and antianxiety drugs to see which work.

•**Surgery.** If the tremor is severe and disabling, doctors may try one of two highly effective surgeries…

•**Focused ultrasound.** Sound waves are used to destroy the patch of brain tissue responsible for the tremor.

•**Deep brain stimulation.** A wire is implanted in the part of the brain called the thalamus and connected to a stimulator placed in the chest. Electrical stimulation helps correct the faulty brain signals that cause tremors.

IS IT PD?

With PD, the hands shake when they are at rest, and it often is accompanied by difficulty walking, reduced voice volume, stiffness in the extremities, slow movements, and reduced facial expression.

If you're concerned about your tremor's underlying cause, see your doctor. He/she likely will refer you to a movement-disorder specialist or a neurologist. For further information about ET, go to EssentialTremor.org. For information about PD, go to Parkinson.org or MichaelJFox.org.

Stay Hydrated to Live Longer

NIH/National Heart, Lung and Blood Institute.

Researchers from the National Institutes of Health found that adults with serum sodium levels at the higher end of a normal range, which suggests low fluid intake, were more likely to develop chronic conditions and show signs of advanced biological aging than those with serum sodium levels that suggest adequate hydration.

Biological aging was based on indicators like metabolic and cardiovascular health, lung function, and inflammation. Adults with serum sodium levels above 142 milliequivalents per liter (mEq/L) had a 10 to 15 percent increased odds of being biologically older than their chronological age and a 64 percent increased risk for developing a chronic disease like heart failure, stroke, atrial fibrillation, peripheral artery disease, chronic lung disease, diabetes, or dementia.

Adults with higher serum sodium levels were also more likely to die at a younger age. Prior research found links between higher ranges of normal serum sodium levels and increased risks for heart failure.

The findings don't prove a causal effect, the researchers noted. Randomized, controlled trials are necessary to determine if optimal hydration can promote healthy aging, prevent disease, and lead to a longer life. However, the associations can still guide personal health behavior.

The National Academies of Medicine suggest that most women drink six to nine cups of fluids daily and that men drink eight to 12 cups.

Don't Scratch That Itch

Consumer Reports.

As people age, immune system changes promote bodywide inflammation, which can cause itchy skin. While scratching may feel good for a moment, it increases inflammation and makes the itch even worse. To prevent itch, bathe with warm, not hot, water, and use a fragrance-free cleanser or soap-free body wash. Avoid exfoliating products. Use a thick moisturizer (if it comes out of a pump, it's not thick enough) that contains hyaluronic acid, lanolin, or shea butter several times per day and after bathing. For itch relief, try an anti-itch cream with hydrocortisone or pramoxine hydrochloride.

We Become Kinder as We Age

Study of more than 100 adults by researchers at Claremont Graduate University, Claremont, California, published in Frontiers in Behavioral Neuroscience.

Seniors spend more of their time volunteering and donate a larger percentage of their income to charity than younger people do.

Likely reason: As we age, our brains release more oxytocin, a neurochemical associated with social bonding, interpersonal trust, generosity, and life satisfaction.

Social Media Helps Seniors

Study of 310 older adults by researchers at University of Texas at Austin, published in Journal of Social and Personal Relationships.

Daily social-media use by older Americans was associated with a more positive mood among those with a small social circle...but not among those with a larger social circle. Social media can help mitigate the effects of a dwindling in-person social network later in life.

Dying on Your Own Terms

Kimberly Callinan, MBA, MPP, certified end-of-life doula and president and CEO of Compassion & Choices, a nonprofit that advocates for the rights of people at the end of their life. CompassionAndChoices.org

Most of us don't readily acknowledge the inevitability of dying—at least not when we presumably still have plenty of time to plan for the peaceful death we are hoping for. It is such an important and deeply personal topic, yet it's rarely examined closely.

The people who have the easiest time with dying are those who have lived their lives to the fullest and have little unfinished business. If they had rifts with loved ones, they mended them...if they had a list of goals, they completed the important ones...and they addressed any regrets along the way.

People who have the most difficulty saying a peaceful good-bye are those with unresolved issues, such as a longstanding fight with a loved one that they now realize wasn't worth having. Resolving any of these "open issues" frees you up to spend the rest of your life in positive ways.

You can prioritize who you want to spend time with and what you want to focus on. You can begin to think about your legacy.

CREATE YOUR LEGACY

People are able to do amazing things when they start to think about their legacy and what they want to leave behind...even when they have little time left.

Example: One man decided to compile a book about his family's history, including how they first came to the U.S., to leave as his legacy. He dictated it to his daughter as a way to make the end of his life meaningful.

Some people decide to write their own obituary or plan their own funeral to define how they want to be remembered.

Example: My father-in-law, a well-known singer from Baton Rouge, planned his funeral service. He requested three choruses he had sung with to perform. He selected the readings and chose who would give the sermon. Acts like this not only allow you to have a say in planning your death but also can help your loved ones cope with your passing—they won't have to guess at what you wanted.

Creating your legacy is a way to document what's important to you—your life story, experiences and values—and leave it for your loved ones. At the same time, it will remind you that your life had meaning. For people living with a terminal condition or facing other difficult circumstances, writing your legacy also can be a way of coping.

Useful Free Apps for Seniors

GoodRx helps save up to 80 percent on prescriptions. Enter your location and prescription, and the app shows which pharmacy has the lowest price. *Medisafe Pill & Med Reminder* helps track medications and warns of potential interactions with other medications and/or foods and beverages. Enter each drug…when it should be taken…and the app will send a reminder. *AARP Now* shows events, discounts, news, and other resources that can be used with an AARP membership. *SmartBP* tracks blood pressure when used with any blood pressure monitor compatible with *Apple Health* or *Google Fit*. *Pacer* tracks activity levels—no need for a Fitbit or smartwatch—and also has plenty of workout ideas to encourage a more active life. All apps are free on Google Play and Apple.

Komando.com

Resource: The Stanford Letter Project (Med. Stanford.edu/letter) has templates and ideas to help you get started.

PREPARE YOUR LOVED ONES

It's important to have good-bye conversations with loved ones so you can express end-of-life issues that are important to you. These talks may be difficult for them, even if your death isn't on the horizon. However, they can be very meaningful. *There's no one right way to approach this conversation, but there are things you can do to make it easier for loved ones…*

•**Give your loved one (or ones) control over when the conversation will take place.** You might say something like, "All of us are going to die, and my time may be near or far away, but I want you to know what's important to me. Can we schedule a time to talk in the next few weeks? When is good for you?"

•**Let them know that you want to have the conversation out of love.** You might say, "When I can no longer make decisions for myself, I want you to make them for me because of how much you mean to me. I'd love to talk

with you about this to be sure you are comfortable in this role and are fully prepared."

•**Let them know it can bring you closure** as well as make your dying easier for them when the time comes.

HELP FOR THE JOURNEY

More and more people are turning to the idea of working with a doula. The dictionary defines a doula as someone who counsels a new mother in the arts of childbirth and early child rearing. An end-of-life doula, also called a death doula, can help you at the terminal phase of your life's journey. This might seem like a new concept, but it has been part of many cultures for centuries to help a dying person control his/her death. An end-of-life doula acts as an extension of you, supporting your wishes surrounding your death and filling a need that goes unmet within the traditional medical system. The doula can help you navigate end-of-life issues and find meaning…assist you with advance care planning and legacy planning…offer relief to your caregivers…and facilitate difficult conversations with your family and let them know what to expect at the end. Most people engage a doula when they are close to dying, but end-of-life doulas can assist you with death planning at any time in your life.

In the U.S., end-of-life doulas often are trained professionals who are certified through a program such as the ones at the University of Vermont and the International End of Life Doula Association. Some offer their services for free…some charge for them. There currently is no regulatory body for end-of-life doulas, so ask for recommendations from your medical providers, a hospice staffer, a patient navigator at your hospital, or even friends.

Also: There is a member directory on the site of the National End-of-Life Doula Alliance at NEDAlliance.org. To find the right fit, always ask the doula about his/her philosophy, training and credentials, and how many people he has helped. Of course, as with any service, you are welcome to ask for references.

CHAPTER 2

Brain Health

Real Breakthroughs in Alzheimer's Disease

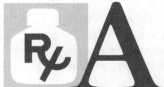**A**pproved in June 2021, *aducanumab* (Aduhelm) was the first new drug for patients with Alzheimer's disease (AD) in 18 years, but the promise of a breakthrough was short-lived. The controversial drug had no compelling evidence supporting its effectiveness. In fact, clinical trials showed that it appeared to cause harm.

This isn't the first time that experts have questioned the efficacy of drugs for AD. Researchers reviewed all the Alzheimer's disease drugs on the market and reported in *Pharmacy & Therapeutics* that they have "limited effectiveness for most patients." They're used only because there aren't "any better alternatives," the authors added.

But there is an alternative for dealing effectively with AD: prevention. The neurochemical changes that lead to AD—principally, the neuroinflammation that drives the disease—develop over the course of 30 to 40 years. By then, it's too late to repair the damage. Preventing or minimizing those changes—even in middle and old age—is the optimal way to deal with the disease.

Prevention may be possible through anti-inflammatory lifestyle habits such as a healthy diet, brain-protecting nutritional supplements, regular exercise, good sleep, and mental stimulation.

MEDITERRANEAN DIET

The classic Mediterranean diet, which is rich in vegetables, fruit, beans, whole grains, fish, and olive oil and low in processed foods, red meat, and dairy products, is highly protective against cognitive decline and AD.

In a study published in the *British Journal of Nutrition*, scientists studied nearly 1,000 peo-

James Greenblatt, M.D., chief medical officer at Walden Behavioral Care, assistant clinical professor at Tufts University and Dartmouth College, and founder of Psychiatry Redefined.

Low-Dose Nutritional Lithium for Alzheimer's Disease

In high doses of 150 to 1,800 milligrams (mg), lithium is a medication for bipolar disorder (BD). But in very low doses of 1 to 20 mg, lithium isn't a pharmaceutical treatment—it's a *nutritional* treatment. And scientific research shows that low-dose nutritional lithium is a uniquely effective therapy for a range of neurological problems, including Alzheimer's disease (AD).

Preventing AD. Brazilian researchers studied 45 seniors with *mild cognitive impairment* (MCI), the stage of memory loss and mental decline that precedes AD. The researchers divided the seniors into two groups, giving one group low-dose lithium and the other a placebo. After one year, more of the people taking lithium had stable cognitive performance and no mental decline. And few of those taking lithium developed AD. Plus, those on low-dose lithium had better memory, more focus, and clearer thinking.

Treating AD. In a study published in *Current Alzheimer's Research*, 113 people with mild to moderate AD were divided into two groups: one received low-dose lithium and the other a placebo. The lithium group had *no cognitive decline* during the 15 months of the study, while mental decline progressed in the placebo group.

Low-dose lithium is equivalent to the amount you could be getting in food and water. (Lithium levels vary geographically.) Take 2 mg of lithium daily for two to three months. If there are no side effects, such as drowsiness, increase to a maintenance dose of 5 mg daily.

In another study published in January in *The American Journal of Clinical Nutrition*, researchers analyzed the diets of 512 people ages 70 and older. Those who ate more foods typical of the Mediterranean diet had less atrophy in the hippocampus section of the brain (the hippocampus shrinks early and severely in Alzheimer's disease) and lower levels of tau protein and beta-amyloid protein, two hallmarks of Alzheimer's. They also performed better on memory tests.

B VITAMINS

Three vitamin supplements—B_{12}, folate, and B_6—protect against mental decline and AD. That's because low levels of these nutrients increase levels of homocysteine, an amino acid that is neurotoxic in elevated amounts.

Studies link elevated homocysteine levels to memory loss and dementia. A study in the journal *Life Sciences* showed that people with the highest levels of homocysteine have a 31 percent higher risk of developing dementia. And research published in the *New England Journal of Medicine* showed that high homocysteine doubles a person's risk of progressive brain atrophy. The evidence linking homocysteine and AD is so strong that in 2018, a group of experts published a consensus statement about homocysteine and AD in the *Journal of Alzheimer's Disease*: "We…conclude that elevated plasma total homocysteine is a modifiable risk factor for the development of cognitive decline, dementia, and Alzheimer's diseases in older persons."

High levels of homocysteine are also linked to heart disease, osteoporosis, depression, and kidney problems.

To modify this risk factor, take a vitamin supplement that includes folate, B_6, and B_{12}. Follow the dosage recommendations on the label.

REGULAR EXERCISE

Many studies link regular exercise with the prevention of AD. In a study published in *Frontiers in Neuroscience*, researchers analyzed health data from more than 163,000 people, comparing those with the lowest levels of physical activity to those with the highest. They found that physical activity reduced

ple for three to 10 years. The researchers traced participants' "subjective cognitive decline" (their own estimation of decline in memory, decision-making, and other mental skills) and gave each participant a Mediterranean Diet Score, ranking their adherence to the diet from 0 to 55. For every yearly 10-point increase in the score, there was a reduction in subjective cognitive decline of nearly 8 percent.

The Aduhelm Controversy

Aducanumab (Aduhelm) was an Alzheimer's "breakthrough" that most Alzheimer's experts said was bogus. On June 7, 2021, for the first time in 18 years, the U.S. Food and Drug Administration approved a new drug for people with mild Alzheimer's-related cognitive decline—even though the agency's independent advisory committee had almost unanimously concluded there was not enough scientific evidence to approve it.

In April 2022, officials at the Centers for Medicare and Medicaid Services took a close look at the drug—an intravenous medication that costs $28,200 a year (reduced from its original price of $56,000, after weak sales)—and made a final decision to restrict coverage, limiting it to participants in randomized controlled trials. This is the first time that Medicare has limited access to an FDA-approved drug.

the risk of AD by 45 percent and dementia (non-Alzheimer's) by 28 percent. Try to engage in at least 20 minutes of walking, dancing, gardening, or any physical activity you enjoy five days a week.

A GOOD NIGHT'S SLEEP

Chronic sleep deprivation causes chronic neuroinflammation—and chronic neuroinflammation is a risk factor for AD. In a 20-year study published in the journal *Nature Communications*, scientists analyzed the sleep patterns of more than 8,000 people ages 50 and older. They found that those who slept six hours or fewer a night were 30 percent more likely to develop dementia than those getting seven hours.

Daily habits for deeper sleep include going to bed and getting up at the same time every day, keeping the bedroom cool and dark while you're sleeping, turning off all screens (cell phones, computers, TVs, video games) one hour before bedtime, and taking a warm bath 30 minutes before bed.

MENTAL STIMULATION

Keeping your brain active is protective against mental decline. A recent study from scientists at Rush University Medical Center in Chicago followed nearly 2,000 people ages 80 and older for seven years. Those who had the highest level of cognitive activity—they regularly read books or played games like checkers, board games, cards, or puzzles—developed dementia an average of five years later than those with the lowest level.

Not All Dementia Is the Same

Zaldy Tan, M.D., director of the Bernard & Maxine Platzer Lynn Family Memory and Healthy Aging Program at Cedars-Sinai Medical Center, Los Angeles. Cedars-Sinai. org

When we hear the word "dementia," most of us think of Alzheimer's disease. But the two terms aren't interchangeable, and in fact, some forms of dementia look quite different from Alzheimer's in terms of symptoms, disease progression, and brain changes.

We asked Zaldy Tan, M.D., director of the Bernard & Maxine Platzer Lynn Family Memory and Healthy Aging Program at Cedars-Sinai Medical Center, to explain non-Alzheimer's dementia and how to reduce your risk for all kinds…

•**Types of dementia.** Defined broadly, dementia is a condition affecting the brain that causes difficulty thinking and remembering, and that increasingly affects the performance of day-to-day functions. Saying someone "has dementia" is like saying they "have cancer"—we know what cancer is, but we acknowledge that there are differences among the various types.

Determining what type of dementia a person has can drive decisions about which treatments to try and provide a set of expectations about how the disease will progress and what the overall prognosis will be.

The four main forms of dementia…

Alzheimer's disease: The reason Alzheimer's commands so much attention is that it's the most common type of dementia, accounting for 50 to 75 percent of cases. While the ultimate cause of Alzheimer's is unknown, its hallmark is the accumulation of a protein called amyloid, which forms plaques, and "neurofibrillary tangles" of tau protein within healthy neurons in the brain. It first affects the hippocampus, the area of the brain responsible for short-term memory. Later, it spreads to other regions affecting attention, concentration, sequencing, motor skills, and long-term memory.

Vascular dementia: This type of dementia is related to tissue damage following loss of blood flow to the brain, usually from a stroke or brain hemorrhages. Its symptoms can resemble those of Alzheimer's but depend on which brain region is impaired. Generally, vascular dementia affects the ability to retrieve new memory, but other symptoms can include apathy, disorganization, confusion, and inability to concentrate. Vascular dementia may come on suddenly, as after a severe stroke, or gradually over the course of years. About 20 to 30 percent of dementia cases are attributed to vascular dementia.

Lewy body dementia (LBD): Actor Robin Williams, who passed away in 2014, had this form of dementia. Like Alzheimer's, LBD is marked by an excess of a protein in the brain, but in this case the protein is *alpha-synuclein*, not amyloid. As alpha-synuclein accumulates, amassing deposits known as Lewy bodies, brain function deteriorates. Besides disrupted thinking and attention, patients can experience hallucinations, delusions, and Parkinson's-like motor problems. In fact, because the loss of motor control looks so similar to Parkinson's, and because there is no blood test that reveals LBD, cases often are misdiagnosed as "Parkinson's dementia," with the Lewy bodies discovered only upon autopsy. From 10 to 25 percent of dementia patients have LBD.

Frontotemporal dementia (FTD): Roughly 10 to 15 percent of dementia cases fall under this umbrella term, which refers to deterioration of the brain's frontal and temporal lobes, responsible for personality, language, and behavior. As the disease sets in, the lobes shrink, diminishing their function. Patients can undergo drastic personality changes and begin to engage in inappropriate behaviors. Some experience reduced ability to use language. Onset of FTD tends to occur earlier than Alzheimer's, between ages 40 and 65. Its cause is unknown.

RISK FACTORS

Various characteristics and behaviors have been associated with increased or decreased risk for dementia. but keep in mind three things when assessing such studies…

•**They almost always express associations (and not causation)** between certain factors and the likelihood of dementia diagnosis.

Example: A recent study by researchers at the University of Plymouth in the U.K. found that being simultaneously prescribed three or more medications—especially for urinary and respiratory infections—was associated with increased dementia risk. But that doesn't mean those medications cause dementia. It could be that the infections themselves drive a later dementia diagnosis…or some underlying condition could make a person prone both to the infections and dementia. Don't draw simple conclusions from such studies.

•**These findings tend to have small effects.**

Example: A study from Southern Medical University in Guangzhou, China, on fish oil and dementia found that people taking supplements were about 9 percent less likely to develop dementia. That's intriguing enough to warrant further investigation, but not a reason to start gobbling fish-oil pills—especially when there are other factors whose significance dwarfs that of fish oil.

•**Risk factors for dementia tend to fall into one of two categories.** In the first category are well-established factors including age, history of head trauma to the point of losing consciousness, family history (dementia in a first-degree relative), stroke, cerebrovascular disease, high blood pressure, African-American race, and Hispanic heritage. Enough research has been done on these factors that little debate remains (although even these still are just associations, not causes). The other category contains less defined or less established factors including poor sleep, smoking, diabetes, high body mass index (BMI), and high triglycerides. These haven't been investigated enough to be considered well-established. Bearing in mind what's established versus what is only associated should help you decide where to focus your efforts to reduce risk.

PREVENTION

Because many well-established risk factors for dementia are beyond an individual's control, taking steps to prevent the condition means making choices within a limited sphere of influence. You can't control your age, your heritage, or whether a parent had dementia—but you can lower your risk for cerebro-vascular disease and high blood pressure.

One thing the science makes clear: What is good for your heart is good for your brain. Diet, exercise, and blood pressure control are the likeliest ways to counteract underlying risk for dementia.

That's especially important given what researchers call the "multiple-hit" hypothesis of dementia risk. Imagine that, thanks to an underlying genetic predisposition, Person A's brain is cluttered with abnormal proteins, and he develops dementia regardless of the lifestyle choices he makes. Meanwhile, most people are more like Person B, who has some accumulation of abnormal proteins but still, in her 80s and 90s, continues to function adequately and live independently. Yet even Person B could develop dementia and lose her independence if she were to suffer a series of small strokes. At that point, the abnormal proteins coupled with the tissue damage from blood deprivation could tip her over the edge.

Getting 150 minutes of moderate to vigorous physical activity each week, plus two days of strength training, is recommended for cardio and brain health. So is following a Mediterranean-style or MIND diet. Both these diets emphasize complex carbohydrates, vegetables, fish, olive oil, and beans, and both are low in salt, red meat, and sweets.

Those two major lifestyle factors will have a greater impact on whether you develop dementia than scrambling after some new behavior (coffee drinking, crossword puzzles) each time a new study comes out.

TREATMENT

There's no cure for dementia, but today's medications lessen the disease's severity, slow its progression, and can help manage its symptoms. *The FDA has approved three classes of drugs…*

•**Acetylcholinesterase inhibitors** such as *donepezil* (Aricept) and *rivastigmine* (Exelon) improve function by increasing the neurotransmitter protein acetylcholine in the junctions that brain cells use to communicate with each other. Although designed for Alzheimer's patients, physicians often try them in LBD and vascular dementia cases, since those patients often have an acetylcholine deficit similar to that seen in Alzheimer's.

•**NMDA receptor antagonists** such as *memantine* (Namenda) help with cognition by blocking the brain receptor NMDA, which becomes overstimulated in dementia cases. These drugs are approved for only moderate- to late-stage Alzheimer's-type dementia, but evidence suggests they can help some vascular dementia patients.

Neither of those classes modifies the disease. They help only with symptoms. But the FDA has approved two monoclonal antibodies, *aducanumab*, and in July 2023, *lecanemab* (Leqembi). Another is in latter-phased trials. These drugs clear the amyloid plaques that cause Alzheimer's. Unfortunately, while they appear effective at removing plaques, their impact on the disease is less impressive.

•**Early diagnosis.** If you notice cognitive problems in yourself or a loved one beyond normal age-related changes, get tested. Today's therapies and the ones coming are promising. And an early diagnosis allows you to plan ahead while you're still able to make decisions about personal goals, money, family, and health care.

The Brain-Protecting Vitamin

Gary Landreth, Ph.D., Martin Professor of Alzheimer's Research, and Miguel Moutinho, Ph.D., PharmD, assistant research professor of anatomy, cell biology, and physiology at the Indiana University Medical School in Indianapolis.

Niacin is shorthand for the two main forms (or *vitamers*) of vitamin B_3: nicotinic acid and nicotinamide. These vitamers work in different ways and have different therapeutic uses. For instance, nicotinic acid, but not nicotinamide, can change the concentration of lipids in the blood in a positive way. This led to the development of Niaspan, a prescription medication that is used to lower LDL ("bad") and increase HDL ("good") blood cholesterol levels.

Both nicotinic acid and nicotinamide are readily available in animal-based foods such as meat, poultry, and fish, and plant-based foods such as nuts, legumes, and grains.

Niacin's classic role is as a building block for nicotinamide adenine dinucleotide (NAD). More than 400 chemical reactions in the body need NAD, from metabolizing all the nutrients in the foods we eat to many functions that happen within the cells, including gene expression and DNA repair. Niacin likely plays significant roles we've yet to uncover.

NIACIN AND THE BRAIN

Studies have shown that people with higher levels of niacin in their diet have a diminished risk for Alzheimer's disease. A prospective study followed 3,718 men and women ages 65 and older for six years, kept questionnaires on their diets, and had periodic cognitive assessments. Researchers reported in the *Journal of Neurology, Neurosurgery, and Psychiatry* that people with the highest niacin intake had lower rates of Alzheimer's disease and cognitive decline, compared with people with the lowest intake. They concluded that niacin may protect against both Alzheimer's and cognitive decline in aging.

The Coronary Artery Risk Development in Young Adults, or "CARDIA" study, with results published in 2017 in *The American Journal of Clinical Nutrition*, followed its participants—3,136 men and women ages 18 to 30 from Chicago, Minneapolis, Oakland, and Birmingham, Alabama—for up to 25 years. The study measured dietary and supplemental B vitamin intake of niacin, folate, vitamin B_6, and vitamin B_{12}, and found that a higher intake of B vitamins, niacin in particular, throughout young adulthood was associated with better cognitive function scores in middle-age years.

A DIFFERENT FOCUS ON ALZHEIMER'S

In contrast to others in the field of Alzheimer's research who are focused directly on amyloid plaques and finding therapeutics that target them, our research centers on the activity of immune cells in the brain and how their *response* to amyloid plaques acts as a central contributor to Alzheimer's disease.

This particular research project began five years ago to build on those earlier findings regarding niacin and Alzheimer's. While *niacin* was used in other models of Alzheimer's, *nicotinic acid* has not. No one before had discerned between the types of niacin. For this research, we used Niaspan and mice specifically engineered to get Alzheimer's disease by modifying certain genes.

WHAT THE STUDY SHOWED

Data from previous studies show that the brain doesn't convert nicotinic acid into NAD as other organs do. Different things happen. Most importantly in terms of Alzheimer's disease, it activates a receptor called HCAR2 in the brain's microglia. Microglia are immune cells that play roles in brain infections and inflammation and have been linked to amyloid plaques.

When niacin activates the receptor, it stimulates beneficial actions from these immune cells. We found protective and therapeutic effects in the mice given Niaspan. The mice who did not receive it had worsening cognitive impairments and greater amyloid deposits. The results suggest that modulating microglia activity through HCAR2—specifically targeting the neuroimmune response to amyloid in the brain—might be effective for preventing or treating Alzheimer's disease.

As exciting as this finding is, it's too early to extrapolate what it means to human beings. All we know for sure right now is that we can reverse the disease effects in a mouse genetically transformed to develop Alzheimer's disease.

Our next goal is to move to a clinical study on people to be sure nicotinic acid has a beneficial effect and to find the right dose. We gave mice a dose equivalent to the one that people are started on to manage blood lipids and lower than the maintenance dose. If you currently take Niaspan for high cholesterol, you may indeed be getting an anti-Alzheimer's benefit.

WHAT CAN YOU DO NOW?

We know that niacin helps with memory, so make sure you're getting it in your diet. According to the Office of Dietary Supplements in the National Institutes of Health, plant-based foods provide about 2 to 5 mg of niacin per serving, mainly as nicotinic acid. It's too soon to say whether you should be supplementing with nicotinic acid to prevent Alzheimer's.

People who take the very high doses of Niaspan must be regularly monitored by a physician. It comes in an extended-release form that allows slower, more gradual absorption and helps avoid side effects of high-dose niacin like flushing.

THE FUTURE OF NIACIN

Our work also includes investigating nicotinic acid's effect on amyloid- and tau-driven disease. At other institutions, it's currently being tested in clinical trials as a possible therapeutic for Parkinson's disease and glioblastoma (an aggressive form of brain cancer), following the thesis that nicotinic acid modulates the brain's immune response.

The New Alzheimer's Drug

Sarah Kremen, M.D., director of the Neurobehavior Program in the Jona Goldrich Center for Alzheimer's and Memory Disorders, Cedars-Sinai, Los Angeles.

Just two years after the *aducanumab* (Aduhelm) controversy, the U.S. Food and Drug Administration has approved anoth-er drug for Alzheimer's disease. This medication, *lecanemab* (Leqembi), certainly fared better in clinical trials, though it's still a far cry from the kind of miracle drug the world is hoping for. Let's take a look at what we know so far.

WHAT IT DOES

In phase III clinical trials, Leqembi significantly cleared amyloid-a protein, which forms plaques and disrupts brain function, and decreased the accumulation of tau protein, which forms tangles inside neurons in the memory centers of the brain.

In practical terms, it slowed the rate of memory loss and functional ability decline in people with early-stage Alzheimer's disease.

"It's important to recognize that this medication does not reverse cognitive decline, it only slows it down," explains Sarah Kremen, M.D., director of the Neurobehavior Program in the Jona Goldrich Center for Alzheimer's and Memory Disorders, and leader of the Alzheimer's Disease Clinical Trial Program at Cedars-Sinai.

It's not yet clear how beneficial that slowing will be in real life. "We see benefits in the data, but we don't yet know how people will be impacted day to day. We're hopeful that it's going to prolong our patients' ability to function, but that might be a difference of as little as three months," she says.

"From the perspective of a scientist, it is exciting that an experimental treatment targeting brain amyloid in Alzheimer's disease appears to slow cognitive decline," Madhav Thambisetty, M.D., a neurologist and a senior investigator at the National Institute on Aging, told the *New York Times*. But "from the perspective of a physician caring for Alzheimer's patients, the difference between lecanemab and placebo is well below what is considered to be a clinically meaningful treatment effect."

HOW LEQEMBI IS DIFFERENT FROM OTHER ALZHEIMER'S MEDICATIONS

"Medications that we have been giving to patients for dementia due to Alzheimer's disease are different from Leqembi because they are not disease modifying," Dr. Kremen says. "This means that they may help memory for some amount of time, but they do not have an effect on the underlying disease process, such as the buildup of amyloid and tau proteins in the brain."

WHO CAN BE TREATED WITH LEQEMBI?

Leqembi is designed for people who have either mild cognitive impairment or mild dementia due to Alzheimer's disease. It's not for people with moderate or severe dementia, where their memory and other cognitive functions are so impacted that they need to rely on other people for help with daily living.

TYPES OF PRE-TREATMENT TESTING PATIENTS WILL NEED

Before taking Leqembi, patients will need a diagnostic evaluation to confirm that their dementia or cognitive impairment is due to Alzheimer's disease, and they will need testing to confirm the presence of amyloid, which is what the medication is designed to treat. This can be done through specialized brain imaging, which is not widely available or covered by insurance, or through spinal fluid tests, Dr. Kremen says.

SAFETY CONCERNS

In the phase III clinical trial, about 17 percent of the participants who were taking Leqembi experienced brain bleeding and 13 percent experienced brain swelling. As such, Leqembi isn't recommended for anyone taking blood thinners, or who has significant brain bleeds, brain swelling, aneurysms, vascular malformation, brain tumors, or an uncontrolled bleeding disorder.

"The side effect we're most concerned about is large brain bleeds, which are fairly rare but can happen," Dr. Kremen says. "So people need to go into this with eyes open, because we're not going to be able to completely mitigate this risk."

People with one or two copies of the APOE4 gene are at increased risk of brain bleeds and swelling and will need to take this into account when deciding whether to be treated.

WHAT THE TREATMENT PROCESS IS LIKE

The medication is given by intravenous infusion over one hour every two weeks. Patients will need to have an MRI before the fifth, seventh, and 14th infusions to check for brain swelling and brain bleeds. The physicians will also monitor for infusion reactions, such as low blood pressure or difficulty breathing.

WHAT LEQEMBI WILL COST

In January 2022, Eisai, the Japanese pharmaceutical company that developed and tested, the drug said the list price would be $26,500 per year.

Leqembi has received full approval from the FDA, so Medicare patients are now eligible for coverage (minus out-of-pocket deductibles).

Lower Dementia Risk by Walking More and Faster

Borja del Pozo Cruz, Ph.D., associate professor in population health at University of Southern Denmark, Odense, and coauthor of a study of 78,340 adults reported in *JAMA Neurology*.

In an eight-year study, adults who walked 3,800 steps daily for almost three years had 25 percent lower risk for dementia…those who walked 9,800 steps per day had 50 percent lower risk. Walking faster is even better—people who walked 9,800 steps per day, including 30 minutes at 112 steps per minute (about three miles per hour), were 62 percent less likely to be diagnosed with dementia.

Curable Condition May Be Misdiagnosed as Dementia

Alzheimer's & Dementia: Translational Research and Clinical Interventions.

Some people who are diagnosed with a type of dementia may instead have a treatable cerebrospinal fluid leak. Cerebrospinal fluid surrounds the brain and spinal

Good Food for a Better Brain

Fiber Fights Dementia

Higher levels of dietary fiber are associated with a lower risk of developing dementia. In a large study, more than 3,500 Japanese adults completed a dietary survey and were followed up for 20 years. Those who ate more fiber, particularly soluble fiber (found in oats and legumes), were less likely to develop dementia. This may be because soluble fiber regulates the composition of gut bacteria, which may affect neuroinflammation, which plays a role in the onset of dementia. Dietary fiber may also reduce other risk factors for dementia, such as lipids, body weight, glucose levels, and blood pressure.

Kazumasa Yamagishi, M.D., Ph.D., professor, faculty of medicine, department of public health medicine, University of Tsukuba, Tsukuba, Japan.

Flavonols in Fruits and Vegetables May Slow Cognitive Decline

People who ate the most foods containing antioxidant and anti-inflammatory flavonols experienced 32 percent slower age-related cognitive decline than those who ate the least.

Especially beneficial: The flavonols *kaempferol* and *myricetin*, found in dark leafy greens such as spinach and kale, onions, tomatoes, pears, and apples. Foods provide greater diversity of nutrients than flavonol supplements.

Thomas Holland, M.D., professor of medicine at Rush University, Chicago, and coauthor of a study of 961 adults published in Neurology.

cord. When it leaks into the body, the brain can sag, causing dementia symptoms.

"Many of these patients experience cognitive, behavioral and personality changes so severe that they are arrested or placed in nursing homes," says Wouter Schievink, M.D., director of the Cerebrospinal Fluid Leak and Microvascular Neurosurgery Program and professor of Neurosurgery at Cedars-Sinai Medical Center. The telltale brain sag can be seen on an MRI,

and people with a leak may have a history of severe headaches that improve when they lie down, significant sleepiness even after adequate nighttime sleep, or a Chiari brain malformation. Brain sagging is often mistaken for a Chiari malformation.

If the source of the leak can be located, the leak can be stopped, and the symptoms reversed. But it can take specialized equipment and training to find them. More research is needed to improve the detection process.

The Miracle of Music in Alzheimer's Disease

Borna Bonakdarpour, M.D., FAAN, associate professor of neurology, Northwestern University Feinberg School of Medicine.

In the documentary "Alive Inside: A Story of Music and Memory," Henry, an elderly man with Alzheimer's disease, sits despondent, barely responding to the people around him. But when his caregiver plays some of Henry's favorite music, Henry comes to life. His eyes open fully. He begins to sing and sway. Even after the music is no longer playing, Henry talks, answers questions, and beautifully sings "I'll Be Home for Christmas."

Listening to just a few minutes of music transformed Henry, seemingly undoing the ravages of Alzheimer's disease. He is not alone in this response. Listening to music taps into many different areas of the brain. It affects emotions, memory, social cognition, and even movement. That means it provides a way to stimulate and connect with a person who was previously cut off by their disease. Even if a person can't speak, they can respond to music.

Part of the benefit comes from simple anatomy: The damage of Alzheimer's disease begins in the back of the brain, where the limbic system, the seat of memory, resides. But music is processed in the front of the brain, which remains largely untouched until very late in the disease. That means that people can retain the ability to dance and sing long after their ability to talk has diminished, explains

Borna Bonakdarpour, M.D., director of the Music and Medicine Program at the Northwestern University Feinberg School of Medicine.

CREATING CONNECTION

Dr. Bonakdarpour recently published the results of a study that showed that music helps patients with dementia connect with loved ones. In the study, an ensemble of chamber musicians and a singer performed songs that appealed to the patients from their younger days. Patients and caregivers received simple instruments such as tambourines and shakers to accompany the music, and music therapists encouraged patients to beat on drums, sing, and dance.

Before the intervention, some of the participants showed only minimal or no communication, but while the music was playing, they started to sing, play, and dance.

In a group conversation after the performance, patients were more socially engaged as evidenced by more eye contact, less distraction, less agitation, and an elevated mood. In comparison, people in the control group, who did not receive the intervention and were exposed to usual daily care and programs, did not show such changes.

"Patients were able to connect with partners through music, a connection that was not available to them verbally," said Dr. Bonakdarpour.

The benefits extended to loved ones, too. "The family and friends of people with dementia also are affected by the disease. It's painful for them when they can't connect with a loved one. When language is no longer possible, music gives them a bridge to each other."

CALMING EFFECTS

Music has calming effects. "People with cognitive disorders can get lost in time and space," Dr. Bonakdarpour says, "but listening to the music they enjoyed as teenagers and in their 20s makes them feel grounded and safe—and that reduces anxiety and agitation."

Music also has a physiological effect. When people listen to slow music, for example, the brain synchronizes and slows down. The heart slows down. Breathing slows down, and the body goes into a resting state where it can recuperate.

The effects seem to linger even after a person is no longer listening to music or singing. Dr. Bonakdarpour works with the Good Memories Choir in Chicago, a choir for people with memory loss and their caregivers. Many of the participants report that their anxiety remains low for up to a day or two after singing in the choir.

SOCIALIZATION BENEFITS

During the early days of the COVID pandemic, when hospitalized people couldn't have visitors, Dr. Bonakdarpour's team invited a music practitioner to perform for patients. Most of those patients reported that the music helped ease the sense of isolation and made them feel better. When the researchers looked at EEGs of people who were in the neurology ward, they could objectively see the effect of music on the brain. The effects were limited to people who reported enjoying music.

ALTERNATIVE TO MEDICATIONS

Music can even reduce the need for medication, Dr. Bonakdarpour notes. Research has shown that people who listen to calming music before surgery or when they are at the dentist need less pain medication. It can even help people who are afraid of MRIs.

"When I see individuals with cognitive disorders in my clinic, we talk about medications, but there are so many other things when it comes to the brain," he says. "If you injure your arm, you don't just take a pill. You need to do rehabilitation to get your function back. It's

Getting Started

Play music from your loved one's teenage years or early 20s. See the list on page 35 for some ideas.

Observe your loved one's response to particular songs. Play more of what they seem to enjoy and avoid anything that appears to create agitation or stir negative memories.

Start by playing music when your loved one seems distant or agitated. If their response is positive, play music on a more frequent basis.

Chart-Topping Songs Over the Years

People respond best to music they enjoyed in their teens and twenties. Here's a look at some of the most popular songs by decade from the 1930s through the 1970s.

1930s
- "In the Mood" by Glenn Miller
- "God Bless America" by Kate Smith
- "Over the Rainbow" by Judy Garland
- "Minnie the Moocher" by Cab Calloway
- "Sing, Sing, Sing" by Benny Goodman

1940s
- "Frenesi" by Artie Shaw
- "I've Heard That Song Before" by Harry James
- "Heartaches" by Ted Weems
- "Near You" by Francis Craig
- "Paper Doll" by Mills Brothers

1950s
- "Goodnight Irene" by Gordon Jenkins and the Weavers
- "Vaya Con Dios" by Les Paul and Mary Ford
- "Don't Be Cruel" by Elvis Presley
- "Cry" by Johnny Ray and the Four Lads
- "The Third Man Theme" by Anton Karas

1960s
- "Mack the Knife" by Bobby Darin
- "Theme from a Summer Place" by Percy Faith
- "Crazy" by Patsy Cline
- "Tossin' and Turnin'" by Bobby Lewis
- "I Want to Hold Your Hand" by The Beatles

1970s
- "You Light Up My Life" by Debby Boone
- "Night Fever" by The Bee Gees
- "Tonight's the Night" by Rod Stewart
- "I'll Be There" by The Jackson 5
- "Bridge Over Troubled Water" by Simon & Garfunkel

the same with the brain. People need memory therapy."

For many people, music fits the bill. For those who don't enjoy music, visiting museums or watching theater are both beneficial.

New Weekly Alzheimer's Patch

Stephen Salloway, M.D., professor of neurology at Brown University, Providence. Brown.edu

The FDA has approved Adlarity, a weekly *donepezil* patch for Alzheimer's dementia. Donepezil has long been available as a daily pill (Aricept) but can cause gastrointestinal side effects, which Adlarity makes less severe. *Rivastigmine* (Exelon), a similar drug, also has been available as a daily patch. Both drugs inhibit an enzyme that breaks down a brain chemical essential for short-term memory.

New Test Can Detect Alzheimer's Disease in Blood

University of Pittsburgh.

Neuroscientists have developed a blood test to detect a marker of Alzheimer's disease neurodegeneration. Currently, to diagnose Alzheimer's disease, clinicians use imaging or cerebrospinal fluid (CSF) samples to detect the presence of three things: amyloid plaques, tau tangles, and neurodegeneration in the brain. Detecting biomarkers in blood is less invasive and requires fewer resources, but the biggest hurdle in using blood samples has been detecting markers of neurodegeneration that are specific to the brain and not influenced by potentially misleading contaminants produced elsewhere in the body. This new test detects a biomarker called BD-tau while avoiding free-floating "big tau" proteins produced by cells outside the brain.

Exercise Improves Cognition

Older adults who exercise regularly have higher levels of a class of proteins that strengthen the connections between neurons that support memory, focus, decision-making, and other aspects of cognition. These exercise-fueled proteins also appear to diminish the toxic effects of amyloid and tau, two proteins strongly associated with Alzheimer's disease. Physical activity also prompts the production of new brain cells and supports healthy circulation.

Alzheimer's & Dementia: The Journal of the Alzheimer's Association.

In experiments, levels of BD-tau detected in blood samples match with levels of tau in the CSF and reliably distinguish Alzheimer's from other neurodegenerative diseases, the researchers reported. They will next study the validity of the test in a wider range of people, including older adults with no biological evidence of Alzheimer's disease.

Regular Exercise Reduces Dementia Risk

Barry Franklin, Ph.D., director, preventive cardiology, Beaumont Health, Royal Oak, Michigan.

There's increasing evidence that consistent physical activity can lower the risk of dementia. But not all exercise is the same. New research published in the prestigious medical journal *The Lancet* suggests that more vigorous exercise may provide more protection.

A BETTER ACTIVITY MEASURE

The Trøndelag Health Study (HUNT) analyzed data on 29,826 people and used a measure called personal activity intelligence (PAI). While current exercise recommendations are based only on time—150 to 300 minutes of moderate activity or 75 to 150 minutes of vigorous activity per week—PAI digs deeper. It considers your sex, age, resting and maximal heart rate, and heart rate fluctuations over time to estimate exercise intensity and energy expenditure. When your heart rate rises, you earn PAI points. The more it rises, the faster those points accrue.

During an average follow-up of 24 years, the people who earned at least 100 points per week at two time periods during the study had a 25 percent lower risk of developing dementia and a 38 percent lower risk of dementia-related mortality when compared with people who had zero PAI points. Among the people who did develop dementia, those with a high PAI score experienced a later onset (2.8 years) and lived 2.4 years longer.

Because you earn more PAI points with vigorous exercise than with moderate activity, adding more heart-pumping workouts into your week is more protective than spending longer periods on lighter workouts.

NOT TOO LATE TO START

The effects weren't limited to long-term exercisers. The investigators compared PAI scores from the first phase of the study (1984 to 1986) with scores from a second phase a decade later (1995 to 1997). People who had scores lower than 100 in the first phase were able to reduce their risk of dementia simply by increasing their PAI score to more than 100 by the second phase. In fact, even small increases in the PAI score showed benefits.

HOW TO MEASURE PAI

You can officially track your PAI with a tool such as a fitness tracker or smart watch. If you have a Fitbit, Apple Watch, Garmin, Polar, or Zepp/Amazfit heart rate monitor, you can measure PAI with the app Memento U, which is available in the App Store and on Google Play.

Once you're geared up to track your progress, you can do any activity you enjoy and that elevates your heart rate. Aim for a combination of moderate and vigorous activity.

If your heart rate is between 60 and 79 percent of your maximum rate, you're exercising at a moderate level. (You can estimate your maximum heart rate by subtracting your age from 220. Use this formula only if you are healthy,

Beyond Dementia

Attaining a weekly PAI score over 100 does more than reduce dementia risk, according to the Norwegian University of Science and Technology. *People who maintain a higher score…*

- live an average of 8 years longer
- have a 30 percent lower risk of cardio-vascular death
- gain less weight than people who are inactive
- have better exercise capacity, sleep, and lower body fat.

These benefits are seen in men and women of all ages, smokers, and people with diabetes, high blood pressure, or overweight.

---

not diabetic, and not taking medications that can affect your heart rate.)

If you get your heart rate to about 80 percent of your maximum, you're in the vigorous zone. The more time you spend in the vigorous zone, the faster your PAI will rise.

The kind of exercise you need to reach those targets is different for everyone. If you are sedentary, going for short walks throughout the week could be enough to elevate your heart rate, but as you get more fit, your heart gets more efficient, and you'll need to work harder to elevate your heart rate. You can start with a smaller goal, like 50 PAI points each week, and gradually work up to 100.

You don't have to be active every day to get to 100. Your total PAI score is calculated over seven days. If you know you can't exercise on some days, you can "bank" your points by earning more points on others.

While exercise is a powerful way to reduce your risk of dementia, it's not the only one. Numerous studies show that eating a healthy diet, avoiding smoking, reducing stress, maintaining a healthy weight, and socializing are all important, too.

Lose Fat to Boost Memory

JAMA Network Open.

In a study of more than 9,000 adults, researchers found that having higher body fat was associated with reduced thinking and memory ability later in life. The findings suggest that there may be pathways linking excess fat to reduced cognitive function separate from what is known about how hypertension or diabetes may affect brain function and thinking skills. While there was no direct cause-and-effect relationship established in the study, researchers did propose that the findings underscore other research that has linked a healthy weight and body fat percentage to healthier cognition and memory.

Five Things You Can Do Today to Keep Your Brain Sharp

Cynthia R. Green, Ph.D., president of Total Brain Health, a company that develops evidence-based brain wellness classes and programs. One of America's foremost experts on brain health, she is founding director of the Memory Enhancement Program at Icahn School of Medicine at Mount Sinai in New York City. TotalBrainHealth.com

By now, you likely know about the go-to tips touted by experts for maintaining your memory as you age—doing crossword puzzles…learning a new language… exercising and eating well. But what about creating daily to-do lists? Or trying to complete the daily Wordle in five minutes or less?

Here are five creative, fun ways to keep your brain sharp, no matter what your age, from brain-health expert Cynthia R. Green, Ph.D.…

1. Play against the clock.

The cognitive areas in the brain that are most challenged by aging include those that allow us to think fast and process information efficiently…that hold or sustain attention…and that think nimbly, which is crucial for multitasking. These all factor into memory, and they tend to wane as we grow older.

Brain booster: Add a time element to some of your usual intellectual pursuits, such as trying to beat the clock when playing *Wordle* or filling out *The New York Times* spelling bee. This forces you to pay attention, work quickly and think flexibly. You can use your own timer for your favorite word games, aiming for a number that feels challenging but doable.

Other suggestions: *The New York Times* online crossword puzzle has a built-in timer, and some word games, such as *Boggle*, include a beat-the-clock element. Or set a timer for one minute, and challenge yourself to name a certain number of winter sports…car models… fruits and veggies…etc.

This sort of play-based training doesn't require a huge time commitment. Even quick five-minute bursts of activity each day can make a difference in your processing time, focus and ability to multitask.

2. Chat with friends.

The pandemic has made it difficult to spend time with friends and loved ones over the last few years, but it's worth the extra effort.

Brain booster: Schedule time to socialize with friends—doing so may cut your risk for memory impairment in half!

Conversing with friends is an opportunity to exercise many thinking skills in an informal way—it hones your ability to focus and keeps you thinking on your toes (there's that nimble thinking again) by requiring you to toggle between speaking and listening. It also challenges your brain to hold pieces of information so you don't constantly interrupt the other person.

The payoff can be almost immediate. In a University of Michigan study, subjects performed better on short-term memory tests after spending just 10 minutes conversing with another person.

Over the long term, enjoying the company of friends and loved ones even may reduce dementia risk for individuals with a genetic predisposition toward it.

Having a friend by your side also can make it easier for you to participate in brain-healthy activities, such as taking long walks or doing other types of exercise…attending a concert or lecture…or traveling to one of your bucket-list destinations.

3. Give the Green Mediterranean diet a go.

By now you've heard a lot about the Mediterranean diet and how effective it is for supporting brain health. This eating plan is heavy on fruits and vegetables…healthy fats such as those found in olive oil, nuts, salmon, and avocados…beans…and whole grains. Also, this diet minimizes consumption of red meat, poultry, and sugar. Dozens of studies, including a 2021 *Neurology* study, found that eating this way preserves memory and prevents shrinkage in the brain's memory centers.

One reason the Mediterranean diet enhances brain health: It is high in polyphenols—anti-inflammatory plant compounds found in berries, green veggies, and other produce that can cross the blood-brain barrier. This means that they physically travel into the brain, including those regions involved in memory. Once there, the polyphenols grab onto health- and memory-damaging free radicals—metabolic byproducts that cause neurons to age faster—and carry them out of the brain.

Brain booster: A new tweak to the brain-healthy diet may render it even more beneficial. A Green Mediterranean diet includes three to four cups of green tea and one-quarter cup of walnuts per day…additional servings of vegetables and fruits…almost no red meat…and more plant-based protein. (Studies usually use *Wolffia globosa*, a high-protein aquatic plant commonly called "duckweed," which is rich in polyphenols.)

Promising findings: In a new Israeli study published in *The American Journal of Clinical Nutrition*, 284 sedentary adults were assigned to follow one of three eating plans—a standard "healthy" calorie-controlled diet…a low-calorie Mediterranean diet…or the Green Mediterranean diet.

Results: After 18 to 24 months, the adults in both Mediterranean-diet groups showed significantly less brain shrinkage, and the effect was even more pronounced in the Green-Med group, especially in participants over 50 years old. Green Mediterranean diet subjects also experienced improved insulin sensitivity, which is linked with decreased risk for dementia in the future.

Walnuts and green tea are rich in polyphenols—the leaves of the tea are minimally processed, leaving more of the beneficial compounds in place. Duckweed is high in polyphenols, too, though not widely available. You can reap similar benefits by incorporating multiple sources of polyphenol-rich foods such as berries, dark leafy green veggies, green tea, walnuts, and olive oil into your daily diet while reducing the amount of red meat you eat.

4. Read more.

Research conducted by the Rush Alzheimer's Disease Center at Chicago's Rush University Medical Center linked lifelong reading with a reduced risk for future cognitive decline, possibly by facilitating the creation of new neural connections. Reading is a wonderful way to engage our brains in creative thought, exploration, planning and problem-solving.

Brain booster: Read more...and read more things on paper. Before the advent of computers and smartphones, people read on paper only. Now, one-third of Americans read a combination of e-books and paper books, according to the Pew Research Center. But reading on electronic devices just isn't the same—it can cause eyestrain, and a 2022 *Scientific Reports* study found that it creates an overactive environment in the brain that reduces reading comprehension.

5. Make lists.

List-making is an excellent cognitive tool. Writing down each task requires you to pay close attention to the information you wish to remember, and placing it in an organizational structure such as a list helps cement it into your memory. To-do lists also help you get more things done, which research shows frees up space in your mind for other plans, tasks, and challenges.

Brain booster: Make lots of lists—for your daily chores, menus, groceries, and other things—and write them out by hand.

Build a Better Memory

Marc Milstein, Ph.D., author of *The Age-Proof Brain*. He is a researcher and speaker.

We all have memory lapses: We forget the name of the person we just met, where we put our keys, or why we walked into the kitchen. These are perfectly normal—they don't signify impending cognitive decline—but they're a nuisance, nonetheless. So we asked memory expert Marc Milstein, Ph.D., how we can improve our recall.

SLOW DOWN

When you process new information, it first enters a "waiting-room" in the brain's hippocampus, where it resides for seven to 10 seconds. If you focus on something for less than seven seconds, it doesn't have a chance to stick, so the first tip to improve memory is to simply give yourself more time before moving on to the next task.

MARK IT AS IMPORTANT

Your brain is constantly deciding if information is important enough to move into longer-term storage or if it can be discarded. You can boost memory, then, by telling your brain what's important.

One way to do this is to recruit different parts of your brain. If you want to remember someone's name, instead of just thinking about the name, try imagining yourself writing it on their forehead. Writing—or imagining it—activates the frontal lobe and helps mark the information as worth remembering.

SAY IT OUT LOUD

Speaking activates parts of the brain used in speech and hearing, so simply saying something out loud helps you better remember it. If you tend to lose your keys or wallet, the next time you put them down, say out loud where you put them. Putting information to music can also activate the motor, emotional, and speech parts of the brain, which all aid in memory.

ADD DETAILS

Your brain loves a story, but a single word, like a name or a password, not so much. So,

Why Memories Change Over Time

Have you ever shared an experience with someone and later realized you have very different memories of the same event? That's because every time you learn something, you make a connection. Every time you revisit it, you break it apart and put it back together, but you don't exactly attach it the same way. Over time, memories can become distorted. The bright side is that therapists can use this process to help traumatic or difficult memories become easier to bear.

add detail to boost your memory. If you are trying to remember that someone's name is George, embellish that information. For example, you might make a mental picture of King George sitting in a pub in England.

USE IT OR LOSE IT

Nowadays, we don't have to work to recall information when we can just Google it. But pushing your brain to find a memory can strengthen your power of recall overall. Play trivia games or join a book club. When the name of an actor in a movie eludes you, don't immediately look it up. Let your brain work on it a bit. When you go shopping, take your list, but also see if you can recall what's on it without looking.

LEARN NEW THINGS

Simply learning something new can boost your brain power and help you practice moving information from your short- to long-term memory. Pick something outside of your expertise, such as painting, a sport, or a new language, as learning new information is one of the best things you can do for your brain.

MANAGE, BUT DON'T AVOID, STRESS

Short bursts of stress are good for the brain. In fact, people with some stress have memories that stay sharper longer. But when that stress tips into being chronic, the hippocampus can actually shrink. To reduce stress and improve memory, exercise, take relaxing breaks, practice mindfulness, and spend some time in nature.

Cleaner Air Slows Cognitive Decline, Improves Brain Age

Keck School of Medicine of USC.

Improving air quality is good for your body and mind. Researchers measured the cognitive function and episodic memory of 2,232 women annually for 10 years and estimated the annual concentration of particulate matter (air pollution) at their home addresses. Women who lived in locations where the air quality improved over 10 years had test scores that were equivalent to the cognitive aging in women who were up to 1.6 years younger.

There are three possible explanations: First, ultrafine particulate matter can bypass the blood-brain barrier and cause direct damage to the brain. Second, particles in the lungs or bloodstream might alert the immune system and trigger inflammation in the brain. Finally, air pollution might cause cerebrovascular damage. Experts recommend minimizing outdoor exercise when air pollution levels are high, avoiding travel times and routes with traffic congestion, and using low-traffic roads when walking or bicycling.

Pets May Protect Cognition

USA Today/Ipsos.

Pets may slow cognitive decline in older adults. An observational study of 1,369 people ages 65 and older found that people who were actively involved with caring for a pet had lower levels of loneliness and depression, and a slower rate of cognitive decline over six years. The study does not prove a cause-and-effect relationship, but it suggests that long-term pet ownership is good for the mind.

Light Drinking May Harm the Brain

Henry Kranzler, Ph.D., director, Penn Center for Studies of Addiction, University of Pennsylvania, Philadelphia.

Researchers analyzed data from more than 36,000 adults and found that as little as one-half of a serving of beer per day is linked to reduced brain volume. Heavier drinking was associated with an even greater toll. People who drink heavily have alterations in brain structure and size that are associated with cognitive impairments.

Early-Stage Alzheimer's Puts Financial Assets at Significant Risk

Study of health and retirement data and Medicare claims over 12 years by researchers at Georgetown University, Washington, D.C., published in *Health Economics*.

In the early stages of dementia—before the condition is even noticed—people often lose their ability to properly manage their finances. Even worse, these financial vulnerabilities can impact a family's ability to pay for care as the disease progresses.

ICU Stays Increase Dementia Risk

Medscape Medical News.

Spending time in an intensive care unit increases the risk of developing dementia, researchers reported at this year's Alzheimer's Association International Conference. In their analysis, ICU hospitalization was associated with a 63 percent higher risk of Alzheimer's dementia and a 71 percent higher risk of all-type dementia. When researchers adjusted for

vascular risk factors and disease, the risk of Alzheimer's disease and dementia doubled.

Ouch! When to Worry About That Bump on the Head

Ashika Jain, M.D., director of the Division of Emergency Trauma at NYU Langone Health in New York City and clinical associate professor in the Ronald O. Perelman Department of Emergency Medicine at NYU Grossman School of Medicine. Dr. Jain's special interests include geriatric head injury, trauma, ultrasound, critical care, and global health. NYULangone.org

It's a common scenario—you stumble, fall, and hit your head...or you bang it on a kitchen cabinet after getting something out of a lower cabinet. Fortunately, you're able to get up on your own or with the help of a friend, and you think that you are relatively unscathed—no cuts, no blood, no giant goose egg.

But how do you know if it's really safe to continue on with your day...or if you should be checked out by a doctor?

We all thought about this same question in the months following comedian Bob Saget's death from head trauma sustained during a fall in his hotel room. He was 65 at the time—noteworthy because adults over age 65 have a 27 percent chance of falling in any given year.

Every year, people ages 65 and up experience 36 million falls—in fact, falls are the most common source of traumatic injury in this age group. One out of five of these falls will result in a serious injury, including head trauma. And these falls usually happen at home and involve tripping over rugs...shoes, boxes, or other things on the floor...pets...cords and wires...or in slippery tubs or showers. And outside, falls can occur on curbs or slippery sidewalks.

What happens when you hit your head: You may develop a visible bump caused by blood, interstitial fluid, or both, sometimes called a goose egg, that can form shortly after the trauma. Patients on blood thinners may notice that the bump, also called a *hemato-*

ma, continues to grow over some hours. Or you may have obvious bleeding, as in a cut or scrape…or hidden bleeding in the brain or the layers of tissue surrounding the brain. Other types of head injuries include skull fractures and concussions, meaning that the brain has been shaken.

A head injury that results in bleeding in the brain or the layers surrounding the brain typically is classified as a subarachnoid hemorrhage…subdural hematoma…epidural hematoma…or intraparenchymal hemorrhage, depending on where in or around the brain the bleeding occurs. All of these injuries are serious and potentially dangerous. Subdural hematomas (bleeding on the surface of the brain) and intraparenchymal hemorrhages (bleeding within the brain itself) are the most common types of brain bleeds in older adults.

Brain bleed symptoms can include confusion, nausea and vomiting, changes in vision, slurred speech, drowsiness and/or a headache that doesn't go away. Without treatment, the bleeding can compromise oxygen flow to the brain, causing oxygen-deprived brain tissue to die and damaging any functions controlled by that particular tissue (breathing, vision, or limb movement, for instance).

Dangerous problem: Brain bleeds don't always have obvious symptoms. Subdural hematomas may not make themselves known for hours or even weeks. And with epidural hematomas, which most often happen as a result of a skull fracture tearing a blood vessel, the injured person usually will lose consciousness immediately after the fall or bump, followed by a period of awareness called the "lucid interval" during which he/she appears to have emerged unscathed. Many people mistake this lucid interval for a sign that no damage has occurred, but the injured person will swiftly deteriorate. This is how actress Natasha Richardson died following a ski accident in 2009.

Symptoms for concussions are similar to those of brain bleeds, along with sensitivity to light and noise, dilated pupils, and mood changes. Loss of consciousness from a concussion is uncommon.

OLDER ADULTS AT GREATER RISK

Several factors conspire against older individuals to make even seemingly minor falls and head injuries dangerous or potentially catastrophic.

•Medications may increase bleeding risk. Several age-related conditions are treated with anticoagulation medications—drugs that thin the blood and help prevent blood clots. While blood thinners can be lifesavers for patients with atrial fibrillation, pulmonary embolism, deep vein thrombosis, and other heart or blood conditions, they increase the chance of severe bleeding. Aspirin is another commonly used medication that has blood-thinning effects.

Fact: As many as 10 percent of elderly patients who show up at urgent-care facilities with a traumatic injury are taking *warfarin* (Coumadin), the most commonly used anticoagulant. Use of newer anticoagulant drugs, such as *dabigatran* (Pradaxa) and *rivaroxaban* (Xarelto), is increasing, too, and has the same risks.

•Age-related brain shrinkage. As we get older, our brains naturally atrophy, or shrink. This occurs even in cognitively healthy adults but is accelerated in people with dementia. As this happens, the space between the *dura*—a

---

Sleep After Hitting Your Head?

We've heard the warning—"Don't fall asleep after hitting your head."

Reality: There's nothing inherently dangerous about sleeping after hitting your head. The problem is that you can't ask a person who is sleeping about his/her symptoms. Or, if the person is alone, he won't realize if his symptoms are worsening.

If you were diagnosed with a concussion at, say, noon, and feel sleepy around 9 or 10 pm, that's perfectly normal and the sleep can help you heal. But if you hit your head and immediately feel drowsy or find it difficult to stay awake, call 911.

—Ashika Jain, M.D.

protective fibrous layer of connective tissue that sheaths the brain—and the brain itself shrinks.

Result: If you hit your head and develop a brain bleed, it may take a while for symptoms such as headache, nausea or vomiting, or tingling, numbness, weakness, or paralysis in a limb or the face to show up, because there is more space for blood to collect before it starts pressing on the brain.

Also, the veins in the membranes between the skull and brain begin to stretch and grow fragile with age. These veins are more likely to tear during a head injury—even a minor one, such as a fall out of a chair onto a carpeted floor.

Reminder: Older adults have more trouble maintaining their balance and poorer vision, both of which increase risk of falling and risk for a head injury.

Even falling and landing on your knees or butt can be enough to rattle the brain inside the skull, as can whiplash from a car accident.

WHEN TO GET ATTENTION

Anyone who falls into the following categories should seek help at your local emergency room...or an urgent-care facility equipped with CT machines...

•**Over age 65 and on a blood-thinning medication.** These medications increase the chances of a dangerous bleed. About one-quarter of older adults on an anticoagulant who develop a brain bleed will die as a result, versus 9 percent of elderly patients who are not on anticoagulation therapy. Even if the exam—usually a head computerized tomography (CT) scan—finds no evidence of a bleed, the patient may be asked to stay at the medical facility for several hours so that a second scan can be performed to check for delayed bleeding.

•**Experiencing clear-cut symptoms of a head injury, brain bleed, or concussion**—a headache that doesn't go away, drowsiness, confusion, nausea and vomiting, changes in vision, and slurred speech.

•**Loses consciousness or experiences a seizure.** Patients may not be certain if they passed out. If so, err on the side of caution and get medical assistance.

Suspected concussions don't usually require a CT scan. The doctor will check your vision,

balance, strength, hearing, reflexes, and memory to determine whether you need a CT scan.

If you don't fall into these categories: Ask yourself, *How do I feel?* Most people realize when something feels off. If you didn't lose consciousness...can stand up from the fall by yourself (or with minimal assistance)... and don't have any concerning symptoms, you likely are in the clear. If your neck, shoulder, hip, or another body part hurts, that could be a sign of a fracture.

TREATMENT FOR A HEAD INJURY

Small bleeds might not require significant treatment—smaller amounts of blood may be slowly reabsorbed by the body without causing complications. In these cases, you may be monitored in the hospital for 24 hours, then sent home to rest. Tylenol typically is prescribed for headache. And patients should follow up with their doctors for medication reassessment and management.

If a CT scan reveals a larger bleed, surgery may be necessary. But not everyone is physically healthy enough to survive a brain operation—your physician will weigh the pros and cons and decide if a wait-and-see approach might be safer.

Concussions usually are not life-threatening, so rest—physical rest as well as resting your brain by avoiding reading, TV, computer screens, and the like—often is sufficient for healing.

Memory Supplements Might Be Misguided

Cell Metabolism.

Supplemental l-serine, an amino acid, is advertised to improve memory and cognitive function and to help stave off Alzheimer's disease (AD), but new findings put its benefit in question. Scientists previously believed that people with AD have too *little* serine in the brain, making supplementation protective, but new research suggests that the opposite may be true.

One of the key enzymes that produce serine is called PHGDH. Researchers found that PHGDH gene expression was higher in the post-mortem brains of people with AD than it was in those without AD. Higher PHGDH suggests higher levels of serine. If people with AD already have elevated levels of serine, supplements offer no benefit. Researchers found a steep increase in PHGDH gene expression in healthy people two years before they were diagnosed with AD. "Anyone looking to recommend or take serine to mitigate Alzheimer's symptoms should exercise caution," concluded researcher Riccardo Calandrelli, Ph.D.

Vitamin D May Help Ward Off Dementia

Elina Hyppönen, Ph.D., director of the Australian Centre for Precision Health within the University of South Australia's Cancer Research Institute.

After analyzing data from 294,514 people, a research team found that those with low levels of vitamin D (25 nmol/L) had a 54 percent higher risk of developing dementia compared with people whose vitamin D levels were normal (50 nmol/L). Exposure to sunlight and dietary modifications may not be enough to boost vitamin D levels and supplementation may be needed. According to the National Institutes of Health, adults ages 69 and younger need 600 international units (IU) of vitamin D daily, and adults ages 70 and older need 800 IU daily.

Flu Vaccine May Protect Against Alzheimer's

Paul E. Schulz, M.D., the Rick McCord Professor in Neurology at McGovern Medical School, UT Health Houston.

People who received at least one influenza vaccine were 40 percent less likely to develop Alzheimer's disease within four years. People who consistently receive the flu vaccine have the lowest risk of all. The study included 935,887 flu-vaccinated patients and 935,887 unvaccinated patients. Over four years, 5.1 percent of flu-vaccinated patients developed Alzheimer's disease, compared with 8.5 percent of unvaccinated patients. There is evidence that other vaccines provide similar protection, so the effects are likely not specific to the flu vaccine, the researchers noted. "Instead, we believe that the immune system is complex, and some alterations, such as pneumonia, may activate it in a way that makes Alzheimer's disease worse. But other things that activate the immune system may do so in a different way—one that protects from Alzheimer's disease," Dr. Shultz said.

COVID-19 May Change the Brain

Gwenaëlle Douaud, Ph.D., associate professor, research fellow, Green Templeton College, University of Oxford, United Kingdom.

A study comparing brain scans from people before and after SARS-CoV-2 infection suggests that even minor cases of COVID-19 may cause a loss of gray matter in the orbitofrontal cortex and parahippocampal gyrus (the regions of the brain associated with smell). Study participants who had COVID-19 also showed a greater cognitive decline between their two scans than people in a control group. The decline was associated with the atrophy of a specific part of the cerebellum linked to cognition.

COVID-19 Linked to Parkinson's Disease

University of Queensland.

COVID-19 activates the same brain inflammation as Parkinson's disease. Infecting laboratory-grown human microglia cells with

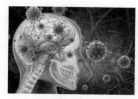 the virus that causes COVID-19 triggers the inflammasome pathway, which kills off neurons, researchers reported. This is the same pathway that Parkinson's and Alzheimer's proteins can activate in disease. If someone is predisposed to Parkinson's or Alzheimer's disease, COVID-19 could increase the risk. But the researchers also found that a type of medication under development for Parkinson's disease —called *UQ-developed inhibitory drugs*— blocked the inflammatory pathway. That could lead to promising new treatments.

Image: © Mohammed Haneefa Nizamudeen—Getty Images

Flavonoids May Prolong Life in People with Parkinson's Disease

Neurology.

Flavonoids, the compounds in colorful foods such as oranges, apples, and red wine, help protect cells against oxidative damage. A study showed that people with Parkinson's disease who ate the most of these foods had a lower chance of dying during the 34-year study period than those who ate the least. After controlling for age, total calorie consumption, and overall diet quality, researchers found that the group of participants in the top 25 percent of flavonoid consumers had a 70 percent greater chance of survival, compared with the lowest group.

Home Device Can Identify Parkinson's

Science Translational Medicine.

Researchers have developed an in-home device that can evaluate a person's Parkinson's disease severity, the progression of the disease, and the patient's response to medication. The device, which is about the size of a Wi-Fi router, gathers data passively using radio signals that reflect off the patient's body as they move around their home. The patient does not need to wear anything.

The researchers found that in-home gait speed (how fast someone walks) can be used to track Parkinson's progression and severity. For instance, declining gait speed suggests the onset of Parkinson's, and intraday fluctuations in gait speed correspond with how a person is responding to their medication. Gait speed may improve after a dose and then begin to decline after a period of time. A clinician could use these data to adjust medication dosage more effectively and accurately.

Weight Change in Early Parkinson's May Be Tied to Changes in Thinking Skills

Jin-Sun Jun, M.D., assistant professor, department of neurology, Kangnam Sacred Heart Hospital in Seoul, Republic of Korea.

More than 350 people who had been diagnosed with Parkinson's disease took a series of cognitive tests over eight years. The people who lost more than 3 percent of their body weight early in the disease had scores that declined 0.19 points faster per year than the scores of people who maintained their weight. The steepest declines were related to verbal fluency skills. Conversely, the people who gained weight had a slower decline in their scores than people who maintained their weight. There was no association between weight change and any other non-motor symptoms. The study does not prove that weight change causes changes in thinking skills. It shows an association only.

Improve Mobility with PD

Parkinson's-related walking difficulties can be mitigated by walking to a beat…counting each step…making wide turns or shifting weight from side to side while turning…using relaxation techniques…not doing other things while walking…mimicking someone else's walk…using your legs other ways such as bike riding.

Anouk Tosserams, M.D., rehabilitation and neurology researcher at Radboud University Medical Center, the Netherlands, and lead author of a study published in *Neurology*.

Parkinson's Is More Prevalent Than Previously Thought

Michael Okun, M.D., medical advisor to the Parkinson's Foundation and chair of neurology and director of Norman Fixel Institute for Neurological Diseases at University of Florida College of Medicine, Gainesville, commenting on a study published in *Nature*.

The most recent estimate of the incidence of new Parkinson's diagnoses is 86,000—up from 60,000 in 2012…and likely linked to an aging population, pesticide exposure, and awareness of the disease. See a neurologist if any of these signs appear—tremor (not always present)…flailing during sleep…loss of smell…constipation…small handwriting…shuffling gait …and depression.

Common Hormone Drug Linked to Brain Tumors

Thomas Santarius, M.D., Ph.D., neurosurgeon at Cambridge University Hospitals, Cambridge, U.K., and coleader of a study of 166,000 patients published in *Scientific Reports*.

Because it blocks the action of male sex hormones, cyproterone acetate (CPA) often is prescribed at high dosages for aggressive prostate cancer, male-to-female gender transitioning, and hirsutism (excess body hair) in women.

Recent finding: High dosages taken for years make patients 20 times more likely to develop brain tumors called meningiomas. Patients prescribed CPA should discuss with their doctor the risk versus the benefits.

CHAPTER 3

Cancer Breakthroughs

Move More to Reduce Cancer Risk

 **I**f you took a walk this morning to improve your heart health or lift your mood, you already know that exercise is good for you. But walking, dancing, stair-climbing, and other kinds of physical activity have an additional health benefit: They can lower your risk of cancer.

In fact, becoming a little more active may be one of the most important things you can do, along with eating a healthy diet and not smoking, to lower cancer risk.

There's strong evidence that physical activity lowers the risk of bladder, breast, colon, endometrial, kidney, and stomach cancers, as well as one kind of esophageal cancer. It might also lower the risk of lung and other cancers. And people who survive some forms of cancer, including breast and colon cancer, appear to face lower recurrence risks if they are physically active.

Just how does moving your body stop cancers from forming, growing, or returning? While scientists are still seeking some answers, there's growing evidence that a complex interplay of physical activity, body fat, and other factors play a variety of roles.

One important clue is that many cancers linked to inactivity also are linked to obesity. For example, according to the National Cancer Institute, a woman's risk of endometrial cancer, which affects the lining of the uterus, is two to four times higher if she is obese or overweight than if she is at a healthy weight. People with obesity have a doubled risk of stomach and kidney cancer and also face heightened risks for colon, pancreatic, and certain esophageal

Anne McTiernan, M.D., Ph.D., internist and professor of epidemiology at Fred Hutchinson Cancer Center, in Seattle, Washington. She was among the scientific advisors who helped develop the most recent Physical Activity Guidelines for Americans. AnneMcTiernan.com cancers. Obese women who are past menopause have an increased risk of breast cancer.

HOW IT WORKS

Decades of research have detailed how physical activity lowers heart disease risk. Research on physical activity and cancer is at an earlier stage, but it has produced compelling evidence for several theories. *Here's the best current thinking on how physical activity lowers cancer risks...*

•**Exercise can reduce levels of sex hormones,** such as estrogen and testosterone, that play roles in several cancers, including breast and endometrial cancer. One reason obesity is linked with breast cancer in older women, but not younger women, may be that body fat becomes a major source of estrogen after menopause. Exercise that reduces body fat lowers hormone levels.

•**Exercise can help the body maintain a healthy insulin level.** High levels of insulin, a hormone that controls blood sugar, are associated with diabetes. But high insulin levels also can promote the growth of cancerous tumors. High insulin levels and other metabolic problems associated with type 2 diabetes are linked with cancers of the breast, colon, pancreas, and uterine lining.

•**Exercise can reduce inflammation.** Inflammation plays an important role in cancer. Physical activity may directly lower inflammation. It also likely reduces inflammation by helping people lose weight and fat. Body fat releases substances that promote inflammation.

Researchers are looking for additional ways physical activity might reduce cancer risks. For example, repeated bouts of exercise might change the immune system in beneficial ways or protect our very DNA from changes that can lead to tumor formation and growth.

WHAT IT MEANS FOR YOU

You don't have to run marathons to reap the cancer-preventing benefits of exercise. Research suggests that every bit of added movement helps, whether that means climbing some extra stairs, spending more time working in your home or garden, or getting in more steps

How Much Activity You Need

Studies have yet to show exactly how much exercise of what kind provides the strongest protection from cancer. But, keeping in mind that every bit counts, you can't go wrong following the U.S. government's physical activity guidelines for adults. *That means you should...*

•**Aim to move more and sit less throughout the day.**

•**Get at least 150 to 300 minutes a week of moderate aerobic activity** (such as brisk walking) or 75 to 150 minutes of vigorous aerobic activity (such as running). You could meet the goal by taking five 30-minute walks or a few long jogs, or by mixing in swimming, biking, dancing, tennis, pickleball, or any other activity that gets your heart beating faster.

•**Do muscle-strengthening activities at least two days a week.** You might lift some weights, use resistance bands, or do exercises such as squats and push-ups. Even carrying heavy groceries or lawn supplies can count.

•**Work on improving your balance if you are over age 65.** Activities such as yoga, tai chi, and ballroom dancing can help.

•**Be as physically active as you can if you have disabilities** or chronic health problems that prevent you from following these general recommendations.

Start slowly and gradually build up your activity levels if you have been inactive for a while.

by driving less often or parking farther from your destinations.

With that said, research suggests that, for some cancers, protection increases with more movement over a longer period of time. So, if you aren't yet meeting the U.S. government's recommendations for physical activity (see sidebar), you might work toward that goal.

Recent studies have found that breast cancer survivors who got about as much physical activity as recommended, the equivalent of a brisk 30-minute walk most days, were significantly less likely to see their cancers return.

Some other takeaways and tips…

• **Weight matters, but it's complicated.** While weight loss might help lower the risk of some cancers, it's better to prevent weight gain in the first place, if you can. For one thing, significant weight loss is hard and virtually impossible to accomplish with exercise alone. Also, some research suggests that people who are already at a healthy weight get a bigger cancer prevention boost from exercise. But studies haven't sorted out the reasons. If you are already overweight or obese, it's good to know that physical activity can lower body fat and increase muscle, even if you lose little or no weight. That improvement in body composition alone appears to offer some protection from cancer.

• **How much you sit may matter, too.** Cancer studies have not yet shown the impact of how much time you spend sitting, lying down, or otherwise moving very little during your waking day. There's no doubt that moving more and sitting less is good for your overall health. So, if you find yourself sitting for long periods, be sure to take breaks to get up and move around.

• **It's never too late to start.** While some evidence suggests that people who are physically active throughout their lives may get the biggest cancer prevention boost, there's also evidence that taking up exercise in later years is beneficial.

---

6 Steps to Prevent Colorectal Cancer

Vi K. Chiu, M.D., Ph.D., director of the Gastrointestinal Oncology and Molecular Precision Programs at Cedars-Sinai The Angeles Clinic and Research Institute, Los Angeles.

Colorectal cancer is the third-leading cause of cancer death in the United States. The American Cancer Society estimates that, in 2022, about 106,180 people will be diagnosed with colon cancer and 44,850 people will be diagnosed with rectal cancer. Vi K. Chiu, M.D., Ph.D., director of the Gastrointestinal Oncology and Molecular Precision Programs at Cedars-Sinai The Angeles Clinic and Research Institute, recommends six steps to lower your risk.

1. Get screened. When detected early, colorectal cancer is highly treatable. Screening can help physicians detect and remove polyps before they become cancer. Adults at average risk for colorectal cancer should begin testing at age 45. Adults with parents, grandparents, or siblings who have had colorectal cancer should begin screening at age 40, or 10 years before the diagnosis of the youngest first-degree relative.

2. Focus on diet. Studies have shown that diets rich in fruits, vegetables, and whole grains, such as oatmeal, brown rice, popcorn, and whole-wheat bread, are linked with a lower risk of colon or rectal cancer, Dr. Chiu notes. It is beneficial to eat only small amounts of beef, pork, and lamb, and eat fewer processed meats. It's also helpful to keep an eye on your vitamin D levels. Analysis of a large, international study found that low levels of vitamin D were associated with a higher risk of getting colorectal cancer.

3. Exercise. Being active may reduce the risk of colorectal cancer by reducing inflammation in the body. People with inflammatory bowel diseases, such as Crohn's disease and ulcerative colitis, are at much higher risk for colon cancer than the general population.

"Exercise may decrease gut inflammation and improve immune surveillance to prevent cancer," Dr. Chiu explains.

Adults should aim for 150 minutes of moderate-intensity aerobic activity each week.

4. Manage weight. Being overweight or obese increases the risk of getting colon or rectal cancer because it can alter the function of hormones, such as insulin and leptin, Dr. Chiu says. Obese people have higher levels of insulin, which regulates blood sugar and can cause irregular cell growth in the colon.

5. Limit alcohol. Limit alcohol consumption to no more than one drink per day.

"Alcohol can cause intestinal damage. It is a toxin whose byproduct can damage DNA," Dr. Chiu says. "The gut may develop inflammation, and the gut immunity is weakened. This can lead to colorectal cancer."

6. Don't smoke. Smoking increases the risk for colorectal cancer because it causes DNA damage and inflammation in the intestine and lungs, Dr. Chiu says. That can cause hypoxia, which, in addition to DNA mutations, may cause aberrant cells to develop in the body and transform into cancer.

A study of more than 4,900 participants, published in the *British Journal of Cancer,* found that current smoking was associated with a 59 percent higher risk of colorectal cancer, and former smoking was associated with a 19 percent increased risk. The risk was not increased among those who stopped smoking more than 20 years prior.

Do Colonoscopies Make a Difference?

Study titled "Effect of Colonoscopy Screening on Risks of Colorectal Cancer and Related Death," by researchers with the Northern-European Initiative on Colorectal Cancer, published in *The New England Journal of Medicine.*

To screen or not to screen for colon cancer...Most doctors advise their patients to begin colonoscopies starting at age 45. A recent study investigated this highly recommended screening with disappointing results.

Colonoscopy is the most commonly used screening exam for colon cancer. During this test, a flexible scope is inserted into the rectum and the whole colon is explored. For people at normal risk for colon cancer, colonoscopies usually start at about age 45 and are continued every 10 years through age 75.

NOT MUCH DIFFERENCE BETWEEN SCREENED AND UNSCREENED

A new study from Europe that compared colonoscopy-screened people to unscreened people found that colonoscopies lowered the risk of colon cancer...but at a disappointing rate. And the screening did not significantly lower the risk of death from colon cancer. The study is from the Northern-European Initiative on Colon Cancer. In this trial, people in Northern Europe were invited to have a colonoscopy screening. After 10 years, these people were compared to a larger group of people who had no screening.

The trial included 84,585 healthy men and women, ages 55 to 64. These people came from Poland, Norway, Sweden, and the Netherlands. Colonoscopy screenings were done between 2009 and 2014. Colon cancer risk and deaths related to colon cancer were recorded at 10 years after colonoscopy. The results are published in *The New England Journal of Medicine. These were the key results...*

- **For people who were screened with colonoscopy,** the risk of a colon cancer diagnosis was about one percent.

- **For people not screened,** the risk of colon cancer diagnosis was 1.2 percent, meaning the risk for these people was 18 percent higher.

- **The risk of death from colon cancer in the screened group was 0.28 percent.**

- **The risk of death from colon cancer in the unscreened group was 0.31 percent.** The researchers interpreted this as not a significant difference.

- **The researchers found that they would need to do 455 colonoscopies to prevent one colon cancer.**

Colonoscopy may prevent colon cancer by removing colon growths called polyps that have the potential to turn cancerous in the future. Although the study did find some prevented cancers, the rate of prevention and the failure to show a significant decrease in deaths due to colon cancer were less than expected and described as disappointing.

REASONS FOR FEWER-THAN-EXPECTED SAVED LIVES

One factor that may have contributed to the disappointing results was the low rate of people who accepted the invitation to colonoscopy. The rate of acceptance was only 42 percent. More colonoscopies may have improved the rate of prevention. The researchers projected that if all the people invited had been screened with colonoscopy, it could have reduced colon cancer diagnosis by 31 percent, but even this number is lower than expected.

Another reason the study did not show a reduction in colon cancer death was that it only followed up for 10 years. Colon cancers may take 15 years to develop.

COLONOSCOPY IS NOT THE ONLY WAY TO FIND CANCER

One interpretation of the study is that colonoscopy may not be substantially better than other screening techniques. *According to the CDC and the U.S. Preventive Services Task Force guidelines, there are several options for colon cancer screening...*

•**Stool tests that look for blood,** cancer DNA, and cancer antibodies can be done once every three years.

•**Flexible sigmoidoscopy,** which is similar to colonoscopy but limits the exam to the rectum and lower colon, can be done every five years.

•**Virtual colonoscopy,** which is an imaging study of the colon displayed on a computer screen, can be done every five years.

•**Colonoscopy,** which has the advantage of examining the entire colon and removing a polyp or early cancer in a polyp, can be done every 10 years.

C. diff. Linked to Colon Cancer

Study led by researchers at Johns Hopkins University School of Medicine, Baltimore, published in *Cancer Discovery*.

Clostridium difficile (*C. diff*) causes severe diarrhea and is difficult to clear—often repeatedly recurring in up to 30 percent of infected patients, including pediatric patients.

Recent finding: Researchers were able to induce colon tumors in mice by exposing them to *C. diff.* bacteria. And in lab experiments, colon cells exposed to the microbe underwent genetic and physiological changes making them more vulnerable to cancer. More research

is needed to confirm these findings in humans and to better understand them.

Self-defense: Be extra vigilant about colon screening if you've ever been diagnosed with *C. diff.*

Throat Cancer Is on the Rise

Carole Fakhry, M.D., MPH, director of the Johns Hopkins Head and Neck Cancer Center and a professor of otolaryngology, head, and neck surgery. Dr. Fakhry is a nationally renowned expert in HPV head and neck cancer and has published multiple peer-reviewed papers in numerous medical journals on the subject.

In the past, cancer of the throat was mainly a disease of heavy tobacco use and drinking. Thanks to a successful public health campaign promoting the dangers of smoking, overall rates of throat cancer have decreased.

But starting in the 1990s, a different type of this cancer began to strike more often, and rates have been increasing ever since. It's called *HPV-positive oropharyngeal cancer* (HPV-OPC), which means cancer of the oropharynx (the middle part of the throat, including the base of the tongue and the tonsils) caused by the human papillomavirus (HPV).

If the acronym HPV sounds familiar, that's because it's the most common sexually transmitted infection in the United States. In fact, the U.S. Centers for Disease Control and Prevention says that nearly every sexually active person will come into contact with the virus at some point in their lifetime.

There are more than 100 strains, or types, of HPV. Some cause genital warts and others can cause cervical, vaginal, penile, anal, or throat cancer. That said, most people will never even know they've been infected, because their immune system clears the virus from their system, usually within two years.

If it doesn't, HPV can cause trouble years, and even decades, after the initial infection. This is what we're now seeing with HPV-OPC. The prevailing theory behind the rise in oral HPV is that oral sex has become much more commonplace, which increased the spread.

Actor Michael Douglas made headlines in 2013 when he was diagnosed with HPV-OPC in his late 60s, and he was outspoken about its oral sex link.

WHO IS MOST AT RISK?

Approximately 20,000 cases of oropharyngeal cancer cases are diagnosed in the United States annually. Of those, about 80 percent are caused by HPV. Men are three times more likely to be diagnosed with HPV-OPC than women. White, middle-aged, and older men (ages 50 to 59) have the highest risk, especially those with a history of multiple oral sex partners and those who smoke.

A specific strain of HPV called HPV16 is responsible for more than 90 percent of HPV-OPCs in the United States. HPV16 is one of the strains targeted by the Gardasil and Cervarix HPV vaccines. (HPV vaccination is recommended starting at age 9 and up until 26. Certain individuals between the ages of 26 and 45 may also be eligible for vaccination, based on their risk factors.)

Widespread vaccination has the potential to decrease rates of cervical and penile cancer and is also thought to protect against HPV-OPC when these vaccinated children, teens, and young adults are older. However, a 2021 *JAMA Oncology* study estimated that it will take more than 25 years until those effects can be seen. But because these vaccines became available only relatively recently, people who are currently in their 50s and older never had the chance to receive them.

WHAT TO LOOK FOR

About 10 percent of men and 4 percent of women have detectable HPV in their mouths at any given time, and rates increase with age. That doesn't mean all of them will go on to develop throat cancer: Most of them will clear the virus from their system before it can cause major trouble. Clinical trials are looking into whether screening may be warranted or effective.

Most people with HPV-OPC don't have symptoms. Typically, patients have a painless lump in the neck (swollen lymph node). Some may have a sore throat, difficulty swallowing, or persistent earache. If you notice any of these, it's time to call your health-care provider.

TREATMENT OPTIONS

Here's some reassuring news: Patients with HPV-positive throat cancer tend to live longer than those with HPV-negative throat cancer, such as that caused by tobacco and/or alcohol use. If found early, the four-year survival rate for HPV-OPC is 87 percent.

Your doctor will test the tumor to determine whether it is HPV+ or HPV-. Treatment typically involves minimally invasive robotic surgery, neck surgery, and possibly radiation or a combination of radiation and chemotherapy. In the future, immunotherapy, a cancer treatment that recruits the body's own immune system to fight cancer, might have a role, though it is still being studied.

A Life-Saving Test for Smokers and Ex-Smokers

Claudia Henschke, Ph.D., M.D., professor of radiology at Icahn School of Medicine at Mt. Sinai, New York City, discussing a study presented at the annual meeting of the Radiological Society of North America (RSNA).

Smokers—a 20-second screening test could add 20 years to your life. Current and former smokers diagnosed via a low-dose CT scan survived lung cancer for 20 years in 80 percent of cases, thanks to advancements in care. Unfortunately, only 15 percent of eligible people undergo this non-invasive scan, resulting in late diagnosis of cancer and an 18.6 percent five-year survival rate. If you're over 50 and have ever smoked, get screened annually.

Beware This Toxin in Dry Shampoo

Study by researchers at the independent laboratory Valisure, New Haven, Connecticut. Valisure.com

---

A test of 134 batches of dry shampoo from 34 companies found that 70 percent had measurable levels of the carcinogen *benzene*, known to cause leukemia and other blood disorders. Some products contained 170 times the FDA-mandated limit of two parts per million. High benzene levels also have been found in other personal-care products, including hand sanitizers, sunscreens, and spray deodorants. Benzene is a byproduct of the propellant used in dry shampoos, including butane, isobutane, and propane. Avoid products with these ingredients on the labels.

Early-Onset Cancers a Possible Global Epidemic

Study titled "Is Early-Onset Cancer an Emerging Global Epidemic? Current Evidence and Future Implications," by researchers at Brigham and Women's Hospital, Boston, published in *Nature Reviews Clinical Oncology*.

Being diagnosed with cancer is no longer a death sentence. Thanks to advances in medicine, survival rates are on the rise. In fact, the National Cancer Institute states that the overall cancer death rate in the United States has declined since the early 1990s. But a disturbing trend concerning cancer appears to be an increase in cases among younger individuals. And this trend is worldwide.

THE BIRTH COHORT EFFECT AND CANCER

According to a study by researchers at Brigham and Women's Hospital in Boston, an extensive global analysis of available studies and data shows a pattern of cancer called the *birth cohort effect*. Starting in 1990, each group (cohort) of people born 10 years later than another cohort shows a higher risk for early-onset cancer. In other words, people born in 1960 have a higher rate of these cancers than people born in 1950 and people born in 1970 have a higher risk than those born in 1960. The researchers say this pattern will probably continue and that it is leading to a global epidemic in early-onset cancers.

Cancers that show the birth cohort effect and have been increasing at epidemic rates in people under age 50 include cancers of the thyroid, stomach, prostate, bone marrow, liver, kidney, head and neck, gall bladder, bile ducts, esophagus, endometrium, colon, rectum, and breast. Finding the early-onset cancers is important, but finding the reason why the increase is happening will hopefully curb the trend. The results of the analysis are published in *Nature Reviews Clinical Oncology*.

THEORIES ON THE INCREASE OF EARLY-ONSET CANCERS

The research team says the exact reason or reasons for the rise in early-onset cancers cannot be determined by their study. To answer that question, researchers will need to design long-term studies that will follow people over time, called *longitudinal studies*. Since cancers can take years to develop, it will be a long time before results are available. For now, the researchers say there are several possible explanations.

Some of the earlier cancers are due to better screening for cancers, causing them to be found at an earlier age. Although routine screening may have been responsible for finding some early cancers, such as breast, colorectal, or prostate cancers, most other cancers do not have screening guidelines. A more important probable cause is early-life exposures that increase cancer risk. Researchers call these exposures the *exposome*. The exposome includes cancer risk factors in early life and young adult years from lifestyle changes, diet changes, obesity, environmental exposures, and changes in the gut bacteria, called the *microbiome*.

Lifestyle changes that have contributed include less sleep and less exercise. Eight of the cancers involve the digestive system, which suggests that diet exposures play a key role. Changes in diet over 50 years include highly processed foods and foods and beverages with added sugars. This may explain other risk factors, such as obesity, a changing microbiome and type 2 diabetes. The early-onset cancer epidemic may just be part of an increasing trend of many other early-developing chronic diseases. Alcohol ingestion is another cancer risk that has increased since the 1950s.

A FUTURE OF BIOBANKING

The research team concludes that it will be important to do longitudinal studies in the future. These studies would start in young children and follow them through life, recording data and taking body and blood samples, called *biobanking*. One of the weaknesses of this study is the lack of data from developing nations. The research team plans to collaborate with international research institutes to monitor global trends in these countries. For now, people need to be aware of the increasing risk and the likely risk factors. Doctors also need to be aware to help patients avoid or control risk factors and to be more aware of possible cancer signs or symptoms in younger adults.

Statins May Slow Cancer Growth

Ulrike Stein, M.D., laboratory group leader at Max Delbrück Center for Molecular Medicine in Berlin, Germany, and leader of a study published in *Clinical and Translational Medicine*.

In mouse models using human tissue, statin drugs successfully stopped the spread of cancer by inhibiting expression of *MACC1*, a gene that helps cancers spread from the original tumor throughout the body. Reviews of patient records also suggest that statins reduce cancer incidence by 50 percent. Human trials are planned before statins can be prescribed to slow cancer spread.

Skip the Sunburn

Jonathan Su, DPT, CSCS, TSAC-F, C-IAYT, physical therapist, yoga therapist, and former U.S. Army officer based in the San Francisco Bay area. Dr. Su is author of *6-Minute Fitness at 60+* and *6-Minute Core Strength*. https://sixminutefitness.com/about/

At least one in five American adults will develop skin cancer by age 70, and more than half of skin cancer-related deaths occur in people over age 65. Yet the

Warning: Multiple Sunburns Doubles Risk of Melanoma

Five or more sunburns over the course of a lifetime doubles risk for melanoma, the most dangerous form of skin cancer. Your chances of getting a sunburn increase if you use skin-care products that remove top skin layers, such as retinoids or glycolic acid…take antibiotics or diuretics…or read on a tablet or other screen outdoors—the screens reflect the sun's ultraviolet light.

Sunburn protection: Use a broad-spectrum sunscreen with SPF 30 or higher…avoid being in the sun altogether from 10 am to 3 pm, when UV rays are strongest.

Skin Cancer Foundation. SkinCancer.org

Centers for Disease Control and Prevention says the majority of older adults neglect to use sun protection when outdoors for an hour or more, even on warm, sunny days.

Sun damage is cumulative, building with every two-mile walk, tennis match, and gardening session. Repeated sunburns are especially dangerous in terms of increasing skin-cancer risk. About half of adults have been sunburned while swimming or playing sports in the past year, and a 2021 *International Journal of Environmental Research and Public Health* study found that nearly 60 percent of adult golfers reported experiencing a painful sunburn in the past year.

Stay safe: Apply a broad-spectrum sunscreen with an SPF of 30 or higher to all exposed skin, including the scalp, face, ears, neck, back, arms, and legs. Reapply every two hours. Sunscreen is important for people of all skin tones.

Bonus: Emerging research suggests wearing sunscreen during outdoor exercise may protect blood vessels, which helps with temperature regulation.

An easier approach is to look for clothing that's been treated or created in a way that limits penetration of damaging ultraviolet (UV) rays. Look for rash guards (high-coverage shirts), shorts, pants, and even sports bras with an ultraviolet protection factor (UPF) rating of 50 or higher. With UPF clothing, you don't need to apply or reapply sunscreen beneath covered areas or worry about missing any spots. Everyday clothing won't cut it, though. A plain white T-shirt allows about 20 percent of rays to sneak through.

Best Way to Apply Sunscreen

NYTimes.com/wirecutter

Apply sunscreen 15 to 20 minutes before going outside, so it has time to soak into your skin. Apply again within your first hour of sun exposure. Use one ounce of sunscreen for each application—about two tablespoons. Don't forget ears and the tops of your feet, which often receive the least protection. For hard-to-reach body areas, such as your back, have someone else help you apply the sunscreen. If you use an aerosol sunscreen for yourself or children, spray for a full two minutes in a windless, well-ventilated area with the spray nozzle close to the skin—even if directions say to keep it four to six inches away. Rub in the sunscreen immediately after spraying, even if directions say rubbing isn't necessary.

Regular Use of Vitamin D May Mean Less Melanoma

Study titled "Regular Use of Vitamin D Supplement Is Associated with Fewer Melanoma Cases Compared to Non-Use," by researchers at University of Eastern Finland and Kuopio University, both in Kuopio, Finland, published in *Melanoma Research*.

Skin cancer is the most common type of cancer. Only one percent of skin cancers are melanoma cancers, but these cancers are the most serious and they cause by far the most deaths from skin cancer. The other cancers are called squamous or basal cell skin cancers. They are much more common and much less dangerous.

Although some recent research has found an association between adequate vitamin D levels and less severe melanoma, previous studies have been inconsistent; some studies show a lower risk of skin cancer with vitamin D, some a higher risk. However, these studies have relied on blood levels of vitamin D, which can vary from skin levels. Some researchers theorize that vitamin D may protect the skin from the sun damage that leads to skin cancer. The skin manufactures vitamin D in response to sun exposure. The vitamin can also be obtained from diet or supplements.

VITAMIN D AND SKIN CANCER

To learn more about the association of vitamin D and skin cancers, a team of researchers from the University of Eastern Finland and Kuopio University (also in Finland) recruited 253 men and 245 women at high risk for skin cancer as research subjects, to see if taking vitamin D supplements might lower that risk. Dermatologists did skin examinations of all the people in the study, whose ages ranged from 21 to 79. They also gathered information about their medical histories, family histories, and vitamin D supplement use. To verify that the supplement use history was accurate, they compared results of reported supplement use and actual vitamin D blood levels.

The research team divided the subjects into three groups of vitamin D supplement use: non-users, occasional users, and regular users. They also divided the subjects by skin cancer risk groups as low, moderate, or high risk. Risk factors for melanoma and other skin cancers include exposure to sunlight, fair skin, personal or family history of skin cancer, the number of moles on the body (nevi), skin growths called actinic keratoses (from sun exposure), and a weak immune system. To test the effects of vitamin D supplements on people with weak immune systems (also called immunocompromised), the team included 96 immunocompromised subjects in the study.

The results of the study are published in the journal *Melanoma Research. These were the key results...*

•**Vitamin D supplements had no effect on aging of the skin from sun exposure,** actinic keratoses, moles, basal cell cancers, or squamous cell cancers.

•**There were lower rates of subjects with a history (past or present)** of melanoma skin cancer in regular vitamin D supplement users (18.1 percent) versus non-users (32.3 percent).

•**The risk of developing melanoma in regular users of vitamin D supplements was less than half the risk for non-users** (a risk reduction of about 55 percent). The researchers used regression analysis (a statistical computation) to come up with this estimation.

•**The results for the patients who were immunocompromised** was not significantly different than in the other subjects.

HOW MUCH VITAMIN D FOR LESS CANCER RISK?

The researchers conclude that regular use of vitamin D is associated with fewer cases of melanoma, when compared to non-use. They caution that association is not the same as cause, and it is unknown if low levels of vitamin D cause skin cancer. Until we have further studies, the researchers suggest that people should follow the recommended daily dietary intake of vitamin D. According to the National Institutes of Health, the recommended daily dietary intake is 600 international units (IU) for ages 1 to 70 and 800 IU for those 70 and over.

New Warning Signs Indicate Pancreatic Cancer Sooner

Study of 24,000 patients by researchers at University of Oxford, U.K., published in *British Journal of General Practice.*

Pancreatic cancer often is diagnosed when it is already advanced and hard to treat.

Recent finding: Thirst and dark urine were identified as symptoms of pancreatic ductal adenocarcinoma (PDAC), the most common type, as early as one year before the disease typically

is diagnosed. Two other serious symptoms—jaundice and gastrointestinal bleeding—already are known to be linked to PDAC and should prompt immediate medical attention.

Game Changer for Cancer Treatment

Anirban Maitra, MBBS, professor of pathology and translational molecular pathology, and scientific director of the Pancreatic Cancer Research Center at The University of Texas MD Anderson Cancer Center, Houston. He is coleader of the MD Anderson's Pre-Cancer Atlas project and the Pancreatic Cancer Moon Shot program. MDAnderson.org

Medical science's approach to treating cancer has always been just that—providing treatment to patients *after* they've received a cancer diagnosis. Of course, preventing cancer before it occurs is a goal, but virtually all cancer-prevention strategies to date have been passive in nature—health-care providers offer advice about lifestyle changes that could reduce patients' odds of later developing cancer, such as "stop smoking" or "use sunscreen."

Exciting news: We're on the cusp of a dramatic paradigm shift—human trials are underway to test medical treatments that could put a halt to certain cancers even before they become cancer. Elizabeth Blackburn, Ph.D., the Nobel Prize–winning past president of the American Association for Cancer Research, has coined the term "cancer interception" for these efforts, drawing a comparison with interceptions on the football field. While most cancer treatments don't begin until the opposition has put points on the board—and the patient's health has suffered—cancer interception would stop the opposition from advancing and potentially provide an opportunity to run the ball back in the other direction.

Treatments that can stop cancer before it becomes cancer already exist in a few very specific circumstances…

•**Vaccines** are available that reduce the odds of developing a small number of cancers that have a known viral component.

Examples: Vaccines that protect against *human papillomavirus* can reduce the odds of developing cervical cancer...and vaccines that protect against hepatitis B can reduce the odds of liver cancer.

•**Removal of precancerous lesions,** also known as an *intraepithelial neoplasia* (IEN), routinely occurs when lesions are identified by imaging or exams.

Examples: When a patient has a polyp removed from the colon during a colonoscopy, that polyp may be a precancerous growth removed to prevent cancer from developing. The same is true for certain types of precancerous skin moles.

But existing cancer preventions are the exceptions. Research underway could soon produce treatments that dramatically reduce the odds of developing a much wider range of cancers, including some of the most common... and deadly.

FROM PRECANCER TO CANCER

By the time someone is diagnosed with cancer, "precancerous cells" might have been lurking in his/her body for decades. These precancerous cells share gene mutations with cancer cells and could develop into cancer, but they are not themselves considered cancerous because they do not invade surrounding tissue or spread throughout the body. Most precancerous cells are eliminated by the immune system before they develop into cancer—and before patients and doctors even realize they exist—but some evade detection by the immune system. The goal of cancer-interception research is to target these precancerous cells with treatments that prevent them from becoming malignant.

Unfortunately, medical science currently has a very limited understanding of how precancers work on the molecular level, much less an ability to identify and treat them. For all of the time and money that has been spent on studying cancers over the years, very little has been devoted to studying precancers.

Exception: Medical science does have a sufficiently strong understanding of the precancerous phase of leukemia and multiple myeloma that doctors can determine when these

cancers might be developing based on blood and bone marrow tests.

Work currently is under way to develop a "precancer atlas"—an in-depth catalog of the biology of a range of precancerous cells and the paths those cells take to develop into cancer. Research teams involved with this project are studying not only the precancerous cells but also the healthy tissues and cells that surround them to understand how the precancerous cells develop and interact with their surroundings. Armed with that information, researchers should be able to identify aspects of the precancer that can be targeted using tools such as vaccines and "immune checkpoint inhibitors"—a type of immunotherapy that could encourage the immune system to continue battling precancerous cells until they are eradicated. Current projects are focused on the precancerous cells that lead to pancreatic cancer, lung cancer, colorectal and endometrial cancers, and head and neck cancers.

CLINICAL TRIALS UNDER WAY

What's especially exciting now is that cancer-interception clinical trials have already begun, including...

•**Colorectal cancer vaccine.** The most common cause of hereditary colorectal cancer is Lynch syndrome—it causes about 3 percent to 5 percent of colorectal cancers. The gene defect that causes *Lynch syndrome* affects the body's ability to repair DNA errors, leading to the accumulation of mutated proteins and increasing the odds of developing colorectal cancer and, to a lesser degree, increasing the risk for endometrial, ovarian, stomach, and brain cancers. It's estimated that one of every 288 people has Lynch syndrome, though most people who have it are not aware that they do.

A genetic counselor can review a patient's family history and look for mutations in germline DNA—but this test currently cannot be self-ordered.

A clinical trial being conducted by Eduardo Vilar-Sanchez, M.D., Ph.D., at The University of Texas MD Anderson Cancer Center is investigating a vaccine that could prevent Lynch syndrome cancers. This vaccine does not have the potential to prevent all colorectal cancers, because many are not linked to Lynch syndrome.

•**Pancreatic cancer vaccine.** Pancreatic cancer is among the leading causes of cancer deaths because it often is not identified until it has reached its late stages. The five-year survival rate is well under 10 percent. A potential pancreatic cancer vaccine developed by Elizabeth Jaffee, M.D., and Neeha Zaidi, M.D., at Johns Hopkins currently is undergoing clinical trials. The hope is that this vaccine will train the immune system to track down and eliminate pancreatic cancer cells before they spread.

WHEN WILL IT BE AVAILABLE?

With clinical trials already under way and the FDA receptive to this area of research, cancer interception is racing forward—but treatments are unlikely to become widely available until the 2030s. Today's clinical trials will have to be followed by large-scale studies to prove that these procedures are safe and effective, and those large-scale studies likely will have to be conducted over periods of five years or longer. When you test a new treatment for an existing cancer, it can be determined relatively quickly whether that treatment has caused the cancer to go into remission...but when you test a vaccine designed to prevent cancer, you have to track your test subjects for years to determine if they are indeed developing the cancer at a lower rate than would otherwise have been expected.

IN THE MEANTIME

If you are at high risk for a particular cancer—based on family history...genetic mutations uncovered by DNA tests...and/or scans revealing high-risk lesions—follow the cancer-screening schedule and lifestyle advice suggested by your health-care providers. And in the years ahead, ask your doctors if they are aware of clinical trials of any new cancer-interception treatments related to the cancer you are at elevated risk of developing. Taking part in such a trial could get you access to the treatment years before it is widely available. If not, watch for these treatments themselves to become available, likely starting in the 2030s.

Robots for Bladder-Cancer Surgery

JAMA.

Robot-assisted bladder-cancer surgery helps patients recover faster than traditional surgery. A study showed that patients who underwent robot-assisted surgery spent 20 percent less time in the hospital and had a 52 percent lower chance of readmission. There was a 77 percent reduction in the prevalence of blood clots compared with open surgery.

Most Cancer Is Caused by Environment, Not Genetics

According to a recent finding, only 10 percent of all cancers can be blamed on the genes a person is born with—the majority of cancers are caused by environmental factors.

Study by researchers at University of Alberta, Canada, published in *Metabolites*.

Eat to Prevent Cancer

Carrie Ali, editor, *Bottom Line Health*.

As skin cancer has become more common and more resistant to chemotherapy and radiation, researchers have looked to plants for possible new treatments. In culture dishes, animal models, and even a few human studies, they have identified phytochemicals that inhibit the development and progression of cancer cells in a variety of ways.

•**Resveratrol** slowed or prevented the spread of cancerous cells into surrounding tissue in mice. It may boost the effects of chemotherapy drugs and decrease melanoma cell viability. *Source:* grapes and peanuts.

•**Caffeic acid phenethyl ester** showed the potential to inhibit melanoma and several other cancers in laboratory and animal testing. *Source:* honey.

●**Genistein** is chemopreventive in melanoma and nonmelanoma skin cancers and has decreased UV-induced sunburn in humans. *Source:* soybeans.

●**Luteolin** can reduce the aggressiveness of skin cancer cells and stop their growth. It can sensitize cells to other anticancer treatments. *Source:* carrots, celery, olives.

●**Curcumin** appears to protect against head and neck squamous cell carcinoma. *Source:* turmeric.

●**Indole-3-carbinol** inhibited the proliferation of human melanoma cells in lab studies. *Source:* broccoli and cauliflower.

●**Caffeic acid.** In a mouse model, topical application inhibited cancer development. *Source:* coffee, fruits, and vegetables.

●**Epigallocatechin-3-gallate (EGCG)** has shown strong potential in human trials to prevent and treat skin cancer. *Source:* four to six cups of green or black tea a day.

●**Allyl sulfides.** Topical use has reduced the incidence and growth of skin cancer in mice. *Source:* garlic.

Scientists are exploring ways to improve bioavailability of these compounds, but you can get started by filling your plate with the healthy foods that contain these promising phytochemicals. Research clearly shows that diets that are high in fruits and vegetables help reduce the risk of developing cancers of any kind.

Parkinson's Drug May Reduce Side Effects from Chemo

Study titled "Istradefylline Protects from Cisplatin-Induced Nephrotoxicity and Peripheral Neuropathy While Preserving Cisplatin Antitumor Effects," by researchers from the University of Lille, France, published in *The Journal of Clinical Investigation*.

The body goes through a lot when it's treated for cancer. Chemotherapy treatments can inflict a heavy blow on the body's healthy cells. *Cisplatin* is a cancer drug developed by Michigan State University researchers more than 50 years ago. Since the 1970s, this drug has been a workhorse drug for cancer and remains the gold standard for many types, including testicular, ovarian, bladder, lung, stomach, and head and neck. Combined with other cancer drugs, cisplatin may also be used to treat cervical and breast cancer. Most cancers that respond to cisplatin are solid tumor cancers.

But for all the good it does, cisplatin often turns into another kind of toxic invader.

HOW CISPLATIN WORKS…AND HURTS

Cisplatin is given as an infusion into a vein or artery over 21 to 28 days. The drug enters rapidly growing cancer cells and disrupts their DNA, causing destruction of the cancer cells. Unfortunately, cisplatin also destroys some normal cells. The higher the dose and the longer the treatment, the more normal cells are destroyed, called adverse effects, or toxicity. This toxicity results in pausing treatment, lowering the dose, or stopping the drug completely. All of these roadblocks increase the risk of cancer spreading.

Cisplatin toxicity causes many uncomfortable side effects that may include nausea, vomiting, loss of appetite, weight loss, diarrhea, and hair loss. More importantly, cisplatin toxicity can cause damage to the nervous system (*neurotoxicity*) and the kidneys (*nephrotoxicity*). The most common sign of neurotoxicity is damage to nerves in the extremities called peripheral neuropathy. Nephrotoxicity can cause kidney failure in up to 35 percent of patients on cisplatin, which may be life threatening.

AN EFFECTIVE ANTIDOTE TO CISPLATIN SIDE EFFECTS

Up until now, the only treatment for cisplatin side effects and toxicity is providing lots of fluids to protect the kidneys. Peripheral neuropathy has been considered an unavoidable risk. Now, an international team of researchers may have discovered a much-needed antidote to cisplatin toxicity. The team has shown that an existing, FDA-approved drug used to treat Parkinson's disease can block many of the adverse effects of cisplatin toxicity. The drug is *istradefylline* (sold as Nourianz).

Istradefylline is an oral drug used along with other Parkinson's disease drugs to reduce muscle stiffness and loss of muscle control. When cisplatin destroys cells, the cells release a chemical naturally found in human cells called adenosine. This chemical causes adverse effects of cell toxicity, and istradefylline blocks these effects. Adenosine plays a major role in kidney injury, so the researchers hoped that blocking adenosine effects could reduce cisplatin nephrotoxicity.

Using mice as subjects, the research team was able to show that adding istradefylline to cisplatin treatments significantly reduced nephrotoxicity, allowing longer treatment at higher doses to kill cancer cells. This type of study working with animals before humans is called preclinical research. The study also found that adding istradefylline reduced peripheral neuropathy and that the combination may actually improve response to cisplatin. The next step will involve human trails to see if these promising preclinical results will help people with cancers that depend on cisplatin.

Cancer Deaths Are Decreasing

Annual Report to the Nation on the Status of Cancer.

Cancer death rates are dropping in every major racial and ethnic group in the United States. From 2015 to 2019, overall cancer death rates decreased by 2.1 percent per year in men and women combined. The declines in death rates were steepest in lung cancer and melanoma (by 4 to 5 percent per year). Death rates increased for cancers of the pancreas, brain, bones, and joints among men, and for cancers of the pancreas and uterus among women. Incidence rates increased for pancreas, kidney, and testis cancers in men and liver, melanoma, kidney, myeloma, pancreas, breast, oral cavity, and pharynx cancer in women.

CHAPTER 4

Cardiovascular Health and Stroke

Are You Taking Heart Health Seriously Enough?

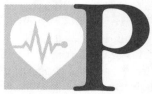

Prepare yourself for a statistic that might make your heart a bit heavier: In the time it will take you to read this paragraph, another American will have suffered a heart attack. That adds up to a yearly total of 805,000 people. And heart disease—which includes heart attacks, arrhythmia, heart failure, and the like—is the No. 1 cause of death in the United States. If you're concerned about health and longevity, you should be concerned about heart disease.

But maybe you're not too concerned because you've never been diagnosed with heart disease. Well, a new study published in *Circulation*, the journal of the American Heart Association, shows it's very possible you have heart disease even if you haven't been diagnosed. The scientists used precise testing on more than 25,000 people ages 50 to 64 without diagnosed heart disease. They found that 42 percent of them had atherosclerosis, the build-up of the fatty plaque that narrows arteries and leads to heart attack. Earlier research from the Cleveland Clinic, which included older participants, showed that people over 50 have an 85 percent likelihood of atherosclerosis.

Bottom line: You should *assume* you have life-threatening heart disease and do everything scientifically proven to prevent a heart attack.

KNOW YOUR NUMBERS

There are several important risk factors for heart disease...

•**Cholesterol.** The blood fat cholesterol is the main component in artery-clogging plaque. For every 40 points you lower total cholesterol, you cut your risk of heart disease by up to 50 percent. Total cholesterol should be less than

---

Barry Franklin, Ph.D., director of Preventive Cardiology and Cardiac Rehabilitation at Beaumont Health, Royal Oak, Michigan. DrBarryFranklin.com

200, and for patients with heart disease, less than 160.

•Blood pressure. High blood pressure damages arteries and is a major risk factor for heart disease. Lowering blood pressure to normal levels can reduce the risk of a heart attack by 64 percent. Normal blood pressure is a systolic (top reading) of less than 120 and a diastolic (bottom reading) of less than 80.

•Resting heart rate. The most protective level is 60 beats per minute (bpm) or less. A patient with heart disease who lowers their resting heart rate from 90 to 60 bpm lowers their risk of a heart attack by 90 percent.

•Hemoglobin A1c. This is a measurement of average blood sugar levels over the previous three months. Higher A1c is strongly linked to a more rapid progression of atherosclerosis. Healthy A1c levels are 4 to 6 percent. People with diabetes and individuals with cardiovascular disease should strive for values *below* 7 percent.

You can modify these risk factors with four simple lifestyle changes: a healthier diet, regular physical activity, losing weight, and not smoking. But if those lifestyle changes don't work, talk to your doctor about the right cardioprotective medications for you. The most effective are cholesterol-lowering statins, beta-blockers to lower high blood pressure and resting heart rate, ACE inhibitors to lower high blood pressure, and aspirin to thin the blood and prevent the blood clots that cause most heart attacks.

DIET

Eating a heart-protective diet is simple…

•Try to get six to seven servings of fruits and vegetables every day. Add some to every meal and snack.

•Reduce your consumption of red meat, particularly processed meats like hot dogs and lunch meat.

•Eat no more than 1 to 2 grams of trans fat per day. Minimize commercial baked goods, like cakes, cookies, fried foods, non-dairy coffee creamer, and stick margarine.

•Limit salt from processed foods by following the 1:1 rule. The food should have approximately the same number or fewer milligrams of salt as calories per serving.

PHYSICAL ACTIVITY

When it comes to protecting your heart, a little physical activity goes a long way. If you're sedentary, don't worry about meeting the government guidelines of 30 minutes of activity most days of the week. Instead, start at a level of activity you'll actually do, like 10 to 15 minutes three days a week. Once you get started, you'll slowly but surely increase your daily activity level. Physical activity is particularly protective against heart disease if you're overweight or obese—and not because it helps you lose weight, but because it improves aerobic fitness.

If you're tracking daily steps, don't worry about getting to 10,000 steps per day. The newest research shows that getting 7,000 steps per day lowers the risk of all-cause mortality (dying from any cause, including heart disease) by 50 to 70 percent compared with those who don't get 7,000 steps daily.

If you want to get even greater cardiovascular benefits from physical activity, monitor your metabolic equivalents (METs)—a measurement of how much energy your body expends. You're at 1 MET when you're sitting still. To protect your heart, you want to achieve a capacity to exercise at five METs—which is attained by exercising regularly above 3 METs. That corresponds to walking on a treadmill at 3 mph on a 0 percent grade or at 2 mph on a 3.5 percent grade. If this is too strenuous, *gradually* achieve that level of activity over time. As a general rule, the exercise should feel "fairly light" to "somewhat hard," and not evoke chest pain or excessive shortness of breath.

WEIGHT CONTROL

People with a body mass index (BMI) of 18.5 to 24.9—so-called normal weight—are at a much lower risk of heart disease than people who are overweight (BMI 25 to 29.9) or obese (BMI 30 or higher). It's particularly important to lose weight if your BMI is 32 or higher, a level that puts you at much higher risk for heart disease. But you don't have to lose a lot of

Lowering Genetic Risk

If your father or mother had a major heart attack at around age 60, you're at double the risk of a heart attack compared with someone without that family history. But a study of more than 50,000 people, published in the *New England Journal of Medicine*, showed that if you have a genetic predisposition for heart disease and adopt a heart-healthy lifestyle—no current smoking, no obesity, regular physical activity, and a healthy diet—you cut that heightened genetic risk in half.

weight to benefit. Losing just 5 percent of your body weight dramatically lowers risk.

DON'T SMOKE

Long-term smoking reduces life expectancy by 10 to 12 years, on average. Cigarette smokers are two to four times more likely to get heart disease than non-smokers. And living with a smoker is bad for you, too. Research shows that frequent exposure to secondhand smoke increases the risk of heart disease by 30 percent.

TAKE PERSONAL CONTROL

Don't rely on your primary care physician to take responsibility for your heart health. Eating right and exercising regularly are your responsibility.

Take a Bath to Protect Your Heart

Jayne Morgan, M.D., executive director of Health and Community Education at Piedmont Health, and the owner and creator of StairwellChronicles.com.

Choosing a bath instead of a shower appears to protect against cardiovascular disease, researchers reported in the journal *Heart BMJ*. In an observational study of 30,076 people, researchers found that bathing almost daily reduced the risk of cardiovascular disease, total strokes, and intracerebral hemorrhage.

Heat may explain the benefits. It increases core body temperature, heart rate, and blood flow, and is associated with a lower risk of high blood pressure. In fact, it has effects that are similar to those of exercise. Repeated bathing or use of a sauna is believed to improve vascular function over the long term. The benefits of bathing remained statistically significant even after adjusting for diet and exercise.

The Easy Artery Health Test

Donald M Lloyd-Jones, M.D., ScM, chair of the department of preventive medicine and professor of preventive medicine, cardiology, and pediatrics at Northwestern University's Feinberg School of Medicine in Chicago. He was also the 2021–2022 president of the American Heart Association.

A painless imaging test can let your doctor peek right into your arteries to see if dangerous plaque deposits (*atherosclerosis*) are putting you at risk for heart disease before you have any signs or symptoms. Here's what you need to know about the coronary artery calcium (CAC) test and if you're a candidate for it.

WHAT IS THE CAC TEST?

The CAC test is a type of CT scan. Using rapid X-rays, it takes cross-sectional images of the blood vessels that supply your heart. A radiologist or technician places electrodes on your chest to monitor your heart activity and takes images between heartbeats. You just need to hold your breath and lie still for the few seconds it takes to capture each image. There are no preparatory or post-activity restrictions; it's non-invasive and painless; and it takes only a few minutes once you're on the exam table.

Your doctor can then look at the images for specks of calcium on the blood vessel walls. (The plaque that deposits on blood vessel walls includes cholesterol and calcium.) Your doctor will count the calcium specks to determine your score and use that number to extrapolate the degree of plaque buildup. (Coronary artery calcium is not the same calcium that's in your bones, and it's not a reflection of the amount of calcium in your diet.)

WHAT DOES YOUR CAC SCORE MEAN?

A higher CAC score means there is more plaque along the artery walls and you have a greater risk of a heart attack. *Here's how the numbers break down...*

•**Zero.** No calcium was detected. You have a low heart attack risk, but if you have a strong family history of atherosclerotic cardiovascular disease (ASCVD), smoke, or have type 2 diabetes, you may be advised to start a cholesterol-lowering drug like a statin.

•**One to 99.** Calcium is starting to accumulate. If you have other cardiovascular risk factors, your doctor may discuss risk-reduction options, including cholesterol-lowering therapy.

•**100 to 300.** You have a moderate amount of plaque deposits and an elevated risk of a heart attack or stroke over the next five to 10 years. Most people in this range need to start on a statin.

•**300 or higher.** This is a sign of very high to severe atherosclerosis and heart attack risk.

Your score will be compared to findings in other men or women in your age group. The average white man will get a nonzero score by age 53. For the average white woman, it's age 62. These stats are similar for people of Asian descent. For African Americans, nonzero scores happen a few years later. If you develop plaque ahead of your peer group, you may need to fast-track treatment.

Though your CAC score isn't the only factor to consider for heart attack prevention, it will inform decision-making about treatments to stop plaque progression and other steps to help prevent heart attack and stroke. These might include following a better diet, getting more exercise, losing weight, and taking medications.

WHO BENEFITS MOST FROM THE TEST?

The CAC test isn't recommended for everyone. It is most helpful for people whose heart attack risk falls in an intermediate zone based

Is the Artery Test for You?

According to guidelines from the American College of Cardiology and the American Heart Association, here are some reasons you may benefit from having a CAC test...

•**You're reluctant to begin statin therapy,** and having a more accurate picture of your heart health will let you know if you'll benefit from the drug.

•**You stopped statin therapy** because of drug side effects and want solid evidence that you really need to restart them.

•**You're between ages 40 and 55** and have a 10-year risk of heart disease that's between 5 percent and 7.5 percent, along with other risk factors.

•**You're a man between ages 55 and 80 or a woman between ages 60 and 80** with intermediate risk with or without elevated risk factors (your age alone could put you in the intermediate risk category) and want to know if you would benefit from statin therapy.

For people over age 80, the decision to have a CAC test (and to start statins) becomes very individualized. There is very little data in people over age 75.

on, in part, the score on an atherosclerotic cardiovascular disease (ASCVD) screening tool. The ASCVD evaluates numbers such as cholesterol levels and blood pressure readings to determine how likely you are to have a heart attack in 10 years. (You can take the test yourself online at https://tools.acc.org).

The CAC test isn't for people who have a 5 percent or lower 10-year heart attack risk and no strong family history of heart disease, because the odds of finding calcium are low. It also isn't deemed necessary for people with a 10-year risk of 20 percent or higher, because it's almost a given that they will have plaque. It makes the most sense for people who have between a 5 and 20 percent risk: Half of people in this group will have calcium deposits and half won't.

Compared with the traditional and imperfect approach of estimating heart disease via risk factors like blood pressure and cholesterol levels, the CAC test directly answers the question of whether you have atherosclerosis. That's why it's so powerful. Since it can also tell if there are no calcium deposits, the result can be reassuring for someone with moderate heart disease risk factors.

The chief drawback to the test is that it may not be covered by your insurance, so it could cost between $100 and $400. The radiation exposure is similar to a mammogram and having the test at a facility with the most up-to-date technology means you'll get the lowest amount of radiation possible.

Cryoablation Is More Protective Than Medication for A-fib

University of British Columbia.

Cryoablation, a minimally invasive procedure that involves guiding a small tube into the heart to kill problematic tissue with cold temperatures, is normally used as a secondary treatment when patients don't respond to medication. But treating patients with cryoablation from the start may prevent progressive changes in the heart and worsening disease. When researchers compared cryoablation with medication for three years, people in the cryoablation group were less likely to progress to persistent A-fib, had lower rates of hospitalization, and experienced fewer serious adverse health events that resulted in death, functional disability, or prolonged hospitalization. Cryoablation treats the cause of the condition, instead of covering-up the symptoms, said lead researcher Jason Andrade, M.D.

Cardiac Valve Disease

Joshua C. Grimm, M.D., assistant professor of cardiac surgery at the Hospital of the University of Pennsylvania.

The "golden years" are meant to be a time of ease and relaxation, of enjoying retirement, and playing with grandchildren, but a stealthy health issue can interfere with those plans: cardiac valve disease. It might start with shortness of breath and feeling tired, or you might feel no symptoms at all. The next thing you know, you could be having chest pains and fainting spells.

Cardiac valve disease, which affects about 13 percent of Americans who were born before 1943, occurs when the valves of the heart don't function properly. Although valve problems can be severe and even life-threatening, the good news is that most are also highly treatable. We spoke with Joshua C. Grimm, M.D., assistant professor of cardiac surgery at the University of Pennsylvania, to learn more.

UNDERSTANDING THE DISEASE

The heart has four valves that open and close to control the flow of blood into and away from it: the mitral, the tricuspid, the pulmonary, and the aortic. Any valve can become diseased, but the aortic valve is most commonly affected. Each valve has flaps, called leaflets, that open and close once per heartbeat. Cardiac valve disease occurs when one or more of those valves doesn't work well.

•**Regurgitation** occurs when diseased valves become "leaky" and don't completely close. Blood leaks back into the chamber it came from and not enough can be pushed through the heart.

•**Stenosis** happens when the opening of the valve is narrowed and stiff, and the valve is unable to open fully when blood tries to pass through.

•**Atresia** refers to instances in which the valve isn't formed, and a solid sheet of tissue blocks the blood flow between the heart chambers.

•**Prolapse** occurs when a valve has improperly closing leaflets.

Risk Factors

• **Older age.** More than one in eight people ages 75 and older have moderate or severe valve disease.

• **History of infections that can affect the heart,** such as endocarditis and rheumatic fever.

• **History of heart disease or heart attack,** including heart failure, atherosclerosis, and thoracic aortic aneurysm.

• **High blood pressure, high cholesterol, diabetes,** and other heart disease risk factors.

• **Heart conditions present at birth.** The most commonly affected valve with a congenital defect is a bicuspid aortic valve, which has only two leaflets rather than three.

SYMPTOMS TO WATCH FOR

In the early stages of valve disease, many of the adverse effects on the heart may be corrected with the right treatment. But left unchecked, the disease can cause complications including heart failure, stroke, blood clots, and death.

"The longer you wait, the more of a deleterious effect valvular pathology will have on your heart," Dr. Grimm says. "By the time you do see a surgeon or a cardiologist, sometimes, that damage is irreversible."

So if you have any of the following symptoms, even if they're mild, check in with your doctor: shortness of breath, particularly when active or lying down, fatigue, chest pain or palpitations, swelling of the abdomen, ankles and feet, dizziness, fainting, or irregular heartbeat. You also might have a symptom you're unaware of—a heart murmur that can be heard when a doctor listens to your heart with a stethoscope.

Dr. Grimm's number-one piece of advice is to listen to your body. "Similar to your car that turns the check-engine light on…there are often signs that things are not going right. If you start developing these signs, don't just say,

'Maybe it's a bad day,' especially if it's persistent over days, weeks, or months." See a doctor as soon as possible.

MEDICAL MANAGEMENT

Treatment depends on which one of your four valves is affected and the type and severity of the disease. If your condition is mild or surgery is not an option, your doctor may prescribe medications to manage your symptoms and help your heart pump blood more efficiently.

• **Antiarrhythmics** control the heart's rhythm.

• **Anticoagulants** (blood thinners) prolong the clotting time of your blood.

• **Beta-blockers** lower high blood pressure, help the heart beat less forcefully, and can decrease palpitations in some patients.

• **Diuretics** remove excess fluid from the tissues and bloodstream.

• **Vasodilators** reduce the heart's workload and encourage blood to flow in a forward direction.

Medications can help your symptoms and reduce further damage, but they can't stop a valve from leaking or open a valve that's constricted.

SURGICAL CONSIDERATIONS

If a valve is seriously diseased and causing more severe symptoms, surgery may be recommended to repair or replace it. *The most common surgery is aortic valve replacement, which is performed in one of two ways…*

• **Conventional open-heart surgery**—or sternotomy—involves making an incision in the chest and opening the heart.

• **Transcatheter aortic valve replacement (TAVR)** is a minimally invasive procedure in which the surgeon works through a catheter that has been inserted in the groin or another access point. TAVR involves a shorter recovery time and is especially suitable for higher-risk patients.

"I know open-heart surgery sounds scary," Dr. Grimm told us, "but we've gotten quite good at it since its inception 60-plus years ago, and patients do quite well." He adds: "You don't have to go to a huge academic center…I think it's a myth that you have to go to some 800-bed hospital to have a good operation."

Early intervention and treatment can help you enjoy a long life.

Everyday Activities Lower Heart Disease Risk

Running, brisk walking, and similar activities are not the only ways to keep the cardiovascular system strong.

Recent finding: Older women who spent at least four hours doing routine activities—called "daily life movement"—had a 43 percent lower risk for heart disease, 30 percent lower stroke risk, and 62 percent reduced risk of dying from cardiovascular disease compared with women who did less than two hours of such activities. Daily life movement activities include housework, gardening, cooking, even self-care such as showering.

Study of 5,416 women ages 63 to 97 by researchers at Herbert Wertheim School of Public Health and Human Longevity Science, University of California San Diego, published in *Journal of the American Heart Association.*

Positivity Protects Your Heart

Glenn N. Levine, M.D., Master Clinician and Professor of Medicine at Baylor College, Houston, Texas.

We've all heard the expression, "It almost gave me a heart attack!" in response to shocking or frightening news. It turns out that this idiom has some scientific backing: Research has definitively shown that extreme negative emotions can be linked to a higher risk of heart disease.

Consider broken-heart syndrome (also called stress or Takotsubo cardiomyopathy), in which a person experiences symptoms that are indistinguishable from those of a heart attack in direct response to stress, grief, anger, or even surprise.

It doesn't even take a dramatic event to influence heart health. Chronic low-level stress, personality traits like pessimism, and even depression are all linked to poorer heart health.

Fortunately, the opposite is true as well: Positive psychological states appear to be heart protective. The link is so strong that the American Heart Association (AHA) released a statement, "Psychological Health, Well-Being, and the Mind-Heart-Body Connection," that summarizes the current body of scientific knowledge.

NEGATIVE EMOTIONS AND CVD

According to the AHA's statement, studies have shown that the risk of cardiovascular disease (CVD) rises from post-traumatic stress disorder (60 percent), social isolation and loneliness (50 percent), work-related stress (40 percent), and high perceived stress (27 percent). That's not all.

Anger and hostility are associated with higher blood pressure, elevated heart rate, and higher rates of heart attack, stroke, and ventricular arrhythmia, according to studies in the *European Heart Journal* and the *Journal of the American College of Cardiology.*

Anxiety appears to be a risk factor for high blood pressure, obesity, and the tendency to smoke, all of which contribute to arterial disease. A study with more than 2 million people that was published in the *American Journal of Cardiology* found that anxiety was associated with a higher risk of stroke, heart failure, and CVD-related death. Depression increases the risk of developing and dying of CVD. It's also associated with a higher risk of heart attack, stroke, and mortality in patients with existing CVD.

Even your personality can affect your heart. Pessimism is a personality trait in which people expect negative outcomes. In an 11-year prospective cohort study, it was found to be a significant predictor of coronary heart disease (CHD) mortality, researchers report in *BMC Public Health.* (CHD, or clogged arteries, is a type of CVD.) The most pessimistic people had double the risk of the least pessimistic.

POSITIVE PSYCHOLOGY

As alarming as these relationships are, research also shows that positive psychological states are heart healthy.

Optimistic people, defined as those who anticipate the best possible outcomes, have lower rates of stroke, CVD, and heart failure. Even people with existing disease benefit from a positive outlook. A study published in *Psychosomatic Medicine* found that women who were more optimistic had slower progression of the buildup of fatty plaques (atherosclerosis) in their carotid arteries. Another study found that higher optimism was associated with decreased risk of hospital cardiac readmission among people with established CVD.

Having a sense of purpose is associated with better cardiovascular health and a 17 percent lower risk of CVD events, such as heart attack and stroke, according to a study published in 2016. It's linked to a longer life, too. Happiness, also called positive affect, was associated with a 22 percent lower risk of incident CHD (such as heart attack, a cardiac revascularization procedure, or death), in a study published in *Australasian Psychiatry*.

Gratitude has been associated with better medication adherence, blood pressure, sleep, inflammatory biomarkers, and heart-rate variability (the variation in time between each heartbeat), according to small clinical trials. And people who practice mindfulness—a nonjudgmental awareness of one's thoughts, emotions, and actions—tend to have less stress, higher levels of well-being, and a heart-healthier lifestyle that includes being a nonsmoker, being free of diabetes, and having healthy blood pressure, cholesterol, and body mass index.

INTERVENTION EFFECTS

While we can't always control the stress we may experience—or the personality traits we're born with—research suggests that we may be able to improve our emotional and cardiovascular responses.

•**Antidepressants.** Some, but not all, studies have found that antidepressant medications are associated with lower rates of heart attack and cardiovascular mortality. The Escitalopram for Depression in Acute Coronary Syndrome trial found that people who took *escitalopram* (Lexapro) had lower rates of major adverse cardiac events. Other trials have shown that the most common type of antidepressants, selective serotonin reuptake inhibitors (SSRIs), improve heart rate variability and mental stress-induced myocardial ischemia (reduced blood flow to the heart as a result of a partial or complete blockage of the coronary arteries). SSRIs have been linked to improvements in inflammatory markers that are associated with improved cardiovascular prognosis.

•**Psychotherapy.** Some programs using psychotherapy or stress management training have improved cardiovascular outcomes in high-risk patients. One trial published in *Circulation* found that adding stress management training to cardiac rehabilitation led to lower rates of major adverse cardiac events, while another found that group-based relaxation and coping skills training improved mortality rates. Yet another study, in *Archives of Internal Medicine*, showed that people who received group-based cognitive behavioral therapy for one year had a 41 percent lower rate of fatal and nonfatal first heart attacks and strokes. But other studies found no benefits.

•**Positive psychology–based programs** that use activities to improve psychological attributes and experiences have been linked to better cardiac outcomes. These programs appear to improve physical activity in patients with or at high risk for heart disease—which lowers risk. However, beneficial effects on cardiac biomarkers have been more limited. Some small studies have found reductions in markers of inflammation in patients with heart failure or coronary artery disease, but minimal effects on other markers.

•**Meditation.** Some studies have found that meditation can decrease perceived stress, anxiety, and depression; increase smoking cessation rates; lower systolic and diastolic blood pressures; and decrease nonfatal heart attacks, cardiovascular mortality, and all-cause mortality. While more studies are needed, medita-

Biology and Behavior

How can your mood and mindset affect you physically? Researchers have identified two drivers: biological changes and behaviors that affect heart health.

•**Biological changes.** Negative emotions launch a cascade of bodily responses. For example, when we're stressed or frightened, the brain releases hormones like adrenaline that prepare us for the fight-or-flight response. While this is beneficial in a short-term situation, chronic stress—and chronic stress hormones—can harm the body. Chronic distress is associated with inflammation, imbalances in cholesterol and triglycerides, impaired glucose control and immune responses, decreased heart rate variability, stiffer arteries, and dysfunction of the membranes that line the inside of the heart and blood vessels. There is strong evidence that depression and PTSD predict higher levels of inflammation, which is associated with an increased risk of plaques and blood clots in the arteries.

Conversely, the ability to regulate emotions effectively is associated with healthier heart rate, heart rate variability, vagal tone, and biological stress responses. Some studies have linked positive psychological factors with better immunity and lower inflammation, too.

•**Behavioral factors.** Psychological health is also associated with behaviors that are strongly linked to heart health. People with negative psychological health are more likely to smoke, be sedentary, eat poorly, and be overweight or obese—all of which are associated with poor heart health. Conversely, people with better psychological health are more likely to avoid smoking, engage in preventive screening, and exercise. Positive psychological health is also linked to better adherence to medications—including those prescribed for heart-related conditions.

tion is a low-cost, low-risk intervention that is worth trying.

•**Stress reduction.** Lowering your stress is good for both body and mind. For some people, that could mean exercising and socializing more, sleeping well, and finding hobbies that distract you from negative thoughts. For others, it could mean retiring from a high-stress job or walking away from avoidable stresses. Something as simple as going for a walk to get a little exercise and clear your mind can help boost your mood, lower your stress, and give your heart a little protection.

Morning Exercise Is Best for Your Heart

Study of 86,657 adults by researchers at Leiden University Medical Center, the Netherlands, published in *European Journal of Preventive Cardiology*.

Physical activity in the morning was associated with a 16 percent lower risk for coronary artery disease and a 17 percent reduction in stroke risk versus the risks of people exercising later in the day.

Heart Failure Drug Treats POTS

Pam Taub, M.D., professor of medicine at UC San Diego Health System, La Jolla, California, commenting on a review of studies in *Cureus*.

The drug *ivabradine*, approved for heart failure, improves symptoms of *postural orthostatic tachycardia syndrome* (POTS)—decreased blood in the brain when standing, leading to dizziness, palpitations, shortness of breath, fatigue, and risk for falls. POTS often follows COVID infection—if you've struggled to recover your energy after COVID, get tested for POTS. Your doctor may prescribe *ivabradine* off-label.

New Drug for Heart Disease

Michelle Kittleson, M.D., Ph.D., director of education in heart failure and transplantation and director of heart failure research at Smidt Heart Institute of Cedars-Sinai Medical Center, Los Angeles.

The FDA has approved the first-ever drug for *obstructive hypertrophic cardiomyopathy* (HCM), characterized by thickened heart muscle and partially blocked blood flow from the left ventricle. *Mavacamten* (Camzyos) targets a protein that controls the strength of heart contractions, the source of HCM symptoms. The drug is best for patients who have problems with traditional beta-blockers and calcium-channel blockers and/or want to avoid surgery.

FDA Approves New Drug for Congestive Heart Failure

U.S. Food and Drug Administration.

The U.S. Food and Drug Administration approved *furosemide* (Furoscix) for the treatment of congestion due to fluid overload in people with New York Heart Association class II/III chronic heart failure. Patients self-administer the subcuteanous (under the skin) diuretic at home with a pre-filled cartridge that attaches to the patient's abdomen for delivery of an 80-mg dose over five hours. Furosemide can cause fluid, electrolyte, and metabolic abnormalities in elderly patients and other groups. Cases of tinnitus and reversible or irreversible hearing impairment and deafness have been reported with this diuretic. The drug manufacturer plans for commercial launch in early 2023.

Sleep Habits Affect Heart Health

Exposure to Light While You Sleep Hurts Your Heart

Just one night of sleeping in a room exposed to moderate light—even just the light from a TV—was associated with a higher heart rate and impaired glucose function the next day.

If you need some light for safety: Place it low to the floor and far from your bed… choose an amber or red/orange light rather than white or blue, which is more stimulating to the brain.

Phyllis Zee, M.D., Ph.D., chief of sleep medicine at Northwestern University Feinberg School of Medicine, Chicago, and lead author of a study published in *PNAS: Proceedings of the National Academy of Sciences of the United States of America*.

Go to Bed Early for Your Heart

A 10 p.m. bedtime is associated with a 12 percent lower risk of heart disease, heart attack, heart failure, and stroke than going to bed at 11 p.m., according to a study of nearly 90,000 people. The risk jumped to 25 percent for people who regularly stayed up past midnight.

European Heart Journal.

Sleep Is the Newest Measure of Cardiovascular Health

Columbia University Mailman School of Public Health.

Sleep duration can predict the risk of cardiovascular disease, researchers from the Columbia University Mailman School of Public Health have concluded. In a sample of more than 2,000 people, those who slept for fewer than seven hours or more than nine were more likely to develop cardiovascular disease. Short sleepers also had a higher prevalence of overweight/obesity, type 2 diabetes, and hypertension, further increasing the risk for heart disease.

"Our results highlight the importance of embracing a holistic vision of sleep health that includes sleep behaviors and…mild sleep problems rather than strictly focusing on sleep *disorders* when assessing an individual's cardiovascular risk," said Nour Makarem, Ph.D., assistant professor of epidemiology.

Whey Protein Helps Your Heart

Study of 25 adults by researchers at Instituto Nacional de Cardiologia, Rio de Janeiro, Brazil, published in *Brazilian Journal of Medical and Biological Research*.

After 12 weeks of supplementation, whey protein improved microvascular circulation in heart failure patients, according to a recent finding. Previous studies have shown that whey protein can help improve blood pressure, arterial stiffness, and other factors that are important for people with cardiovascular disease. Whey protein powder, available online and in many grocery and other retail stores, can be added to food or beverages.

New Cholesterol Drug Is a Game Changer

Steven Nissen, M.D., chief academic officer at the Sydell and Arnold Miller Family Heart, Vascular & Thoracic Institute, Cleveland Clinic, commenting on a study published in *The New England Journal of Medicine*.

Inclisiran (Leqvio), a twice-yearly injection, reduced low-density lipoprotein cholesterol (LDL-C) levels by up to 52 percent in a recent study. The drug uses *small-interfering RNA therapy* (siRNA) to improve the liver's natural ability to regulate cholesterol levels. Inclisiran is meant to work with statins for patients who are unable to control cholesterol at statins' maximum doses. Side effects were mild.

Common Cough Syrup May Treat a Rare Heart Condition

Study led by researchers at Columbia University, New York City, published in *Nature Cardiovascular Research*.

Dextromethorphan, a cough suppressant, in OTC medicines such as Robitussin and Delsym, normalized heart cells in people with long QT syndrome. Long QT is marked by sudden, fast, chaotic heart rhythm and can cause fainting, seizures, and death.

Staying Hydrated Protects Your Heart

Study of 5,000 adults by researchers at the National Heart, Lung, and Blood Institute, Bethesda, Maryland, published in *European Heart Journal*.

According to a recent study, people with high levels of serum sodium, an indication of dehydration, during middle age were 54 percent more likely to develop heart failure in later years than people whose middle-age serum sodium levels were in the normal range. Those with the highest serum sodium levels also were 102 percent more likely to develop left ventricular hypertrophy, a condition in which the heart muscle becomes thickened and the heart pumps blood less efficiently. The human body requires adequate fluids to support many functions, including circulation.

Recommended: Most healthy people need about four to six glasses of water daily, adjusted for body size, physical activity, health conditions, and temperature of the environment. Fluid does not have to be water—milk, juice, herbal teas, tea and coffee (including caffeinated and decaffeinated), and many fruits and vegetables also are hydrating.

Coffee and Alcohol: The Good and the Bad

Krishna Aragam, M.D., MS, cardiologist at Massachusetts General Hospital and associate scientist at Broad Institute of Harvard and MIT, and senior author of the alcohol study...and Peter Kistler, Ph.D., head of clinical electrophysiology research at Baker Heart and Diabetes Institute, professor of medicine at University of Melbourne and senior author of the coffee studies.

There's bad news and good news about beverages and heart disease...

Bad news: A glass of wine with dinner won't help your heart. Earlier studies had suggested that moderate alcohol consumption might reduce rates of heart disease. But when researchers used modern statistical techniques to analyze more than 370,000 adults, they found that isn't so. Moderate drinkers tend to have low heart disease rates, but that's because they tend to exercise, eat vegetables, and live healthy lives. Drinking about one drink per day or less has minimal impact...but more substantial drinking dramatically increases risk for heart problems.

Good news: Coffee consumption is associated with lower risk for heart disease and longer life span. Previously, there had been concerns that the temporary heart-rate increases caused by caffeine meant that coffee posed a health risk. But when researchers tracked more than 382,000 adults for a decade or longer, they found that drinking two to three cups of coffee per day seems to lower risk for coronary heart disease, heart failure, and other heart issues by 10 to 15 percent. Coffee also *benefits* people who already suffer from cardiovascular disease—they were less likely to die during the study period if they drank two to three cups of coffee per day.

What to do: If you're in good health and enjoy an alcoholic drink every so often, keep it on the light side. If you like coffee, go on drinking it...and if you have a history of heart disease, ask your doctor whether coffee might be beneficial.

Most People Should Not Take Aspirin Daily to Prevent Heart Problems

Steven Nissen, M.D., chief academic officer at Sydell and Arnold Miller Family Heart, Vascular & Thoracic Institute, Cleveland Clinic, commenting on U.S. Preventive Services Task Force guidelines published in *JAMA*.

New recommendations: For most people, risk for internal bleeding from aspirin outweighs the possible health benefits. People ages 40 to 59 should consider daily aspirin only if they have a 10 percent or higher risk for cardiovascular disease based on factors such as cholesterol levels, blood pressure, diabetes, and smoking status.

Caution: Don't stop taking aspirin without consulting your doctor.

More Electronics Pose a Danger to Implanted Defibrillators

Corentin Féry, MSc, research associate at University of Applied Sciences and Arts Northwestern Switzerland in Muttenz and leader of a study published in *Circulation: Arrhythmia and Electrophysiology*.

When held within an inch, magnets in the iPhone 12 ProMax, Apple's Air Pods Pro charging case, Microsoft Surface Pen, and Apple Pencil Second Generation disrupted implantable cardioverter-defibrillators (ICDs) that regulate heartbeat in people with heart-rhythm disorders.

If you have an ICD: Never rest any electronic device on your chest or carry one in a chest pocket.

Warning for People on Heart Medications

Study by researchers at Lahey Hospital and Medical Center in Burlington, Massachusetts, published in *Journal of the American College of Cardiology*.

The COVID treatment Paxlovid, a combination of the antivirals *nirmatrelvir* and *ritonavir*, can cause a dangerous interaction with many medications used to treat heart disease.

Examples: Interactions with certain blood thinners can increase risk for bleeding...certain cholesterol medications including statins can be toxic to the liver...and certain blood pressure medications can cause low blood pressure and swelling. Some medications that potentially interact with Paxlovid can be safely stopped short-term or their dosage temporarily adjusted...but others cannot be stopped, and doctors will have to decide the best treatment options.

Note: Aspirin and certain other medications are safe to take with Paxlovid.

Best Time to Measure Blood Pressure

Blood pressure rises and falls in natural cycles throughout the day. Measurements taken at different times of day are less useful than measuring at the same time every day, which can alert you to meaningful changes.

Good times to measure: In the morning, 30 to 60 minutes after waking up, before eating breakfast or taking medicines... or in the evening, an hour after dinner at a time when you feel relaxed.

Nicholas Ruthmann, M.D., staff cardiologist, Heart, Vascular & Thoracic Institute, Cleveland Clinic. ClevelandClinic.org

Acetaminophen Affects Blood Pressure

Study of 110 adults by researchers at Royal Infirmary of Edinburgh, Scotland, published in *Circulation*.

According to a recent study, taking 1,000 milligrams (mg) of *acetaminophen* (Tylenol) four times a day for two weeks raised blood pressure by an average of five points—enough of a change to affect blood pressure medication dosage as well as whether medication is needed at all. Researchers have known that other nonsteroidal anti-inflammatory drugs (NSAIDs) such as *ibuprofen* (Advil, Motrin) and *naproxen* (Aleve) also raise blood pressure. If you need to take a pain reliever, take the lowest possible dose for the shortest possible time.

More Older Adults Should Check Blood Pressure at Home

University of Michigan.

Only 48 percent of people ages 50 to 80 who take blood pressure medications or have a health condition that's affected by hypertension regularly check their blood pressure at home or other places, a new study finds. Regular home monitoring can help with blood pressure control, and better control can mean reduced risk of death, cardiovascular events including strokes and heart attacks, and cognitive impairment and dementia. People who own a monitor are more than 10 times more likely to check their blood pressure outside of health-care settings than those who don't own one.

Limit Coffee to One Cup a Day If You Have Severe Hypertension

Hiroyasu Iso, M.D., Ph.D., MPH, director of the Institute for Global Health Policy Research, Bureau of International Health Cooperation, National Center for Global Health and Medicine in Tokyo, Japan, and professor emeritus at Osaka University.

People with severe high blood pressure (higher than 160/100 mmhg) should limit coffee consumption to one cup per day. While one daily cup of coffee may lower the risk of death after a heart attack and may prevent heart attacks or strokes, just two cups is associated with double the risk of cardiovascular disease-related death. (People with blood pressure under 160/100 mmHg showed no elevated risk of cardiovascular death when drinking two daily cups of coffee.) If you have high blood pressure, try green tea instead. It isn't associated with elevated risk at any level of consumption, possibly because it contains micronutrients with antioxidant and anti-inflammatory properties.

How to Eat a Low-Salt Diet

Allison Tallman, MS, RDN, CNSC, registered dietitian who has worked in health-care corporate wellness, nutrition communications, and sports nutrition.

If you're age 65 or older, your doctor may have told you to follow a low-salt diet. A low-salt diet, also known as a low-sodium diet, is essential to prevent and manage heart disease. *Here are some tips to try...*

•**Avoid or limit high-salt foods** such as potato chips, frozen meals, packaged products, and canned products.

•**Many high-sodium foods don't even taste salty.** For example, a vanilla milkshake (11 oz.) has close to 300 mg of sodium, while 3 ounces of imitation Alaska king crab made from surimi has 715 mg. A croissant clocks in at more than 400 mg, according to the University of Maine Cooperative Extension.

•**Read nutrition labels** and avoid any foods that have 400 mg or more of sodium per serving.

•**Instead, eat more fresh and raw foods** like fruits, vegetables, and meat.

•**There are many low-salt snacks or prepackaged products.** To find them, look for information on the label such as "no salt added" or "low-sodium." (When reading food labels, low sodium is defined as 140 mg of sodium or less per serving.)

•**Reduce the amount of salt you cook with.** Instead use other spices, garlic, vinegar, and herbs for flavor.

•**Watch out for medications, too.** Medications that fizz when added to water, such as Alka Seltzer, are high in sodium.

Intensive Blood Pressure Lowering After Stroke Appears to Be Harmful

Rockefeller University.

Around 85 percent of strokes are caused by the loss of blood flow to an area of the brain due to a blockage in a blood vessel. *Endovascular thrombectomy* is a nonsurgical treatment in which thin tubes visible under X-rays are inserted into the blood clot to dissolve it. The rapid return of blood supply to an area that has been deprived of oxygen can cause tissue damage known as *reperfusion injury*, so physicians sometimes lower blood pressure to a systolic target of less than 120 mm Hg after clot removal. A new study, however, shows that this intensive blood pressure reduction can lead to deterioration in surrounding brain tissue and higher rates of disability, compared with less intensive treatment. While the study showed that intensive blood pressure control can be harmful, the optimal level of control is yet to be defined.

Gout, Heart Attack, and Stroke

JAMA.

People with gout have a higher risk of heart attacks and strokes in the four months after a gout flare. In an analysis of data on more than 62,000 people, researchers found that gout patients who suffered a heart attack or stroke were twice as likely to have had a gout flare in the 60 days prior to the event, and one-and-a-half times more likely to have a gout flare in the preceding 61 to 120 days. If you have recurrent gout flares, consider long-term treatment with a urate-lowering medication, such as *allopurinol*, treatment with an anti-inflammatory medication, such as *colchicine*, and the adoption of a healthy lifestyle.

Transient Ischemic Attack

Louise D. McCullough, M.D., Ph.D., professor, and Huffington chair of the department of neurology at UTHealth Houston, and chief of neurology at Memorial Hermann Hospital at the Texas Medical Center.

A transient ischemic attack (TIA) is a temporary blockage of blood flow to the brain. To dismiss it as a mini-stroke, as it's often referred to, is a big mistake. "Mini-stroke" implies that a TIA is not dangerous when, in fact, it can be a warning that a full-blown stroke is ahead.

WHAT IS A TIA?

A TIA is a short-lived reaction to a clot or other form of blockage in the brain. It's considered temporary because the clot either dissolves or dislodges on its own. (With a full-blown stroke, on the other hand, emergency clot-dissolving medication is often needed.)

An underlying TIA trigger is often the buildup of plaque along the walls of an artery or artery branch that feeds the brain. Plaque slows the nutrient-rich flow of blood to the brain and can itself cause a clot.

Though people associate strokes with older age, a TIA can happen to anyone, and they're occurring in younger and middle-aged adults more frequently than in the past.

A TIA is particularly concerning because it is often a warning sign, sounding the alarm for additional TIAs, a full-blown stroke, or other cardiovascular problems to come. About 15 percent of all strokes are preceded by a TIA.

Looked at another way, close to one-third of people who experience a TIA will have a stroke within the following year. That means taking immediate steps to reduce stroke risk is vital.

RECOGNIZING A TIA

The symptoms of a TIA are the same as a full stroke and include double vision or loss of vision in one or both eyes, slurred speech, unsteadiness, and sudden changes on one side of the body, from numbness or weakness to paralysis.

On average, the symptoms of a TIA last for less than five minutes, but they can go on for longer. A sudden severe headache can be a sign of bleeding within or around the brain, most commonly linked to high blood pressure or an aneurysm. The symptoms usually do not go away. Getting to the hospital is just as important, especially if symptoms like weakness or vision changes are present.

ACT QUICKLY

If you or someone with you experiences any of these symptoms, get help immediately—*even if the symptoms go away*. Check the time as you call 911 so you'll be able to tell the EMTs and doctors in the emergency room when the symptoms first appeared.

Also, bring a list of your medications with you. This is important because certain medications are needed right away, and some medications such as blood thinners may be dangerous in that setting.

An immediate medical work-up is needed to determine whether you had a TIA, a more significant stroke, or something

"Close to one-third of people who experience a TIA will have a stroke within the following year. That means taking immediate steps to reduce stroke risk is vital."

entirely different, such as a complex migraine or a seizure. Some strokes that seem to be TIAs are not.

Doctors will try to determine where the blockage originated and whether damage was done to the brain, the determining factor in whether this was a TIA or a more serious stroke. A workup is likely to include blood tests and one or more imaging tests, such as a CT scan or MRI. A TIA may involve other tests in younger people.

IF IT WAS A TIA

A TIA, by definition, means that you will completely return to your baseline condition in 24 hours. No damage will be seen on imaging tests. With a true TIA, your body was probably able to restore blood flow to the brain before any anatomical changes or damage could occur. It's important for your doctors to determine what might have led to the TIA to prevent another one or a larger stroke.

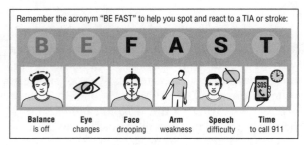

Remember the acronym "BE FAST" to help you spot and react to a TIA or stroke:

B	E	F	A	S	T
Balance is off	**Eye** changes	**Face** drooping	**Arm** weakness	**Speech** difficulty	**Time** to call 911

IF IT WAS A STROKE

Even though your symptoms may go away, damage can sometimes be seen on imaging tests, especially on an MRI. If that occurs, you have had a stroke. It's important to know what type of stroke you had and where it came from so you can prevent a larger one that does lead to permanent symptoms. Even a small stroke can cause ongoing issues, including gait and memory problems.

Your doctor may perform an echocardiogram on your heart to look for clots. If an irregular heart rhythm, such as atrial fibrillation, is suspected, you may need a temporary implantable monitor placed under your skin to look for it. Recent studies suggest that wearing an external 30-day portable monitor

often misses atrial fibrillation, which takes closer to 80 days to detect. You might benefit from treatment with an anticoagulant drug like *apixaban* (Eliquis) or *coumadin* (Warfarin), which can reduce the risk of a stroke by 60 to 80 percent.

You might undergo a carotid ultrasound or cerebral angiogram to look for a blockage in the carotid artery in your neck. For a minor blockage, antiplatelets like aspirin and statins may be prescribed or, if there's more than 70 percent blockage, you may need a procedure to correct it.

Doctors may perform a CT angiogram to see how the blood vessels supplying your brain look. If you have plaque in the arteries within the brain, they may have caused a stroke in one of the smaller vessels (called a lacunar stroke). These will show up on MRI. You might be prescribed an antiplatelet drug, such as *clopidogrel* (Plavix) or aspirin as part of a management strategy.

PREVENTING A TIA OR STROKE

Most TIAs (and strokes) can be prevented by managing risk factors that are within your control…

•**Get and keep hypertension under control.** It's a leading contributor to vascular disease, which affects all blood vessels, leading to heart attacks and stroke. When blood pressure increases beyond 130/80 mmHg, so does stroke risk. Talk to your doctor about taking blood-pressure readings at home between office visits, fine-tuning medications, and cutting down on salt.

•**Manage other chronic conditions** such as high cholesterol, diabetes, and any type of heart disease.

•**Lose weight.** Obesity, especially belly fat, increases stroke risk.

•**Stop smoking.** It's a triple risk factor because it contributes to blood clots, high blood pressure, and plaque buildup in arteries.

•**Limit foods that are high in cholesterol and fat,** such as red and processed meats, to reduce plaque buildup.

•**Boost your diet by eating lots of fruits and vegetables.**

•**Exercise for 30 minutes a day.** Aim for moderate-intensity exercise to lower blood pressure and burn extra calories.

•**If you drink alcohol,** it should be fewer than one drink a day for women and two for men.

Seated Tai Chi Is as Effective as Traditional Stroke Rehab

In a recent study, researchers developed a tai chi routine that people who had hand and arm weakness or partial paralysis from a recent ischemic stroke could do from a chair or wheelchair. Half of the 160 study participants followed the routine and the other half followed a standard stroke rehabilitation program. At three months, the people in the tai chi group had equal or greater improvement in balance control, hand and arm strength, shoulder range of motion, activities of daily living, and symptoms of depression. The American Heart Association's/American Stroke Association's Guidelines for the Early Management of Patients with Acute Ischemic Stroke recommend that people start stroke rehabilitation within seven days and continue for up to six months after a stroke. Sitting tai chi can be practiced in a chair or wheelchair, requires no special equipment, and costs almost nothing.

Jia Zhao, Ph.D., lecturer at Yunnan University of Traditional Chinese Medicine in Yunnan, China.

Anti-Nausea Meds Increase Stroke Risk

BMJ.

Drugs that are widely used for nausea and vomiting, called *antidopaminergic antiemetics*, have been associated with an in-creased risk of ischemic stroke. Researchers found a 3.62-fold increase with *metopimazine* (Nortrip, Vogalen, Vogalene) and a 3.53-fold increase with *metoclopramide* (Reglan, Metozolv). Patients with cancer were excluded from the study. The researchers noted that the study was observational, so it doesn't prove causation.

Singing Helps Stroke Rehab

University of Helsinki.

Singing-based rehabilitation can improve language and well-being after having a stroke. Approximately 40 percent of stroke survivors experience difficulty understanding or producing spoken or written language (a condition called *aphasia*). In half of these cases, the impairment persists for at least one year. But even in the presence of severe aphasia, many people retain the ability to sing.

Now, researchers have discovered that singing-based group rehabilitation has a variety of benefits. In a University of Helsinki study, a trained music therapist and a trained choir conductor led rehabilitation sessions that included choral singing, tablet-assisted singing training, and melodic intonation therapy. In five months, the intervention improved communication and speech production, enhanced patients' social participation, and reduced caregiver burden.

Statins Protect Against Brain Bleeding and Stroke

Study titled "Association Between Statin Use and Intracerebral Hemorrhage Location: A Nested Case-Control Registry Study," led by researchers at the University of Southern Denmark, Odense, published in *Neurology*.

When statins first came out 35 years ago, they were prescribed for people with high levels of LDL "bad" cholesterol to prevent heart disease and heart attacks. Over time, it became apparent that statin drugs also reduce the risk of strokes caused by a blood clot, called ischemic strokes. Recently, a new study has found that statins also reduce the risk of strokes caused by bleeding in the brain, known as hemorrhagic strokes. Statins are one of the most frequently prescribed medications, used by more than 200 million people worldwide.

HEMORRHAGIC STROKES ARE MORE DANGEROUS THAN ISCHEMIC

Multiple studies have shown that statins reduce ischemic stroke risk, but the evidence for reducing hemorrhagic stroke has been less apparent. The new study found a significant risk reduction for hemorrhagic stroke that improves the longer a person takes a statin drug. This is important because hemorrhagic strokes tend to be more dangerous than ischemic strokes. They make up 10 to 20 percent of all strokes, but they are fatal in 40 percent of cases, compared to about 15 to 30 percent for ischemic stokes.

The new study, which is from the University of Southern Denmark, is published in *Neurology*. The research team used Danish health records to identify more than 2,000 patients ages 55 or older who were diagnosed with a first-ever hemorrhagic stroke between 2009 and 2018. As a control group, the researchers identified more than 85,000 people who never had a stroke. To find out about statin use, they used a nationwide prescription registry.

Stroke patients were matched to control group patients for sex and age. Using a method called conditional logistic regression, the team calculated the odds of having a first hemorrhagic stroke between patients on statins and not on statins. *These were the key findings…*

•**Statin use reduced the overall risk of hemorrhagic stroke by 16 to 17 percent.**

•**Statin use for five years or more reduced the risk of hemorrhagic stroke by 33 to 38 percent.**

HOW STATINS WORK

Statin drugs work by reducing the amount of cholesterol made in the body. In early years of statin use, people were placed on statins primarily due to their cholesterol numbers. Further research found that statins can remove bad cholesterol from plaques inside arteries that supply blood to the brain and the heart, even for people with normal cholesterol numbers. Today statins may be used by people with high risk of stroke or heart attack, even without high levels of bad cholesterol.

Studies continue to show that the benefits of statin drugs are high compared to the risks, which are low. This new study adds more benefits. People in the study were recruited from Southern Denmark, an area of 1.2 million people. The researchers would like to see more studies to confirm their findings in a more diverse group of people, since their sample was heavily European.

CHAPTER 5

Consumer Health Alerts

Beware: 6 Common Health Coverage Misconceptions

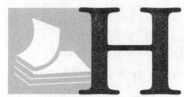How well do you understand your health coverage? In the world of health insurance and, to a lesser extent, Medicare, a single misstep can trigger massive out-of-pocket costs. We asked patient advocate Maura Carley, MPH, CIC, to share some of the coverage misconceptions she has encountered.

MEDICARE MATTERS

•**One spouse transitioning onto Medicare can reset the other spouse's deductible.** A couple obtained health insurance together through the individual market until the older spouse switched to Medicare at age 65. The insurance company told the not-yet-Medicare-eligible spouse that she would have to enroll in a new plan when the older spouse enrolled in Medicare.

Problem: She had already met her annual deductible, so if she enrolled in a new plan, she would have to meet a new deductible.

What to do: Couples enrolling in individual coverage together in years leading up to Medicare eligibility should have the younger spouse serve as the "subscriber." If your insurer tries to reset your deductible, contact your state's insurance department for advice.

•**Medicare's 100 days of nursing home-care doesn't mean what you think it means.** A Medicare recipient's ability to care for himself was rapidly deteriorating, and a move to a nursing home seemed inevitable. His adult children examined their father's Medicare benefits and discovered that Part A provides up to

---

Maura Carley, MPH, CIC, CEO of Healthcare Navigation, LLC, a patient advocacy and consulting company based in Darien, Connecticut, and host of the company's YouTube video series. She previously held senior management positions with Kaiser Permanente, Stamford Hospital, and Yale-New Haven Hospital. HealthCare Navigation.com

100 days of nursing home coverage—but they mistakenly thought this meant Medicare would pay dad's nursing home claims for 100 days.

Problem: Medicare will not pay for a nursing home stay needed just because the recipient cannot safely take care of himself. Medicare's nursing home benefit is available only immediately following a hospital stay of at least three days…and only if the patient requires "skilled services" in an inpatient setting to treat medical issues related to that hospital stay. Even if those conditions are met, Medicare covers nursing home costs only as long as those inpatient skilled services are needed—100 days is the maximum, not a guaranteed coverage duration.

Also, days 21 to 100 of this coverage with original Medicare have $194.50-per-day co-pays. Many but not all Medicare Supplement plans provide coverage for these co-pays. Medicare Advantage plan members should check with their plans to understand what is covered.

What to do: Don't expect Medicare to be the answer to the question, *How are we going to pay ongoing nursing home bills when it is not safe for the individual to live alone?* Medicare coverage in a nursing home is for patients who are receiving skilled services, such as physical or speech therapy, and are recovering from illness or injury. The main payment options for long-term care (LTC) in a nursing home are paying out of pocket…having LTC insurance… or having hybrid life insurance featuring an LTC component—but policies must be obtained while the policyholder is healthy. Many individuals in nursing homes spend down assets until they are eligible for Medicaid, which is coverage for individuals who have little income and/or assets.

•**The death of a spouse can affect a 65-or-older widow/widower's coverage in unexpected ways if he is not yet on Medicare.** A man in his late 60s obtained health coverage as a dependent through his wife's employer's group plan—then his wife died. He received a letter from the employer's benefits department offering him the option of remaining on the company's plan by paying out of

pocket for COBRA coverage. He liked the coverage and had met his annual deductible, so he chose the COBRA coverage option.

Problem: COBRA is secondary coverage for people who are Medicare eligible—it will pay as though Medicare paid first even if that individual is not enrolled in Medicare. If a person in this situation is not enrolled in Medicare Part B, he is likely to be responsible for the amount that Medicare would have paid.

What to do: If you lose access to a group plan after age 65, you almost certainly should decline COBRA and enroll in Medicare immediately.

Even better: Sign up for Medicare Part A as soon as you reach 65 even if you don't need it right away, unless you have a plan with a Health Savings Account (HSA) and want to continue contributing to that HSA.

If you have active group coverage through your or your spouse's work and the employer has 20 or more employees, Part A will be secondary to the group coverage. If you continue working beyond age 65 or are married to a spouse with active group coverage through an employer with 20 or more employees, you are not required to enroll in Medicare Part B.

Rules for people working beyond age 65 who work for employers with fewer than 20 employees vary by state and plan, so you need to know whether you are required to enroll in Medicare Parts A and B. Your employer and/ or the broker should know what is required.

GROUP AND INDIVIDUAL COVERAGE

If you're not yet on Medicare…

•**In-network providers might insist that you pay more up front than you owe.** An ophthalmologist's office insisted that a patient pay $100 at time of service even though this patient's insurance plan had a $35 co-pay. Weeks later, the patient received an Explanation of Benefits (EOB) statement from her insurer confirming that she was responsible for only the $35 co-pay.

Problem: When this patient called the ophthalmologist's billing staff to ask for a refund, they dragged their feet about returning her money.

It has become common for health-care providers to overcharge in-network patients. Sometimes this happens accidentally—insurance coverage can be difficult even for health-care providers to understand. But sometimes it's intentional—providers don't like to wait to receive payment from insurers and don't want to risk not getting paid if an insurer rejects the claim. Overcharges are especially common with high-deductible plans…and/or when patients have met their plans' out-of-pocket maximums. Once this maximum is met, the patient should no longer have to pay co-pays to in-network providers.

What to do: Know what your deductible and co-pay are and whether you've met your out-of-pocket maximum. Push back if a provider asks you to pay more. If a provider insists on an overpayment, pay with a credit card—it often is easier to challenge an overpayment through the credit card issuer than wait for a refund from the provider. After the claim is processed, review the EOB from your insurer. If you were overcharged, contact the provider and insist that a refund be issued immediately. If you don't receive the refund promptly, contact the credit card issuer to dispute the overcharge. Act quickly—your legal right to dispute a credit card overcharge extends for only 60 days after that charge appears on your credit card statement.

•**Enrolled in coverage doesn't necessarily mean *entitled* to coverage.** A woman had been divorced for years but continued to obtain coverage as a dependent on her ex's employer's group plan—her ex didn't report the divorce to his employer. The insurer sent this woman an insurance card each year and paid her claims.

Problem: She was not entitled to the coverage. If the insurer discovered this, it could refuse to pay her future claims and sue her to recoup the years of claims it had paid following the divorce. This isn't the only way people can end up enrolled in coverage that they aren't entitled to—people who obtain coverage on the individual market sometimes relocate outside their plan's coverage area but fail to change plans.

What to do: Never interpret an insurer sending you an ID card and/or accepting your premium payments as evidence that you can remain on a plan following a divorce or a move—that might just mean the insurer hasn't yet noticed that you're now ineligible. Plan in advance of divorce or relocation so you will know when to enroll in a new plan. You should qualify for a "special enrollment period" when you face the loss of coverage, but if you miss that window, you risk having no coverage until the next open-enrollment period.

•**Nontraditional coverage options can be risky.** A woman signed up for a "limited benefit" health plan after confirming that her preferred hospital was in its network.

Problem: When she spent five days in that in-network hospital following a stroke, the plan contributed only $15,000 toward a bill of $175,685.

Problem: "Limited benefit plans," "short-term health plans," "association plans," and "Christian cooperatives" often have lower premiums than coverage through Affordable Care Act (ACA) exchanges. But these plans often fail to protect enrollees against the risk of financial ruin. Not only might the plan cover a smaller percentage of medical bills than an ACA plan, it might not have negotiated rates with the in-network providers, leaving enrollees to pay potentially exorbitant rates. There also have been cases of Christian cooperatives going bankrupt, leaving enrollees with unpaid claims.

What to do: When you need individual coverage, buy it through your state or federal marketplace or directly through a reputable insurer. You want the coverage and consumer protections associated with an ACA-compliant plan.

The Inflation Reduction Act and Your Health Care

Caitlin Donovan, senior director of public relations, National Patient Advocate Foundation, Washington, D.C. NPAF.org

On August 16, 2022, President Biden signed the more than $700 billion Inflation Reduction Act, a sprawling piece of legislation affecting policy related to climate change, taxes, and health care. What-ever you think about its other provisions, the parts of the Act that deal with Medicare are indisputably good news for seniors—and even may have positive spillover effects for younger health-care consumers. *Here's a breakdown of the changes this Act will bring to our health-care system over the next decade…*

PRESCRIPTION DRUG CHANGES

•**Medicare will be required to negotiate drug prices.** In 2003, when Congress passed the Medicare Prescription Drug, Improvement and Modernization Act and established Medicare Part D for handling prescription-drug coverage, it prohibited Medicare from negotiating with pharmaceutical companies on pricing. Seniors would enroll in a Medicare Part D program through a private insurance company such as Humana or Blue Cross Blue Shield. Those individual insurers (or their intermediaries, known as Pharmacy Benefit Managers, or PBMs) would negotiate prices with the drug companies—but Medicare as a whole did not have a seat at the table.

Good news: The Inflation Reduction Act changes that. The Medicare system now will be negotiating with pharma, flexing its heft as an 800-pound gorilla to arrive at a "lowest maximum fair price."

Result: Significantly lower prices across the board for seniors on Part D programs.

Even better: This may result in lower drug prices for consumers outside of Medicare. What happens in Medicare and Medicaid often spills over into the rest of the health-care market, and some observers expect that to happen. Others, however, anticipate that pharmaceutical companies might raise prices outside of Medicare to make up for the shortfall. It's impossible to say who's right—but certainly Medicare patients should expect to see lower drug prices thanks to the system's new negotiating power.

This provision won't kick in until 2026, when Medicare will begin negotiating prices on 10 of the highest-spending Medicare-covered drugs. Fifteen more drugs will follow in 2027…another 15 in 2028…and finally 20 more in 2029. Which drugs will comprise the first batch of 10 (or subsequent batches) has not yet been determined. The Centers for Medicare and Medicaid Services (CMS) has until September of 2023 to select them.

•**Out-of-pocket drug expenses will be curbed, then capped, for Medicare beneficiaries.** Until now, a few unlucky seniors—often the most vulnerable, with serious medical conditions such as cancer or multiple sclerosis—were hit with astronomical out-of-pocket drug costs.

Good news: The Inflation Reduction Act contains a provision that sets an annual cap of $2,000. This is a very big deal. Although most seniors will not reach the cap, it will be a game changer for those who must take multiple expensive meds. The $2,000-cap provision will take effect in 2025.

Even sooner, in 2024, the Act will curb out-of-pocket medication costs by eliminating the 5 percent co-insurance fee enrollees are forced to pay if they exceed the catastrophic coverage amount of $7,050. More than one million patients likely will save about $2,700 per year, on average, on brand-name drugs.

•**Price hikes can't outpace inflation.**

Good news: Starting in 2023, pharma companies that decide to raise prices on their drugs at a rate higher than inflation will be forced to pay rebates to Medicare. The specifics differ according to whether the drugs fall under Medicare Part B or Part D, but generally speaking, they'll be based on how many units are sold at a cost that puts the rate of the price increase higher than a 2021 benchmark figure adjusted for inflation.

Oversimplified example: If a drug company sold 10 units of a heart medication at a cost that was $2 higher than its 2021 price when adjusted for inflation, it would have to pay 10 x $2 = $20 to the trust fund.

Also: This provision includes language indicating that, for certain drugs, seniors on Medicare won't have to pay more than 20 percent of a drug company's price increase adjusted for inflation. So if the company increases its drug cost from $200 to $250 but the inflation-adjusted price is $225, a senior would pay only 20 percent of that $225, or $45—and the company would pay Medicare a $25 rebate for each sale. Because prices that go into these formulas are not limited to what Medicare pays but rather what's charged in commercial markets, this provision will likely rein in excessive price hikes across the board.

•**The out-of-pocket cost of insulin will be capped for Medicare enrollees.** On average, the roughly 3.3 million seniors who use Medicare Parts B or D to obtain insulin have been paying about $54 per month. That's just the average—some are coughing up more than $100…or going without because they can't afford the medication.

Good news: As of 2023, Medicare enrollees' out-of-pocket monthly insulin cost will be capped at $35. Even if the manufacturer increases the cost of insulin, Medicare patients will continue paying their locked-in rate of $35 a month.

•**Adult vaccines will cost seniors nothing.** Most vaccines already are relatively inexpensive—but the Inflation Reduction Act improves even on that.

Good news: This provision, set to take effect in 2023, removes all cost for any adult vaccine, including COVID, shingles, influenza, and monkeypox. It extends to Medicare enrollees as well as those on Medicaid and the Children's Health Insurance Program (CHIP).

This is good news not just for the millions of direct beneficiaries of the policy but for public health in general. The removal of any disincentive to get vaccinated means fewer people getting sick, lowering the overall health-care burden.

Overall result: Taking all of the prescription-drug provisions together, the Congressional Budget Office estimates that the federal deficit would be lowered by $288 billion over 10 years.

INSURANCE CHANGES

•**Medicare subsidies will become more accessible.** In the past, seniors whose incomes fell between 135 percent and 150 percent of the federal poverty line received only partially subsidized Part D benefits.

Good news: The Inflation Reduction Act not only raises the income level for Medicare subsidies to 150 percent of the poverty line

but also eliminates partial benefits. In other words, eligible seniors will pay no Part D premiums and no deductibles and only modest copayments up to the catastrophic threshold, after which they will pay nothing. This provision, which starts in 2024, will save financially fragile seniors about $300, on average, in annual payments—a meaningful amount for those hovering just above the poverty level.

•**ACA subsidies will be extended.** This provision does not relate to Medicare but rather to people who receive federal subsidies on private insurance plans under the Affordable Care Act and subsequent legislation—many of whom are not yet retirees but approaching retirement age and who can pay up to three times more for insurance than younger people.

The ACA, of course, established subsidies to help low-income Americans purchase insurance over "the Marketplace" (either Healthcare.gov or a state Health Insurance Marketplace). The cutoff for receiving such subsidies was 400 percent or less of the federal poverty line, which would amount to $54,360 in 2022. If you earned even $1 more than that—$54,361—you were on your own.

During the pandemic, it became clear that many Americans needed even more help obtaining insurance, so, through the American Rescue Plan Act (ARPA), Congress authorized temporary changes to the income requirements. Instead of using an absolute income figure with a hard cutoff (400 percent of the poverty line), ARPA temporarily re-established eligibility according to the percentage of one's income spent on insurance. No one would be required to pay more than 8.5 percent of their annual income on insurance purchased on the Marketplace.

That piece of legislation was set to expire at the end of 2022, which would have left an estimated 13 million Americans either paying up to 50 percent more for insurance or losing coverage. Such a scenario would have been nothing less than catastrophic for millions of families and for the country's health-care burden.

Good news: The Inflation Reduction Act contains a provision extending those ACA subsidies. They are set to expire in 2025. Congress will need to vote to extend them again or pass legislation making the subsidies permanent. Thanks to the extension, many struggling pre-retirees could save about $2,000 on their premiums annually.

Medicare Penalties and How to Avoid Them

MoneyTalksNews.com

Post-Medicare contributions to a health savings account (HSA) are not allowed—if you do contribute to an HSA, that amount is counted as gross income for tax purposes and subject to a 6 percent penalty. *Late enrollment in Medicare Part A*—the hospital-insurance portion—can cost you a 10 percent penalty for twice the number of years during which you did not sign up, which you are supposed to do as soon as you are eligible. *Late enrollment in Medicare Part B*—the part covering doctors and outpatient and home health care—brings a lifetime penalty of 10 percent for each year you should have signed up but did not. *Late enrollment in Medicare Part D*—prescription drug coverage—can bring a penalty of 12 percent a year that continues as long as you have Part D coverage.

To avoid all penalties: Study Medicare rules carefully before becoming eligible, and go to Medicare.gov for details on how and when to sign up.

How to Appeal Medicare Surcharges

MedicareWire.com and SSA.gov.

About 7 percent of Medicare beneficiaries—4.4 million people—pay more than standard premiums for Part B outpatient care and Part D prescription drugs. The added costs are based on beneficiaries' tax returns from two years earlier. Surcharges were assessed on individuals with modified adjusted gross income (MAGI) above $97,000…or $194,000 for married couples filing jointly (2023 figures).

To appeal a surcharge: Fill out Form SSA-44, *Income-Related Monthly Adjustment Amount—Life-Changing Event*. Eligible events include marriage, divorce, death of a spouse, retirement from work, reduction in work hours, and loss of pension.

To be reassessed: Provide evidence that your current-year income is significantly lower than the one that led to the surcharge.

Medicare Advantage vs. Medigap

Danielle K. Roberts, founding partner of Boomer Benefits, Fort Worth, Texas. She is a Medicare Supplement Accredited Advisor and author of *10 Costly Medicare Mistakes You Can't Afford to Make*. BoomerBenefits.com

Should you sign up for a Medigap plan, a Medicare Advantage plan, or neither when you become eligible at age 65? *Consider these factors…*

PREMIUMS

•**Medicare Advantage plans typically have low or no monthly premiums.**

But: Enrollees generally still pay the Medicare Part B premium, which has been $163.40 for 2023 per month for most participants.

•**Medigap monthly premiums usually fall between $50 and $250,** depending on the plan, local health-care costs, and other factors—plus that Part B premium.

ADDITIONAL OUT-OF-POCKET COSTS

•**Medicare Advantage participants face co-pays and co-insurance**—a $10 co-pay to see a primary care physician…a $50 co-pay to see a specialist…a $300 per-night co-pay for hospital stays. Co-insurance for treatments such as chemotherapy often is 20 percent of what the provider charges. Read the "benefits summaries" to determine out-of-pocket costs. Annual out-of-pocket maximums can be as high as $7,550. These plans change coverage details from year to year.

•**Most Medigap plans cover most or all of the co-pays,** co-insurance, and other gaps in Original Medicare...and that doesn't change from year to year.

Example: Medigap plans cover Medicare Part A co-insurance and hospital costs up to 365 days beyond the Medicare benefit limits...and most Medigap plans cover all Medicare Part B co-insurance and co-pays.

ENROLLMENT

•**Medicare Advantage.** You can sign up for a Medicare Advantage plan during the seven-month stretch that includes the month you turn 65 plus the three months before and after. Once you've reached age 65, you also can sign up in any year during Medicare's October 15 through December 7 open-enrollment period...and if you're enrolled in an Advantage plan, you can switch plans or switch to Original Medicare from January 1 to March 31. Advantage plans cannot decline coverage or increase rates because of preexisting conditions.

•**Medigap.** You can sign up for a Medigap plan during the six-month window that begins the month you enroll in Medicare Part B. You also can apply for Medigap plans after this window closes, but you could be charged extra or declined coverage based on a preexisting condition.

Exceptions: It might be possible to sign up for a Medigap plan after the enrollment window if you live in a state with broad "guaranteed issue" rules, such as Connecticut, Massachusetts, and New York, and/or you lose health coverage.

PROVIDER NETWORKS

•**Medicare Advantage plans come in two types**—HMO plans, which often provide little coverage outside the plan's network of doctors and hospitals in non-emergency situations... and PPO plans, which provide some coverage but with higher out-of-pocket costs.

•**Medigap plans do not have provider network restrictions**—participants can obtain treatment from any doctor or hospital that accepts Medicare's rates.

PRESCRIPTION DRUG COVERAGE

•**Medicare Advantage.** Most of the plans include prescription coverage.

•**Medigap plans do not include prescription coverage**—a Medicare Part D plan should be purchased separately.

Faster Disability-Claim Processing

Social Security Administration. SSA.gov

The Social Security Administration says that it will make decisions within a few days on claims involving more than 250 conditions, including certain cancers, adult brain disorders, and some rare disorders that affect children. Find the list and other information at Social Security.gov/compassionateallowances.

Medicare Genetic-Testing Scam Warning

Kathleen Pursell, director, Arkansas Department of Human Services' Senior Medicare Patrol. HumanServices.Arkansas.gov

How it works: Fraudsters find out the name of a victim's doctor and spoof the office phone number to call or text the victim and offer a "free" cheek-swab genetic test. Crooks then send test kits to victims—and file claims with Medicare to get paid. Most claims are caught and blocked, but enough get through to make the scam worth pursuing.

Worst case for Medicare recipients: Medicare denies a claim and bills the patient for the unapproved test, requiring the recipient to go through a complex appeal to Medicare to void the charge.

Self-defense: Hang up on any call claiming to offer a free genetic test—and do not respond to any text making that kind of offer. Also, check your Medicare Summary Notice (explanation of benefits) for words such as "gene analysis" or "molecular pathology," which could indicate charges for questionable genetic testing.

You Now Can Buy Hearing Aids Over the Counter—and for Far Less

Karl Strom, editor-in-chief of the hearing health-care website HearingTracker.com.

The FDA permits the sale of OTC hearing aids to adults with mild-to-moderate hearing loss without a prescription.

Cost: About $300 to $2,200 for a pair—far less than prescription aids, which can run more than $5,000.

New hearing aid users: While you don't need a prescription, it's worth getting a hearing test from a specialist (covered by Medicare) to have a baseline so you can self-program an OTC hearing aid. Also, pay attention to warranties, trial periods, and return policies.

Low-Cost Senior Dental Care

ThePennyHoarder.com

Dental Lifeline Network (DentalLifeline.org), a program of the American Dental Association, offers free, comprehensive care in limited areas for people below certain income levels, but wait lists are very long. *Community health clinics* (FindAHealthCenter.hrsa.gov) are federally funded and offer free or reduced-cost dental care to people with low incomes. *Dental schools* sometimes offer reduced-cost cleanings and other care. Find a school in your area at CODA.ADA.org. *NeedyMeds.com* has a list of dental offices with sliding-scale payment options. *Dental savings plans* (DentalPlans.com) charge annual fees and offer discounts on services performed by participating dentists.

Why Your Prescriptions Are So Expensive

Siva B. Mohan, M.D., FACC, FSCAI, interventional cardiologist at Emory Healthcare and the president and chief medical officer of RazorMetrics. Tom Dorsett is the CEO of RazorMetrics.

Have you ever been in line at the pharmacy, staring at the display of reading glasses and eye-care solutions, only to overhear an awkward conversation at the front of the line about the prescription being too expensive? Have you been the person at the front of the line trying to have this conversation?

This is a point of failure for the health-care industry. The time to have a conversation about medication cost is before leaving the physician's office, but that rarely happens.

The problem is that your doctor likely has no idea how much a medication costs for you—because there are a wide range of prices for every drug. *There are any variables that affect the drug price for each of us…*

•**Formulary.** Formularies are the list of drugs that a health plan or employer develops to get medications at a lower price for their constituents. It's negotiated and specific to each company. These prices are not public information because the formulary protects confidentiality of the companies. Formularies are redesigned every year and often get mid-year changes, which affects drug prices for individuals. Also, the formulary assigns drugs into tiers, which determines the copay or coinsurance to be paid at the register. Tier 1 drugs cost the least, and the prices go up with the tiers.

•**Specialty drugs.** Specialty drugs are a small class of drugs that typically get the label based on three factors: high cost, high complexity, and high touch. High cost is usually anything that costs $1,500 or more per month. High complexity means the medication is technically difficult to produce. High touch refers to any medication that requires more professional handling, shipping, or storing.

•**Generic.** Does the medication prescribed have a generic version? Is the generic available? Generic medications are chemically equivalent to the brand name but are a fraction of the price. When the exclusive provisions run out for a particular drug, other manufacturers can get the formula and start producing and selling it. Unfortunately, not all markets or pharmacies carry all the generics available, meaning there could be a generic for the prescription, but the local pharmacy doesn't carry it.

•**Pharmacy.** Pharmacies do not charge the same price for the same drugs. The difference in price can be an order of magnitude, especially if the pharmacy accepts a discount card like GoodRx. For example, insulin aspart (NovoLog), used to treat type I and type II diabetes, has a variety of retail prices (see table).

The *manufacturing* cost may be the same for every vial of insulin, but fees are added on to the medication at each step in the distribution chain. Also, the end pharmacy can assess a markup on the medication, which may or may not be in line with the cost at other pharmacies.

An independent survey of retail pharmacy representatives found that only 16 percent of reps tried to offer the lowest cost, while 93 percent were focused on offering a "competitive price." The issue with pharmacy price shopping is that the final cost is not easily comparable.

•**Rebates.** A rebate is a negotiated discount for drugs. The decrease in price is shared between the negotiator (health plan, pharmacy benefit manager, or employer) and the consumer. Rebates help get new, expensive medications to people who could not otherwise afford them.

EDUCATING PHYSICIANS

For patients to get the drugs they need at prices they can afford, physicians need patient-specific information. Physicians are, unfortunately, a large source of high drug costs, and it is because they are forced to prescribe with blinders on. This is where health-care tech companies are bridging the transparency gap. Health-care technology removes those blinders and gives physicians visibility into the real cost of each prescription for each individual patient.

MANAGE YOUR COSTS

In the meantime, here's what you can do to manage your medication costs.

•**Check your insurance card for your plan name,** and then head to your insurance company's website to look up the formulary. You can also call and ask them to mail you a copy. Remember that the formulary can change, so be sure to update your records, and take a copy with you to your doctor's appointments.

•**If your doctor recommends a drug that is listed on a higher tier,** ask about generic or other lower-cost alternatives. Sometimes, simply changing the brand can make a big difference.

•**If you need a specific drug that is not on the formulary,** you can file an appeal with your insurance company to request that it be added.

•**If you are changing insurance plans,** check the formulary to see if your current medications are covered before making the switch.

•**If you're taking a pricey medication,** visit the drug company's website to look for rebates.

•**Shop around for pharmacies to find the best deals for your medications.** There can be significant price differences among pharmacies.

Table. Insulin Aspart Costs

PHARMACY	RETAIL	WITH DISCOUNT
Walgreens	$174	$57.33
HEB	$173	$120.95
Costco	$194	$161.14

Four Insurance Secrets They Don't Want You to Know

Amy Finkelstein, Ph.D., professor of economics at Massachusetts Institute of Technology, Cambridge, and co-director of the Health Care Program at the National Bureau of Economic Research. She is coauthor of *Risky Business: Why Insurance Markets Fail and What to Do About It.* Web.MIT.edu

Americans spend more than $1 trillion every year to insure their health, their homes, their cars and more. And each year, many of those Americans are left wondering why their insurance adds interesting perks but won't cover their claims…their rates keep rising…and no insurer seems to offer reasonable coverage for certain risks. Insurance is supposed to protect us against financial risks and provide peace of mind—but instead, policies often leave people perplexed and infuriated. *Here are four insurance-sector secrets that you should know about…*

1. That gym membership included in your health insurance isn't to keep you healthy. Many health insurance and Medicare Advantage plans include free or heavily discounted gym memberships.

But: Insurers don't do this to help enrollees become healthier and incur fewer medical bills. In fact, monetary-based employer incentives such as gym memberships don't usually help people start going to the gym.

Reality: Insurers offer this because the insurance shoppers most likely to be enticed by free gym memberships are already fit and healthy.

What to do: Lean toward health insurance options that include gym memberships, all else being equal—even if you suspect you'll never go to the gym. These insurers can afford to offer policyholders better benefits than other plans because they tend to attract healthy applicants, who are cheaper to insure.

2. Pet insurance is never very good. Take a close look at a policy that promises to provide health coverage for your pet, and you're likely to conclude that it isn't worth the cost.

Extreme example: A policy for a 12-year-old bulldog costs more than $4,300 annually but pays out only $5,000 per year.

Insurance is economical only when consumers buy coverage even though they don't expect to use it often, as they do with homeowners and auto insurance. But that's not the case with pet insurance, which suffers from a problem called "selection" within the industry. Many pet owners who buy pet insurance have unhealthy pets and/or are willing to try any treatment option that offers even a slim chance of extending their pets' lives.

Result: Pet-insurance providers price their policies as if everyone who enrolls is one of these expensive-to-insure customers. The only way insurers can offer pet policies with affordable premiums is to include low coverage limits, massive coverage gaps, long waiting periods, and other restrictions.

What to do: Pet insurance might be worth its high cost if you believe that your pet is likely to endure lots of expensive health issues and/or you will do everything possible to keep your pet alive. If not, take the money you would have used to pay premiums and fund a savings account to cover the vet bills.

3. Dental insurance is doomed to disappoint. It doesn't seem like dental insurance should suffer from a selection problem—virtually everyone is at risk of incurring sizable dental bills. The problem is that many expensive dental procedures can be delayed for months, so people often wait to enroll in dental coverage until their dentists warn them that expensive procedures are on the horizon.

Result: Many dental policies cover routine cleanings and inexpensive procedures fairly well…but pricey and less common procedures very poorly, if at all. That is exactly the opposite of what insurance is supposed to do.

What to do: Dental insurance offered by an employer might be worth its price if it's well-subsidized by the employer. But read the details carefully before signing up so you understand what is and isn't covered and what waiting periods and other restrictions apply. If dental coverage that does cover big bills fairly well is available to you but is expensive, schedule your dental exams for shortly before your insurance annual open-enrollment period and ask your dentist to give you as much advance warning as possible about procedures that you might need down the road. Depending on the policy's terms and your dental needs, you might be able to sign up for coverage and wait out its waiting periods without endangering your dental health.

4. Life insurance and annuities are priced for life span outliers. If you've ever applied for life insurance, you likely were subjected to medical tests and were required to fill out a lengthy questionnaire about your health history, hobbies, and habits. After all those tests and questions, you probably thought that the insurer must have all the info necessary to predict your longevity and price your life insurance policy accordingly. But surprisingly, it didn't.

When an economist now at Swarthmore College examined the data, she discovered that, despite all the information life insurers collect and statisticians and software they use to analyze it, life insurance consumers still somehow have a better sense of their own likely longevity than insurers do.

Result: Based on her research, consumers who decide to buy life insurance tend to somehow know that they're likely to die sooner than the insurers expect.

Result: Insurers know this issue, so to protect themselves, they set premiums on the assumption that every applicant will die somewhat sooner than the medical tests and questions predict. This makes insurance overpriced for consumers who simply want it for peace of mind or financial-planning purposes.

This problem is more pronounced for insurance companies that sell annuities, which provide monthly payments as long as the policyholder is alive. The longer an annuity buyer lives, the greater the odds that the insurance company will take a financial loss—but insurance companies typically price annuities based only on the applicant's age and gender, without any medical tests or lengthy questionnaires. Thus, an annuity buyer who comes from a very long-lived family and/or who lives a safe, healthy lifestyle has a huge advantage over annuity sellers. So annuity sellers price their annuities on the assumption that every buyer will outlive the actuarial tables.

What to do: If you want life insurance but don't expect to die anytime soon…or you want an annuity but don't expect to live exceptionally long…lean toward the policies and annuities that longevity-outlier consumers tend to shun.

Examples: An annuity buyer might select a "period certain" annuity that's guaranteed to make payments for a predetermined number of years rather than based on life span—a buyer who expects to live a very long life wouldn't choose that option. Or a life insurance shopper

might select a policy that has a long waiting period before death benefits begin. Insurance products such as these often offer better terms.

Similar: Choosing policies that signal insurers that you don't expect to make many claims can lead to significantly lower rates with other forms of insurance, too.

Example: Insurers tend to offer the best terms to home and auto insurance shoppers who select policies that have large deductibles. Not only do these deductibles save insurers money, people who buy these policies send the message that they don't expect to make claims.

Long-Term Care Insurance: The Pros…the Cons…and the Alternatives

Glenn S. Daily, CFP, ChFC, CLU, a fee-only insurance consultant in New York City and cofounder of Tell Us the Odds, LLC, an LTCI policy evaluation service. TellUsTheOdds.com

---

Traditional long-term-care insurance (LTCI) has been in a long-term decline. Fewer than 50,000 policies were issued in 2020, a small fraction of the more than 500,000 sold each year a few decades ago. Many insurers have stopped issuing traditional LTCI policies altogether because they were losing money on them. Meanwhile, consumers have been frightened off by rate increases imposed on earlier LTCI policyholders, and they don't want to pay thousands of dollars in premiums for insurance that may never provide any benefits.

Are those consumer concerns warranted? Is traditional LTCI still worth considering? And what are the alternatives for financing long-term care? *Here's a look at LTCI and other long-term-care coverage options today…*

WEIGHING THE OPTIONS

Long-term care can cost $50,000 to more than $150,000 a year, depending on where you live and the type of care that you require. This is more than most retirees could afford to pay out of pocket for long without devastating their savings. Options for covering these bills include traditional LTCI…"hybrid" or "linked-benefit" policies that combine elements of LTCI and life insurance or annuities…LTC riders on life insurance policies…and Medicaid.

•**Traditional LTCI.** The sector's worst pricing problems are behind it—but is anyone even paying attention? People who purchased LTCI many years ago often have horror stories about massive premium increases. Notices arrive in the mailbox one day informing them of a rate increase of 30…50 percent…or even more. These policyholders feel trapped—they don't want to lose the coverage that they have been faithfully funding for years, but the rate hikes strain their retirement budgets. Insurers offer options to reduce the hikes by reducing the maximum daily benefit, the benefit period, or the inflation adjustment, but it is hard to know which option to choose.

What happened: In the beginning, LTCI was a relatively new insurance, and insurers had to make guesses about how much to charge for early policies. Every major pricing assumption turned out to be too optimistic. Insurers assumed that many policyholders would let their policies lapse over the years—but most people continued to pay premiums. Also, fewer people died than expected. These two factors led to more claims. Insurers underestimated the length of nursing home stays due to neurodegenerative diseases. Finally, insurers were counting on significant earnings from their investments in bonds and mortgages, but interest rates have remained low.

Good news: Policies sold today are far less likely to face major rate increases due to more conservative pricing assumptions and better oversight by state insurance regulators. Insurers that remain in the sector today aren't making those early mistakes, and state insurance regulators have made it more difficult for insurers to justify future rate hikes.

The rates you're quoted will vary based on your age, health, gender, amount of coverage you want, and specific policy terms including its inflation protection—adding significant inflation protection can more than double a policy's premiums.

Examples: A healthy 55-year-old man might pay $950 in annual premiums for a policy with no inflation protection that provides $165,000 in benefits…a healthy 55-year-old woman, $1,500…a healthy 55-year-old married couple, $2,080 combined, according to the American Association for Long-Term Care Insurance's 2022 Price Index survey. But add 3 percent annual benefit growth to protect against inflation, and that man will pay $2,200…the woman, $3,700…and the couple, $5,025.

More good news: Traditional LTCI enjoys tax subsidies. If you're self-employed and file a Schedule C, *Profit or Loss from Business*, you likely can deduct the cost of your LTCI premiums (subject to a dollar limit based on your age) for yourself and/or your spouse up to the total amount of your Schedule C income.

Exception: You can't claim this tax break if a subsidized LTCI plan is available to you and/or your spouse through an employer.

If you don't file a Schedule C, you still might be able to deduct LTCI premiums to the extent that those premiums together with your other unreimbursed medical expenses exceed 7.5 percent of your adjusted gross income (AGI). To take advantage, you'll have to file a Schedule A, *Itemized Deductions*, rather than claim the standard deduction.

Note that LTCI premiums are deductible only for "qualified" policies that meet a list of criteria—ask your insurance agent to confirm that a policy is qualified before purchasing it. There also are caps on the size of the annual LTCI premiums that can be deducted—as of 2023, those caps are $480 for taxpayers age 40 and younger, but they climb to $5,960 for taxpayers age 71 and older. These caps are doubled for married couples when both spouses have LTCI coverage.

Some states offer significant tax breaks for LTCI premiums as well.

Example: In New York, taxpayers who have AGIs less than $250,000 can receive annual nonrefundable state tax credits worth either 20 percent of the total amount paid in premiums or $1,500, whichever is less.

Those state tax credits, together with the federal deductions above, sometimes slash the after-tax actuarial cost of premiums to less than the actuarial value of the policy's benefits. In other words, once taxes are factored in, New Yorkers who file a Schedule C may, on average, receive more back from traditional LTCI policies than they pay into them. Consult your tax adviser for advice.

Important: At the first sign that you may have a need for long-term care, consult your agent or other knowledgeable professional to review the claims process for your policy. Some advance planning will increase your odds of getting the benefits that you have paid for.

•**Hybrid policies.** These policies use life insurance and annuities as a base for providing LTC benefits.

Example: A $100,000 single premium buys a hybrid life/LTC policy with a $102,000 death benefit. A long-term-care claim will draw down the death benefit by $3,050 per month for 33 months. After 33 months, another pool of money will provide a lifetime $3,050 LTC benefit with 3 percent inflation. The policy also has a cash value that grows to $102,000 at age 121 if you have no claims.

To understand what you are getting, you need to do an actuarial valuation of each benefit. However, it's clear that some of your money is buying life insurance, not LTCI, so this policy is likely to be less useful than traditional LTCI if your goal is to pay for long-term-care expenses.

A hybrid policy is designed to provide the comfort of knowing that some benefit will be paid whether or not you need long-term care, but that comfort is just an illusion if you don't know the value of the benefits.

Annuity/LTC hybrids use the annuity's cash value and an additional pool of money to provide long-term-care benefits. If you own an annuity with a large taxable gain, you can turn the taxable gain into tax-free long-term-care benefits by doing a tax-free exchange ("Section 1035 exchange") from your existing annuity to the hybrid.

The hybrid advantage: People who cannot get traditional LTCI at affordable rates due to poor health may be able to find an affordable hybrid policy.

•**LTC riders.** LTC riders are an add-on to a life insurance policy that you are buying for a known purpose, such as leaving a legacy for your heirs. The long-term-care benefits reduce the policy's death benefit, subject to a minimum. The rider increases the usefulness of the policy while possibly jeopardizing the policy's primary purpose.

•**Medicaid.** The eligibility rules are unpalatable—and they could get worse. Most Americans don't buy any variety of LTCI—if they require long-term care that they can't pay for out of pocket, they expect the government to pick up the bill. But qualifying for Medicaid long-term-care coverage requires spending down almost all of your assets and living as a virtual ward of the state.

And there's no guarantee that these rules won't be even less appealing years from now when you might need nursing home care. Federal government debt skyrocketed during the pandemic, and Medicaid long-term-care coverage could be curtailed if future politicians are looking for ways to trim spending.

On the other hand, some politicians have proposed greatly expanding government coverage of long-term care. So can we count on the government to pay for our long-term care when we need it…or can't we? Any answer to that question is little more than guesswork—which means any financial planning that depends on government assistance in this area is risky at best.

Possible solution: Many experts have advocated combining LTCI with lifetime income, provided by an annuity, redesigned pensions or Social Security.

Example: You get $1,000 each month when you're healthy and that increases to $2,000, $3,000, or more when you need long-term care. Income annuity/LTC hybrids would provide two benefits that many people need—income they can't outlive and money for long-term care.

Yes, You Can Self-Fund Your Own Long-Term Care

Christine Benz, director of personal finance and retirement planning for Morningstar, Inc., an investment research firm based in Chicago that tracks 621,000 investment offerings. Morningstar.com

The price of long-term care (LTC) is staggeringly high and steadily increasing. Yet for some people, the best option for financing these fearsome future bills might be to pay out of pocket.

Frightening facts: The average annual cost of a private room in a nursing home recently rose above $108,000, according to a study by insurance company Genworth. As expensive as that might sound, it's a bargain compared to what you might have to pay if you need LTC down the road—Genworth expects this annual price tag to sail past $150,000 in 10 years...and past $200,000 in 20 years.

Those figures have left many people wondering, *How am I ever going to pay those prices?*

Many people have decided that an LTC insurance policy is not the answer. Sales of these policies have plummeted in recent years, with consumers scared off by steep prices and the sector's history of springing unexpected premium increases on existing policyholders.

Hybrid policies that combine elements of life insurance and LTC coverage are somewhat more popular, but still only a fraction of people in or approaching retirement have purchased these policies.

Medicaid is another option for financing LTC, but it is by no means appealing—this government program won't pick up your LTC bills until you've spent down virtually all of your assets and are essentially living in poverty.

One major option remains: Save enough to pay any future LTC bills out of your own pocket. It's a viable strategy for many Americans despite the daunting cost of care. *Here's how to make it work for you...*

HOW MUCH DO I NEED?

The conventional wisdom about self-funding future LTC expenses holds that if a retiree has a nest egg of $2 million or more, his/her savings should be sufficient to support this strategy.

But that's not necessarily true—if you enter retirement with a nest egg of $2 million but spend $100,000 a year, you could easily end up without enough assets to pay LTC bills when the time comes.

For self-funding LTC to be a viable option: You must have a nest egg of seven figures or more...and be able to pay your bills through age 90...and still have a surplus that's comfortably into six figures to pay for LTC. A retirement calculator, such as Vanguard's Retirement Nest Egg calculator (Vanguard.com/nesteggcalculator), can help with this math.

•**How much should you set aside?** For most retirees, it isn't feasible to prepare for LTC worst-case scenarios—a diagnosis of dementia that leads to a decade-plus nursing home stay could easily produce bills of $1 million to $2 million or more...and a married couple would have to plan for the possibility that both spouses could require such extended care.

More realistic savings target: The amount needed to pay for the average nursing home stay—for men, the average is 2.2 years...for women, it is 3.7 years. Nursing home costs, currently just north of $100,000 per year, are climbing fast, so it's reasonable for an individual to set aside $300,000 for LTC expenses...and for a couple to target twice that amount.

That still sounds like a lot of money to set aside for LTC that might never be needed, so don't look at this money as only for LTC costs. It serves three worthy purposes—paying LTC costs if you do in fact require a nursing home stay...a hedge against longevity risk, so you won't have to live in poverty if you outlive your other retirement savings...and/or if the money isn't needed for either of the possibilities above, a legacy for your heirs or your favorite charity.

Warning: The data in this article is largely based on national averages, which might not fit your circumstances. *When you are deciding how much to save for LTC, factor in the following...*

•*Where you live*—the cost of LTC is dramatically higher in expensive coastal regions than in many middle-America locales. *Examples:* The current annual cost of a private room in a nursing home in Missouri is $71,175...but $182,044 in Connecticut.

•*Family health history and personal health history.* If you and/or your spouse have been diagnosed with dementia or have a family history of dementia, significantly more LTC savings are warranted. In fact, a family history of dementia could be a strong motivation to apply for LTC insurance or a hybrid policy that includes LTC coverage rather than planning to pay for LTC out of pocket. *But keep in mind:* Someone with a dementia diagnosis probably would not qualify for LTC insurance...and even someone with a family history of dementia may be limited in the type of coverage he can buy.

Of course, if your LTC savings target is based on the average length of a nursing home stay, there's a reasonable chance that your LTC bills will exceed those savings. *Have an emergency backup plan in mind in case that occurs...*

•**Tap your home equity.** This could be done by selling your home...taking out a reverse mortgage...or taking out a home-equity line of credit. Many retirees don't want to take equity out of their homes or sell their homes, but emergency backup plans aren't about what we want—they're about making do in difficult circumstances.

•**Spend down assets to qualify for Medicaid or the U.S. Department of Veterans Affairs "Aid and Attendance" benefits.** These government programs pay LTC bills only for applicants who have extremely limited assets. That makes them unappealing but still worth considering in emergency situations.

•**Family-provided care.** No one wants to be a burden to a spouse or descendants, but seeking familial assistance can dramatically reduce the number of years spent paying for

LTC. Spouses are major providers of care and often the first line of defense for individuals with LTC needs. Someone who is diagnosed with dementia might live with loved ones for as long as possible before moving into a nursing home, for example. Such arrangements are extremely common—83 percent of the assistance provided to older adults in the U.S. comes from family members, friends, and/or other unpaid caregivers, according to the Alzheimer's Association.

INVESTMENT VEHICLES AND DECISIONS

If you decide to self-fund LTC, put money earmarked for those future bills into an account other than your retirement funds to reduce the odds that the money will be misspent.

Assets earmarked to pay future LTC costs should be invested fairly aggressively even during the early years of retirement. The typical nursing home stay doesn't begin until around age 80, so someone in his late 60s probably won't need the money for more than a decade—and that's usually sufficient time to ride out any stock market fluctuations. These assets might be slowly transitioned into a more conservative allocation comparable to that of a retiree's other retirement savings as he approaches his mid-70s.

Best vehicle for these savings: A traditional IRA. That might seem counterintuitive—other savings vehicles such as Roth IRAs and Health Savings Accounts (HSAs) offer tax-free withdrawals, a wonderful benefit that traditional IRAs lack. But that isn't a massive advantage when it comes to paying for LTC costs.

Reason: Most LTC expenses qualify as health-care expenses...and health-care expenses that exceed 7.5 percent of adjusted gross income are tax-deductible. Thus, any taxes generated by withdrawing money from a traditional IRA to pay LTC bills likely will be mostly offset by the resulting deduction. Factor in that pretax dollars are used to fund a traditional IRA, and it's an excellent savings vehicle for LTC costs.

Beware For-Profit Hospice

Private-equity firms are buying up hospice agencies, and that could have a negative effect on patients as the firms cut back on care to maximize profits. Researchers reported in *JAMA Internal Medicine* that for-profit hospices hire fewer employees than non-profits and rely more on lower-cost licensed practical nurses and nursing aides than registered nurses. Further, the U.S. Government Accountability Office reported that patients in for-profit hospices are less likely to receive any hospice visits in the last three days of life—when their needs are highest. A report in the *Journal of Palliative Care* noted that for-profit hospices have more deficiencies and complaints, and send patients to rooms and hospitals more often. To find a nonprofit hospice, visit https://www.hospice innovations.org/find-a-not-for-profit-hospice-care-provider/.

Clinical Advisor.

How to Tell If Your Doc Is a Quack

Charles B. Inlander, consumer advocate and healthcare consultant based in Fogelsville, Pennsylvania.

Trust between patient and doctor is essential, but sometimes you need to be skeptical of a diagnosis or proposed treatment. *Whether it's skullduggery or out-and-out quackery, the warning signs and steps to take are the same...*

When to be suspicious...

•**If a practitioner tries to sell you something**—a procedure or a product—especially if he/she owns the facility or company involved. It's a red flag if you hear, "I want you to take a supplement, but the only good one is the one I sell" or "It's a new operation, and I'm the only person performing it."

•**If a practitioner offers services beyond his/her area of expertise.** This could be an effort to boost his income, such as an ob-gyn who adds cosmetic services.

What to do...

•**While you're still at your appointment,** say, "I want to think about this" or "I'm not ready to take action yet." Once you're home, research the doctor and/or the treatment.

•**Check the Open Payments Page at the Centers for Medicare & Medicaid Services website (OpenPaymentsData.cms.gov)** to see if the doctor is receiving incentives to promote a drug or a medical device. Medical companies are required to disclose this, and the site compiles the information.

•**If the doctor claims to be a true pioneer in a new treatment,** do an online search using "[doctor's name] + research." Then look to see if there are any studies in bona fide publications. Confirm that a publication is bona fide by looking it up on NCBI.nlm.nih.gov, a website of the National Library of Medicine.

•**Check your state licensing board for complaints against the doctor.** Also check for board certification—and confirm that he is certified in the area of medicine in question. Research if he is affiliated with a leading hospital or medical school—these institutions are likely to weed out bad players.

•**Get a second or even third opinion.** According to a well-reported 2017 study, 21 percent of patients who sought a second opinion at the Mayo Clinic left with a completely new diagnosis...and 66 percent of the diagnoses were deemed to be only partly correct and needed to be refined or completely redefined. Get an independent second opinion from a respected institution, not someone in the same practice as the first doctor or from anyone he suggests.

If, after all this, your trust has been eroded, look for a new doctor.

Medical Malpractice: How to Protect Yourself and Your Loved Ones

Stephan Landsman, JD, Clifford Professor of Tort Law and Social Policy, Emeritus, at DePaul University College of Law in Chicago and coauthor of *Closing Death's Door: Legal Innovations to End the Epidemic of Healthcare Harm*. Landsman has successfully argued before the U.S. Supreme Court and is a member of the leadership of the American Bar Association Litigation Section. Law.DePaul.edu

I njury or infection caused by medical treatment is one of the leading causes of death in the U.S. In fact, most of us will experience a diagnostic error at some point in our lives, according to "Improving Diagnosis in Health Care," a report from the Institute of Medicine.

These errors are equal-opportunity killers, affecting patients regardless of gender, race, and socioeconomic status.

Examples: Receiving the wrong medication…contracting an infection in the hospital… having surgery performed on the wrong body part…and more.

Three case studies of medical errors and what you can learn from them…

CASE #1: In 2012, astronaut Neil Armstrong underwent coronary bypass surgery at Cincinnati's Mercy Health Fairfield Hospital. The procedure included having a temporary pacemaker implanted to regulate his heartbeat. It was successful, but soon after, Armstrong began bleeding internally and his blood pressure dropped. He needed immediate surgical intervention but instead was taken to the catheterization lab, where minimally invasive procedures are performed. By the time he got to the operating room, it was too late. He passed away a week later.

Result: The hospital awarded Armstrong's family $6 million in a wrongful death settlement, according to Harvard T.H. Chan School of Public Health.

What went wrong: Armstrong had chosen a local medical facility rather than a larger, renowned institution for the procedure. For a serious procedure—a stent in your heart, knee replacement, treatment of chronic obstructive pulmonary disease—select a facility where the procedure is done frequently. A 2015 *U.S. News & World Report* analysis of hospital outcomes for these procedures and two others between 2010 and 2012 showed that more cases equal fewer deaths. And according to a 2019 *Journal of Orthopaedic Surgery and Research* meta-analysis, patients undergoing hip arthroplasty had superior outcomes when the surgery was done in a high-volume hospital.

That's not to say you can't get quality care at a low-volume hospital—but expect improved outcomes with hospitals that often handle your procedure…are equipped to handle problems that might arise…and are staffed by experienced health-care providers who are knowledgeable about your condition.

What to ask before moving ahead…

•**How many of these procedures do you do a day/week/month?** You want large numbers. Ask how the number compares to that of other providers.

•**What are the potential complications, and how often do they occur?** Data on complication rates depends on state and locality. You can contact several institutions to compare the stats. Also check LeapFrog (LeapFrogGroup.org), which collects, analyzes, and publishes data on the safety and quality of health care.

•**Will you be performing my procedure?** Make sure your provider is not just supervising—as is often the case in teaching hospitals.

CASE #2: A grave mistake was made in 1994 when two patients—*Boston Globe* health reporter Betsy Lehman and teacher Maureen Bateman—both were being treated for breast cancer at Dana-Farber Cancer Institute. They were given huge overdoses of their experimental chemotherapy medication. Lehman died immediately. Bateman recovered, but her heart was severely damaged and she died in 1997 from several cancers.

Result: Both families were awarded undisclosed settlements from the hospital, according to *AP News*. The doctor responsible for prescribing the overdoses was suspended for three years by the Massachusetts Board of Registration in Medicine, and the hospital initiated a patient-safety campaign that continues to this day.

What went wrong: Health-care workers are overworked and overscheduled these days. You should always know what medication and dose you are receiving…and ask for it to be double-checked by a health-care professional. Inquiring is an added layer of protection. This is especially important for treatment that has potentially dangerous side effects, such as chemotherapy and kidney dialysis.

What to ask before receiving any medication…

•**Can you double-check that the medication and dose are correct?** If this feels intimidating, lighten it up a bit by saying, "Humor me! I just need a little reassurance." Before you are sedated for a medical procedure, ask what procedure is to be performed and make sure the correct body part is clearly marked.

•**I regularly receive this medication. Does everything look the same, prescription-wise?** The best health-care organizations welcome these questions from patients.

•**Are you and the institution QOPI certified for cancer treatment?** The American Society for Clinical Oncology introduced the voluntary Quality Oncology Practice Initiative (QOPI) in 2006 to enhance patient safety for cancer patients. Participation in the QOPI Certification Program allows medical practices to measure the quality of their oncology care against 100+ measures and compare their performance with other practices nationwide. An interactive map of QOPI-certified practices can be accessed from Practice.asco.org (follow the drop-down menus under the "Quality Improvement" tab).

CASE #3: When Christina Flach called her husband's doctor's office on March 7, 2018, saying that her husband was experiencing chest pain, fever, weakness, and fatigue, a nurse trained to triage patients scheduled a telehealth visit with Ken Flach's physician for four hours later. During that three-minute appointment, the doctor recommended Flach try multiple over-the-counter and prescription medications and call back if his condition worsened. It did worsen, and early the next morning, Flach—a

former Olympic and Wimbledon doubles champ—went to the emergency room, where he was diagnosed with pneumonia, a *methicillin-resistant Staphylococcus aureus* (MRSA) infection, acute respiratory failure, renal failure, septic shock, hemoptysis (coughing up blood), and more. Despite treatment, he died several days later.

Result: The Flach family won a medical malpractice lawsuit against Kaiser Permanente Medical Group.

What went wrong: Telehealth visits can provide health-care access for patients and reduce cost, but they come with greater risk for missed diagnoses. According to CRICO, the risk-management branch of Harvard Medical Institutions, 66 percent of telehealth-related malpractice claims between 2014 and 2018 were related to missed diagnoses. According to malpractice-insurance carrier the Doctors Company Group, these missed diagnoses tend to be related to cancer, stroke, and infection. Misdiagnoses are not unique to telehealth. But while certain fields of medicine, such as psychiatry and dermatology, lend themselves to telehealth, it may be more difficult to identify system-wide infections.

What to ask yourself before choosing telemedicine…

•**How sick am I?** In some situations—especially if you feel like you're at death's door—being seen in person may be wise. Physicians have tools for improving virtual assessments, but if you have chest or abdominal pain, shortness of breath, or swelling in the legs, an in-office visit is best.

•**Do I have the right setup for telehealth?** You'll need a private space and strong Wi-Fi connection. Lighting is key, allowing your provider to accurately gauge your coloring and see any rashes, bumps, or other similar concerns. Sit with your back to a wall and not a sunny window. Be on time so you can spend as much of your visit as possible on important health-related matters.

Beware Medication Thieves

Federal Trade Commission.

Thieves can take a pill bottle out of your trash and have your name, prescription, pharmacy, and refill date in an instant. They can use that information to refill your prescription, use your name or health insurance numbers to see a doctor, and steal your identity. There have also been cases of thieves breaking into people's homes looking for pain medications after they found empty pill bottles in the trash.

To stay safe, use these tips…

1. Always strip the labels off the bottles before you throw them away. If it's something that comes in an envelope, cut it up so you can't tell what it is.

2. Shred the papers that come with the prescription. They may contain codes or information that can be traced back to you.

3. Likewise, shred your health insurance enrollment forms, health insurance cards, billing statements from your doctor or other medical provider, and explanation of benefits statements from your health insurance company.

4. Don't tell just anyone that you are on pain medication or another controlled substance.

5. Keep your medication somewhere no one would think to look. Don't keep controlled medications out in the open or with your other medications or in the medicine cabinet.

Mycotoxin Danger from Common Foods

Gregory A. Plotnikoff, M.D., MTS, integrative medicine physician, founder and medical director of Minnesota Personalized Medicine in Minneapolis. MNPersonalized Medicine.com

Mycotoxins, naturally occurring toxins produced by molds in certain foods, can cause shortness of breath, chest pain, sinusitis, cognitive impairment, anxiety, and depression.

Risky foods: Corn, cereals, ground and tree nuts, spices, dried fruits, fresh fruits, and coffee beans.

Self-defense: Buy grains and nuts in small batches, and consume within six months…don't store foods in high-moisture areas…eat mycotoxin-prone foods in moderation.

Grieving Makes You Vulnerable

Joshua Slocum, executive director of Funeral Consumers Alliance in South Burlington, Vermont. Heart 2Soul.com

Grieving makes you vulnerable to unscrupulous funeral directors. Watch out for upselling.

Example: Rubber casket seals to "protect your loved one from the elements." You have the right to select items à la carte rather than purchasing a package…and if a funeral director tells you that one of your choices is against the law, ask to see that law in writing.

Fake COVID Home Test Kit Warning

U.S. Food and Drug Administration (FDA). FDA.gov

The FDA has issued a warning about fake COVID-19 test kits that are sold over-the-counter and look like legitimate ones.

To spot a counterfeit: Look for poor print quality…missing information on the box, such as a missing lot number, expiration date, or bar code…grammatical or spelling errors…kit components that do not match the content description.

Self-defense: Use only tests on the FDA's approved list of home test kits. Go to FDA.gov and enter "At-home OTC COVID-19 diagnostic tests" into the search box.

Drive Better...Eat Better...Save on Insurance

The Wall Street Journal. WSJ.com

Allowing the insurer Allstate to track your driving habits, such as speeding and braking, through its "Drivewise" program can earn a premium discount of up to 25 percent. Hancock's Vitality life insurance policies give a premium discount of up to 25 percent for buyers who fulfill requirements such as exercising, buying more healthful foods, and getting mammograms.

New joint venture: Drivewise policyholders who have earned Safe Driver status can earn points for premium discounts at Hancock. However, it doesn't work the other way—drivers with healthy lifestyle habits at Hancock do not get Allstate discounts.

Free Ways to Work Out at Home

MoneyTalksNews.com

Find *free yoga videos* at CorePowerYoga.com. *Download the free Planet Fitness workout app* (available from Apple and Google Play)...or the free *FitOn* app that lets you stream videos on your TV, computer or smartphone. Go to *Orangetheory Fitness* YouTube channel for a variety of workouts—you do not have to be a member. *Add exercise bands* to your regular workout exercises, keeping tension on the band throughout the workout. *For weight-based training,* use common household items, such as canned food or drinks for bicep curls...*do interval training with the stairs in your home* by moving up them as quickly as possible, then walking slowly back down to catch your breath, and repeating several times.

CHAPTER 6

Diabetes Breakthroughs

Mind-Body Practices Can Help Beat Type 2 Diabetes

Along with medication and lifestyle changes, about 66 percent of Americans with diabetes include some type of mind-body practice in their daily care to help them control or lower their blood sugar.

Studies do exist on mind-body practice for type 2 diabetes, but there's no consensus on how much these practices help control and lower blood sugar. A new review of studies by researchers at the University of Southern California's Keck School of Medicine finds that mindful disciplines (such as yoga and meditation) do help, and the amount of help was surprising to the research team.

WHAT MIND-BODY PRACTICES WERE STUDIED

The research team reviewed randomized controlled trials—the highest level of research trials—from across the globe between 1993 and 2022. They selected 28 trials that compared treatment with a diabetes medication alone to treatment with medication plus a mind-body practice. This was the first trial to include a range of mind-body practices such as meditation, yoga, qigong, and mindfulness-based stress reduction. The researchers calculated the effect of these practices on fasting blood sugar and hemoglobin A1c.

Like yoga, qigong is an ancient mind-body exercise that combines breathing, meditation, and movement. Mindfulness-based stress reduction was developed at the University of

Study titled "Mind- and Body-Based Interventions Improve Glycemic Control in Patients with Type 2 Diabetes: A Systematic Review and Meta-Analysis," by researchers at Keck School of Medicine of USC, Los Angeles, published in the *Journal of Integrative and Complementary Medicine.*

Massachusetts Medical Center in 1979. It combines meditation, meditative exercise, gentle and mindful movement (including yoga), and loving-kindness meditation (which involves repeating positive phrases expressing compassion for yourself and others).

HOW TO KNOW YOU HAVE DIABETES...AND WHAT HELPS

Hemoglobin A1c is a blood test that measures your average blood sugar over the past two to three months. This test is a good way to tell how well type 2 diabetes is being managed. The result is given as a percentage. A result of 6.5 percent or above indicates diabetes. People with type 2 diabetes should have an A1c below 7.

The results of the review are published in the *Journal of Integrative and Complementary Medicine. These were their key findings...*

•**All mind-body practices taken together lowered hemoglobin A1c** by almost a full percentage point (0.84 percent) more than medication alone.

•**All the mind-body practices lowered A1c,** but the most effective practice was yoga, which lowered A1c by a full percentage point. The benefit increased as the number of yoga sessions increased.

•**All mind-body practices together lowered blood sugar** by almost 23 milligrams more than medication alone.

Lowering A1c by one percentage point is very significant because only about 50 percent of people with type 2 diabetes can keep their A1c under 7. The most prescribed medication—metformin—lowers A1c by an average of 1.1 percent, indicating that a mind-body practice is almost as effective as medication.

MIND-BODY PRACTICES ARE HEALTHFUL FOR EVERYBODY

Although prevention of type 2 diabetes was not part of the study, the results suggest that mind-body practice could help people with prediabetes reduce their risk for future type 2 diabetes.

And according to the CDC, most people have prediabetes before they have type 2 diabetes. Close to 100 million adults in the U.S. have pre-

diabetes—unfortunately, more than 80 percent are not aware of it. A yoga and/or a meditation habit can be very effective for people with prediabetes—a condition that is reversible with lifestyle changes.

The Glycemic Index (GI) Is Not Reliable for Controlling Blood Sugar

The GI assigns a score to foods to indicate their supposed effect on glucose levels.

But: The GI's math is based on faulty assumptions—individual glucose responses to identical foods can vary.

Better: Focus on foods rich in fiber (about 3 grams per serving) such as fruits, vegetables, and whole grains, which reduce the share of carbohydrates that your body absorbs.

Katherine Beals, Ph.D., RD, associate professor of nutrition at University of Utah in Salt Lake City, commenting on a study published in *The American Journal of Clinical Nutrition.*

COVID Boosts Diabetes Risk

Ziyad Al-Aly, M.D., chief of research at VA St. Louis Health Care System, Missouri, and leader of a study of 181,000 veterans published in *The Lancet: Diabetes and Endocrinology.*

According to a recent study, recovering from COVID-19 is associated with a 40 percent higher risk of being newly diagnosed with diabetes. One theory is that the SARS-CoV-2's spike protein may dysregulate pancreatic cells responsible for producing insulin. If one out of every 100 people with COVID develops diabetes, that could be significant for public health—1 percent of 80 million U.S. cases equals 800,000 new diabetes diagnoses.

Exercise May Treat COVID-Induced Diabetes and Depression

Candida Rebello, Ph.D., RD, postdoctoral researcher at Louisiana State University.

John Kirwan, Ph.D., director of the Integrated Physiology and Molecular Metabolism Laboratory, Louisiana State University.

Even after recovering from a minor COVID-19 infection, some people experience a vicious cycle of inflammation that can lead to diabetes and depression months after the original infection subsides. Exercise may counter this effect by breaking the chain reaction of inflammation that leads to high blood sugar levels, and then to the development or progression of type 2 diabetes. Walking slowly for 30 minutes each day is ideal, but even a 15-minute walk is beneficial.

The Latest Findings About Fat...and What They Mean for You

Paul Cohen, M.D., Ph.D., head of the Laboratory of Molecular Metabolism at The Rockefeller University, New York City. He is coauthor of the recent article "Brown adipose tissue is associated with cardiometabolic health" published in *Nature Medicine*. CohenLab.Rockefeller.edu

Fat is widely viewed as an enemy of our health. Obesity increases the odds of developing a host of problems, including heart disease, type 2 diabetes, hypertension, and many types of cancer. Troublingly, obesity rates now top 40 percent in the U.S. But researchers recently have uncovered some interesting findings about fat—findings that could help reduce the health risks posed by obesity...and perhaps even lower obesity rates themselves. Among the surprises—the *quality* of one's fat might matter more than the *quantity*.

GOOD FAT, BAD FAT

When people picture fat, they imagine white fat, the most common and familiar form of flab.

Teatime to Stop Diabetes

Tea Drinking May Cut Diabetes Risk

Drinking at least four cups a day of black, green, or Oolong tea is associated with a 17 percent lower chance of developing type 2 diabetes during a 10-year period.

Likely reason: Tea contains healthful antioxidant, anti-inflammatory, and anti-cancer compounds.

Meta-analysis of 19 studies of more than one million adults by researchers at Wuhan University of Science and Technology, China, published in *Diabetologia*.

Green Tea Extract Improves Blood Sugar and Gut Health

People who took a green tea extract supplement for one month had lower blood sugar, less gut inflammation, and reduced small intestine permeability than those in a control group. The effects were seen in both healthy people and those with metabolic syndrome (a combination of excess belly fat, high blood pressure, low HDL "good" cholesterol, and high levels of fasting blood glucose and triglycerides). The benefits suggest that it may be possible to alleviate or even reverse the inflammation that is linked to cardiometabolic disorders. The dosage was equal to five cups of green tea.

Richard Bruno, Ph.D., RD, professor of human nutrition and director of the Bionutrition Core Laboratory, Ohio State University, Columbus, Ohio.

But mammals, including humans, also have a second type of fat known as brown fat—and brown fat functions differently than white fat in some fundamental and significant ways.

White fat stores energy in case it's needed later. Brown fat converts energy into heat through the process of *mitochondrial uncoupling* of certain proteins. Our ancestors likely developed brown fat as a defense against hypothermia, which was a major threat to early humans.

The fact that humans have some brown fat is not news, but until recently, the scientific consensus was that brown fat played a meaningful role only for newborn babies.

Recent finding: Brown fat has a meaningful effect on our health throughout our lives. A 2021 study by a team of researchers at The Rockefeller University and Memorial Sloan Kettering Cancer Center examined the PET scans of more than 52,000 patients and confirmed what many smaller studies already had suggested—people who have significant levels of brown fat have much lower rates of many obesity-related health problems, including type 2 diabetes, coronary artery disease, cerebrovascular disease, congestive heart failure, and hypertension, versus similar people who lack significant amounts of brown fat. Brown fat's health benefits appear to be most pronounced among individuals who are overweight or obese. In fact, type 2 diabetes rates among people who are obese but who have brown fat are similar to those of people who are not obese but lack brown fat.

Theories on how brown fat protects against obesity-related health risks…

•**Brown fat might burn potentially toxic metabolites,** such as glucose, free fatty acids, and branched-chain amino acids, as fuel.

•**Brown fat might influence where the body stores white fat,** leading to relatively more "subcutaneous" fat, located under the skin…and less "visceral" fat, also called belly fat, located around the interior organs.

•**Brown fat might secrete beneficial hormones that affect insulin sensitivity and appetite regulation.**

•**Brown fat might provide some protection against obesity itself,** not just obesity-related health problems. Mouse studies have found strong associations between increased brown-fat activity and reductions in obesity. It's not yet clear if humans have sufficient brown fat to experience these weight-loss benefits, but this does create a compelling possibility—that this type of fat might one day help keep us thin.

ACTIVATING BROWN FAT

Mammals have two types of brown fat—the brown fat they're born with…and inducible brown fat, also called "beige fat." The *inducible brown-fat cells* activate their thermogenic properties in response to stimuli that may include cold temperatures, certain drugs, and exercise.

Does this mean that people can reduce their risk for obesity-related health issues by intentionally increasing their exposure to these brown-fat–activating stimuli? *There isn't yet sufficient evidence to recommend that—larger and longer-term studies are needed—but some early results are promising…*

•**Cold.** Numerous small studies have found that brown fat can be activated by exposure to cold temperatures. In one study by researchers at Maastricht University, 23 of 24 participants showed evidence of brown-fat activity when exposed to cold temperatures. Notably, exposure to extreme cold does not appear to be necessary to activate brown fat—these participants were subjected to a cool-but-far-from-frigid 61°F (16°C) for two hours. Another small study by Maastricht University researchers found that exposure to cool temperatures appears to significantly increase insulin sensitivity among people with type 2 diabetes, so perhaps turning down the furnace to activate brown fat could become a diabetes treatment in the not-too-distant future.

•**Pharmaceuticals.** Drugs could one day activate brown fat without the mild discomfort of cool temperatures. In fact, one drug does this already—in a small study, the medication *mirabegron*, approved in the U.S. for bladder control, has been shown by researchers at the National Institutes of Health to both activate brown fat and increase insulin sensitivity.

But there are risks: Mirabegron could elevate heart rate and blood pressure. Based on this finding, though, other drugs that can activate brown fat without this risk could be developed.

•**Exercise.** Studies conducted on mice have found that aerobic activity such as running on a treadmill can activate brown fat. But a recent study involving human subjects was less encouraging—researchers at Spain's University of Granada found no evidence that 24 weeks of exercise training increased brown-fat activity in previously sedentary adults. But further research is needed before this possibility is discarded.

•**Genetics.** There likely is a genetic component to the varying levels of brown-fat activity observed in different people and population groups. One study by Leiden University Medical Centre researchers found that South Asians living in the Netherlands tend to have less brown-fat activity than Caucasians who live there, for example. That might help explain why South Asians, in general, have significantly higher incidence of type 2 diabetes than Caucasians. Finding that a genetic component does exist could open the door to future gene therapy.

How much brown fat activity do you currently have? There's no easy way to know—currently this can be determined only by examining PET scans. But studies have uncovered certain trends—brown-fat activity tends to be more prevalent in women than men…in younger people than older ones…and in people with lower body mass indexes than higher ones.

The Protein Cure for Obesity and Diabetes

Study titled "Macronutrient (Im)Balance Drives Energy Intake in an Obesogenic Food Environment: An Ecological Analysis," by researchers at the Charles Perkins Centre, University of Sydney, Australia, published in *Obesity*.

Y ou'd think it'd be all about super-sized portions…but there are actually multiple factors concerning the epidemic of obesity, a trend that has led to a corresponding increase in heart disease and type 2 diabetes. Researchers continue to actively study a variety of possible causes. Evidence has been mounting for one theory called the *protein leverage hypothesis*. A new study from researchers at University of Sydney's Charles Perkins Centre in Australia gives more support for this hypothesis.

SEARCHING FOR PROTEIN IN PROCESSED FOODS

There are two parts to the protein leverage hypothesis. The first part is that the human evolution has favored a diet that primarily regulates protein. Protein is the basic building block for human cells. Cell growth and repair are based on having enough protein in the diet. The second part is that if you don't get enough protein in your diet, you'll start to crave energy-dense foods.

In the diets of developed countries like the U.S. and Australia (usually referred to as the Western Diet), calories often come from highly processed foods. To get enough protein from these foods you need to eat a lot of calories and that means lots of fats and carbohydrates. Excess calories from these protein-diluted foods lead to obesity. The protein leverage theory suggests that the search for proteins in processed foods contributes significantly to obesity, heart disease, and diabetes.

PROTEIN FOR BREAKFAST IS KEY

The University of Sydney study is published in the journal *Obesity*. The research team looked at one year of diet history in 9,341 people with an average age of 46. They used diet histories from the Australian National Nutrition and Physical Activity Survey. The study found that these people got about 18 percent of their calories from protein, 43.5 percent from carbohydrates, and about 31 percent from fats. The study also found that people who consumed more protein for breakfast (first meal of the day) needed to take in less calories during the rest of the day. Those who ate less protein for their first meal of the day ate more food during the day to make up for the deficit. These foods were calorie and energy dense foods high in saturated fats, sugars, salt, or alcohol. Because these foods lack protein, they ate more calories to reach the body's protein demand.

The study suggests that the first meal of the day should be higher in protein from foods including milk, eggs, fish, lean meat, soy, legumes, and beans. These are also the best sources for protein at any meal. Processed foods are often favored over these foods because they are high in flavor and calories for energy. They are also heavily marketed, convenient, and often less expensive compared to whole foods. Marketers and manufacturers know that a diet high in processed foods increases overall appetite and consumption.

Intermittent Fasting Fights Diabetes

Dongbo Liu, Ph.D., is professor of subhealth intervention technology at Hunan Agricultural University, Changsha, China, and lead author of a study published in *Journal of Clinical Endocrinology & Metabolism*.

Intermittent fasting can lead to diabetes remission.

Recent finding: 44 percent of people with type 2 diabetes who fasted intermittently for three months went into medication-free remission that lasted for one year.

Intermittent fasting protocol: Cycles of 10-day periods of normal eating with five-day "fasts" where consumption was limited to 800 calories daily. Talk to your doctor before making any changes to your diet.

Vitamin D Might Prevent Chronic Inflammation That Leads to Diabetes

International Journal of Epidemiology.

A study that examined the genetic data of 294,970 participants showed a direct link between low levels of vitamin D and high levels of inflammation. Increasing vitamin D in people with deficiencies may reduce that inflammation and lessen the risk or severity of chronic illnesses with an inflammatory component, such as cardiovascular disease, diabetes, and autoimmune diseases. It might also mitigate the ill effects of obesity.

Options to Insulin Shots

George King, M.D., chief scientific officer at Joslin Diabetes Center in Boston. Joslin.org

Type-2 diabetes patients have more options beyond lifestyle changes and insulin shots. A class of drugs called GLP-1 receptor agonists—such as *dulaglutide* (Trulicity), *albiglutide* (Tanzeum), and *liraglutide* (Victoza)—mimic a natural hormone that enhances insulin release, slows food absorption, and suppresses appetite. *Pramlintide* (SymlinPen), an amylin analogue, works similarly. These drugs are effective for blood sugar control and weight loss.

Oral Insulin May Be on the Way

University of British Columbia.

Researchers have developed a dissolving oral insulin tablet that provides insulin to the liver for two to four hours—about the same time as a rapid-acting insulin injection. The tablet is intended to reduce the cost of insulin per dose, be easier to transport, and eliminate the need for injections. It's currently in animal trials.

Best Diabetes Drugs to Supplement Metformin

Study titled "Glycemia Reduction in Type 2 Diabetes—Glycemic Outcomes," led by researchers at the National Institute of Diabetes and Digestive and Kidney Disease, Bethesda, Maryland, published in *The New England Journal of Medicine*.

Up to 95 percent of people with diabetes have type 2 diabetes, which includes approximately 37 million Americans. Once diagnosed, these individuals have to keep an eye on their blood sugar (or blood glucose). Treatment usually begins with exercise, diet, and *metformin*, an oral drug that decreases the amount of sugar the body absorbs from food and processes in the liver.

Insulin is a hormone that moves the sugar you need for energy from your blood into your cells. Type 2 diabetes occurs when the pancreas is unable to create enough insulin—or

Type 1 Diabetes Breakthroughs

First Type 1 Diabetes Preventive Treatment Has Been Approved

Teplizumab (Tzield), a 14-day course of infusions, delays clinical diabetes onset by two to three years, on average, in people with "stage 2" type 1 diabetes—the stage before obvious symptoms. Tzield costs $193,900 for a typical course, potentially covered by insurance. Screening is required and can be started through physicians' offices...participation in research including T1DTrialNet (Trialnet.org) or an at-home test kit such as JDRF "T1Detect" ($55, JDRF.org/t1d-resources/t1detect).

Jason Gaglia, M.D., physician with Joslin Diabetes Center, Boston, and assistant professor of medicine at Harvard Medical School. Joslin.org

New Treatment for Type 1 Diabetes

Insulin-producing pancreas cells were successfully transplanted in mice without requiring immunosuppressive drugs, which have serious side effects, including increasing risk for cancer. The experimental approach stops the body from recognizing the transplanted cells as a threat. Human testing is planned.

Animal study led by researchers at University of Missouri–Columbia, published in *Science Advances*.

resistance occurs from the body's cells to use insulin. People with diabetes have too much sugar (glucose) in their blood.

When blood sugar is not controlled well enough with exercise, diet, and metformin, most people will need another diabetes drug added to their treatment regimen. However, there isn't a consensus among doctors concerning which drug is the best. A new study from the National Institute of Diabetes and Digestive and Kidney Disease gives doctors and patients more information to use when making this choice.

SEARCHING FOR THE BEST ADD-ON DIABETES DRUG

The study is called the Glycemia Reduction Approaches in Diabetes: A Comparative Effec-

tiveness (GRADE) Study. Researchers began the GRADE study in 2013 at 36 U.S. sites. It included over 5,000 patients with type 2 diabetes who were already on metformin. The primary goal of the study was to find out which added medication would be best at keeping glycated hemoglobin—also called A1c—at target range of 7 percent. A1c is a measurement of the average blood sugar level over about three months. An A1c of 7 is considered adequate blood sugar control to reduce complications from the disease, such as kidney, eye, or nerve damage or cardiovascular disease. *The added drugs tested were...*

- **Glargine U-100,** a long-acting insulin injection
- *Glimepiride* **(Amaryl),** an oral drug that increases release of insulin by the pancreas
- *Liraglutide* **(Victoza),** an injection drug that decreases appetite and increases insulin release
- *Sitagliptin* **(Januvia),** an oral drug that decreases absorption of insulin from the gut

All the participants had been diagnosed with type 2 diabetes for less than 10 years. They were randomly assigned to one of the four drugs. *The results of the study after about four years are reported in The New England Journal of Medicine...*

- **All four drugs improved A1c.**
- **Both Glargine and Victoza lowered A1c modestly** but significantly more than the other drugs.
- **Treatment effects did not differ** based on age, sex, race, or ethnicity.
- **Patients who had the highest A1c at the start of the study** had the most benefit from Glargine, Victoza, and Amaryl, and the least benefit from Januvia.
- **The side effect of low blood sugar (hypoglycemia)** was most common with Amaryl at about 2 percent of patients. The drug least likely to cause hypoglycemia was Januvia at less than one percent.
- **Gastrointestinal side effects were more common with Victoza.**
- **All four drugs increased weight loss, which helps stabilize blood sugar.** Victoza

and Januvia caused the most weight loss with averages of four to seven pounds.

Conclusion: After an average of four years of follow-up, participants taking *metformin* plus *liraglutide* (Victoza) or insulin glargine achieved and maintained their target blood levels for the longest time compared with sitagliptin or glimepiride.

NEWER DRUGS IN THE MIX

Despite the benefit of adding another drug, only about 25 percent of the patients were able to maintain their A1c in the target range during the length of the study. The research team concludes that their findings can help patients and doctors make the best choice for adding another type 2 diabetes drug, but more work needs to be done to find the best way to maintain target A1c over time.

One shortcoming of the study was that it started before a new class of drugs called SGLT2 inhibitors was approved by the U.S. Food and Drug Administration. These drugs lower blood glucose levels by blocking the absorption of sugar from the blood. Further research that includes new drug options will be needed to recommend the best evidence-based drug choices for the treatment of type 2 diabetes.

Metformin Reduces Risk of Joint Replacement

Canadian Medical Association Journal.

The medication *metformin* may help people with type 2 diabetes avoid total joint replacement. In a study with more than 40,000 patients, metformin was associated with a 30 percent lower risk for total knee and hip replacement. More research is needed to tease out whether it could have the same joint-protective effect in people without diabetes.

Device Provides Lasting Pain Relief from Diabetic Neuropathy

Journal of Neurosurgery: Spine.

A spinal cord stimulation device provided lasting pain relief from diabetic neuropathy. Adding 10 kilohertz (kHz) of high-frequency spinal cord stimulation to conventional medication management reduced diabetic neuropathy pain by up to 73 percent in a clinical trial. Patients also reported improvements in numbness, burning, tingling, and cold feet. Close to 64 percent of patients saw improvements in motor, sensory, or reflex functioning.

New Research Reveals Why You Must Cut Back on Sugar

Jacob Teitelbaum, M.D., author of *The Complete Guide to Beating Sugar Addiction*. Vitality101.com

If you want to make one fundamental change to dramatically improve your health and protect yourself from chronic disease and premature death, cut back on sugar. That's the conclusion of a new study published in *Circulation*, the journal of the American Heart Association.

The study used a wide range of scientific data—from nutritional surveys to studies linking sugar with disease—to develop a detailed model of the likely health effects of sugar reduction in processed foods. *The model showed that cutting 20 percent of sugar from packaged foods and 40 percent from beverages could prevent American adults from suffering...*

- **2.5 million cardiovascular events like heart attacks and strokes**
- **490,000 cardiovascular deaths and**
- **750,000 cases of diabetes.**

WHY SUGAR IS BAD FOR YOU

The average American consumes about 22 teaspoons of "added" sugar a day (sugar that is added as an ingredient to processed foods). That's more than three times the amount recommended by the American Heart Association for women and more than six times the amount for men. *Added sugar negatively affects health in many ways…*

•**It is an empty calorie,** devoid of health-giving nutrients. Sugary calories replace more nutritious calories.

•**It has no fiber,** a nutrient that balances blood sugar and regulates appetite. A low-fiber diet can lead to chronically high blood sugar and obesity.

•**It directly weakens immune cells,** allowing viruses, bacteria, and fungi to flourish.

•**Sugar triggers high blood pressure,** high cholesterol, and inflammation, three key drivers of heart disease.

•**Sugar affects the brain.** It drives the addictive desire for more sugar, working in much the same way as other addictive substances, like cocaine. And it damages brain cells in ways that lead to negative emotions like depression, anxiety, and hostility.

FOUR TYPES OF SUGAR ADDICTION

You can break your addiction to added sugar.

The trick: understanding the four main types of sugar addiction and customizing your sugar-reducing strategy to your type.

TYPE 1: The Energy Loan Shark

If you're tired all the time and use quick hits of sugary foods (and caffeine) to restore your energy, this is likely your type. Other signs of type 1 include the constant feeling that there is never enough time in the day to get everything done, a midafternoon slump nearly every afternoon, and frequent headaches.

If you're type 1, use these strategies to reduce sugar intake…

•**Take a good multivitamin supplement.** A steady supply of energy depends on nutrients like the B vitamins and minerals like magnesium. To make sure you're getting them, take a multivitamin supplement that supplies much more than the RDAs (which are calculated to prevent deficiency, not to optimize health).

•**Forget sugary energy drinks; take an energy supplement.** Many herbal supplements now include adaptogens—herbs that energize cells, like Rhodiola, ashwagandha, and ginseng. Preliminary results from a clinical trial showed that taking a supplement containing the adaptogens Rhodiola, ashwagandha, Schisandra, and green tea extract increased daily energy levels by 70 percent.

•**Practice energy fundamentals.** Get eight hours of sleep, exercise regularly, eliminate junk food, and stay hydrated. These fundamentals—along with a good multivitamin supplement—are useful for all four types of sugar addicts.

TYPE 2: Feed Me Now or Else

Modern life delivers 24/7 stress and the worry and tension that go along with it. This non-stop stress can exhaust your adrenal glands, the organs that generate the hormones cortisol and adrenaline in response to stress. Adrenal exhaust has two main symptoms: You get irritable when you're hungry (cleverly called being hangry) and you crash under stress. Type 2 uses sugar to compensate. *If you're a type 2, try these strategies…*

•**You can't eliminate stress from your life,** but you can cultivate a realistic framework for worry and tension. When you start feeling anxious and stressed out, ask yourself, "Am I in imminent danger?" If you aren't (and almost always the answer will be "no"), simply taking a moment to realize this will turn off the "fight or flight" reaction and allow your adrenals to relax. If you still feel stressed, take three deep breaths.

•**Nourish your adrenals.** The adrenal glands need specific nutrients to function. Supplement your diet with vitamin C (300 to 1,000 milligrams [mg] daily), vitamin B$_5$ (100 to 300 mg daily), and the mineral chromium (200 micrograms daily). Also take licorice extract, which slows the breakdown of adrenal hormones (200 to 400 mg daily, standardized to contain 5 percent of the active agent glycyrrhizin).

•**Don't let yourself get too hungry.** Eating small, frequent, high-protein, low-sugar meals as opposed to the usual three large ones can make a huge difference.

•**Snacking is also important.** Snack on high-protein foods like mixed nuts and cheeses two to three hours after lunch and at bedtime. Hard-boiled eggs make great snacks, too.

TYPE 3: The Happy Ho-Ho Hunter

You crave sugar, but you're not tired or irritable: You're just happily searching for a sugary snack. This type of craving is often caused by intestinal overgrowth of candida, a yeast that feeds on sugar. If you're type 3, you also likely suffer from one or more of the conditions linked to excess candida, like chronic nasal congestion, chronic sinusitis, and irritable bowel syndrome. *For type 3, treating yeast overgrowth is the best strategy...*

•**Eliminate all sugar and use sugar substitutes instead.** Among the healthiest are *stevia* (PureVia) and *erythritol* (Truvia). If you don't like the taste of this substitute, try *saccharine* (Sweet'N Low; pink packet), which has a long history of use and safety. Avoid *aspartame* (Nutrasweet; blue packet) and *sucralose* (Splenda; yellow packet), which have poor safety records and can cause digestive problems.

•**Take natural antifungals.** Many natural herbs and products can kill yeast, and the most effective approach is to take a low dose of several natural antifungals.

Try this daily regimen for six months: 240 mg coconut oil powder with 50 percent caprylic acid, 200 mg oregano powder extract, 120 mg uva-ursi extract, 160 mg grapefruit seed extract, 200 to 500 mg berberine sulfate three times daily, and 200 mg olive leaf extract.

•**Take a probiotic.** As you kill the yeast in the gut, it's important to replace the yeast with friendly bacteria, or the yeast will simply grow back. Take a probiotic supplement or eat a cup of sugar-free, probiotic-rich yogurt daily.

TYPE 4: Depressed and Craving Carbs

Your cravings may be caused by hormonal fluctuations. If your sugar cravings are more intense around your menstrual cycle, if they increased when you entered perimenopause, or if you're a middle-aged man with the signs of andropause like depression, lack of motivation, and excess abdominal fat, the following strategies are right for you...

•**Eat edamame.** Women in menopause who have low estrogen can benefit from eating a daily handful of soybean pods (edamame). If you're perimenopausal, you may find it helpful to eat edamame around your period.

•**Enjoy chocolate.** Chocolate in moderation—especially dark chocolate, which is rich in antioxidants and low in sugar—is a potent mood elevator and antidepressant. Chocolate also contains a mild stimulant called theobromine, which provides an energy boost. Aim for 1 ounce daily.

•**Exercise for 30 to 60 minutes daily, preferably outside.** Not getting enough vitamin D can increase the risk of depression and increase sugar cravings. More than 90 percent of our vitamin D comes from sunshine. (Avoid sunburn, not sunshine.)

Exercising daily also boosts serotonin and endorphins, biochemicals that help alleviate depression and improve mood. Again, daily exercise is a good strategy for all four types.

•**Consider bioidentical hormones.** Hormone replacement therapy (HRT) with natural (bioidentical) rather than synthetic hormones can improve low estrogen and progesterone levels in women and low testosterone in men. Bioidentical HRT boosts energy and overall well-being and helps curb sugar cravings.

ONE STRATEGY FOR ALL FOUR TYPES

Several strategies apply to all four types of sugar addicts, but the most important one is to stop eating foods with added sugar. Eating added sugar fans the fires of your addiction and, as with any addiction, you have to cut out the addictive substance to start healing.

The major sources of added sugars are soda, candy, cakes, cupcakes, cookies, pies, fruit drinks, desserts, various dairy products (like ice cream and yogurt), and nondessert grain-based products like cereal and waffles.

Many foods have hidden sugars, so read labels carefully and avoid foods with sucrose, glucose, fructose, dextrose, maltose, and other words ending in "ose." Also be on the lookout for high-fructose corn syrup, fruit juice concentrates, corn sweetener, cane sugar, raw sugar, syrup, and molasses.

CHAPTER 7

Emotional Rescue

Is Long-Ago Trauma Causing Today's Health Problem?

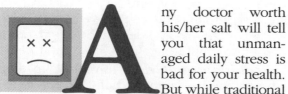

Any doctor worth his/her salt will tell you that unmanaged daily stress is bad for your health. But while traditional mind-body research continues to focus on this link, a much lesser known yet very important connection exists between severe stress, trauma or abuse encountered long ago and the development, even years or decades later, of any of a number of chronic medical conditions. Losing a parent at a young age…growing up amid a dysfunctional family…even surviving a serious accident or disease are just a few examples of experiences that can affect our health decades down the line—without our even realizing it.

We spoke with Samuel J. Mann, M.D., professor of clinical medicine at New York Presbyterian Hospital–Weill Cornell Medical Center.

He has spent years studying how powerful emotions related to past stress or trauma that have been repressed can cause or contribute to current health conditions such as hypertension, inflammatory bowel disease, chronic migraine, chronic fatigue syndrome, fibromyalgia (chronic widespread pain), and more…

OFTEN-OVERLOOKED CONNECTION

Health-care providers rarely consider the relationship between long-ago stress or trauma and a patient's current health.

Reason: Physicians generally don't inquire about adverse events from the past, and patients who have repressed those emotions don't feel or report the emotional effects related to them.

It is surprising how many patients, no matter how rough their stories, feel they are doing just

Samuel J. Mann, M.D., professor of clinical medicine in the division of nephrology and hypertension at New York Presbyterian Hospital–Weill Cornell Medical Center, New York City. He is author of *Hidden Within Us: A Radical New Understanding of the Mind/Body Condition.* Dr. Mann is board-certified in internal medicine and certified by the American Society of Hypertension as a hypertension specialist. NYP.org fine…believe they have experienced no lasting psychological consequences…and have never considered a possible link between their past experiences and their current ills. For many, recognizing this link offers a new direction in successfully treating many chronic medical conditions.

Physical *and* emotional stress stimulate the sympathetic nervous system (SNS)—the "fight-or-flight" branch of the nervous system that pumps *adrenaline* (epinephrine) into the blood. This is helpful when confronting a threat. But during periods of prolonged stress—such as during a divorce, an illness, or while grieving the loss of a loved one—our stress hormones can contribute to insomnia, anxiety, tension headaches, stomachaches, and more. This is one aspect of the mind-body connection that we often hear about.

What is rarely recognized, though, is that many of us make it through severe stress or trauma without experiencing overwhelming emotional distress. We do that by repressing… and not being aware of…those powerful and potentially overwhelming emotions. This may sound unhealthy, but it's actually a miraculous coping mechanism—a gift of evolution—that allows us to focus on survival.

Problem: Even though we are unaware of them, these powerful repressed emotions persist within us and can cause otherwise unexplained hormonal and other effects, such as elevation of SNS activity or inflammation, that can manifest sooner or later…even decades later…and they eventually can lead to all manner of chronic health conditions.

Here are examples of how these repressed emotions can fuel the development of medical conditions whose causes have otherwise remained poorly understood…

HIGH BLOOD PRESSURE

More than 100 million Americans have hypertension, a disorder that many incorrectly think is related to day-to-day stress. In most patients today, it can be attributed to genetics and/or poor health habits such as high sodium intake, being overweight, and/or lack of exercise. But recent clinical observations suggest that long-repressed emotions can be the unsus-

pected cause in perhaps 5 percent to 10 percent of patients with any of three atypical forms of hypertension—paroxysmal (episodic) hypertension…severe resistant hypertension…and unexplained hypertension in young patients.

Real-life example: For five years, Cindy, age 56, had been experiencing sudden, severe headaches and skyrocketing blood pressure every few weeks. Despite multiple ER visits and physician consultations for her paroxysmal hypertension, no cause was found and antihypertensive drugs failed to prevent the recurring attacks.

When asked about her personal history at a doctor appointment, Cindy mentioned a divorce from a "drinker and drug user who never grew up." Though happily remarried, she had spent years struggling as a single parent while working two jobs and finishing college. When asked if she ever cried or felt depressed during those tough years, she said, "Never"—she'd simply soldiered on.

Result: At her follow-up visit a month later, Cindy reported having cried every day about those tumultuous years. Remarkably, without medication, she has suffered no further hypertensive attacks.

Diagnosis: Repression of those emotions had served Cindy well, but ultimately they were causing her hypertensive attacks. Allowing herself to experience those emotions now, when her life was in order, enabled both emotional and physical healing.

Real-life example: A 48-year-old patient who suffered uncontrolled and severe "resistant" hypertension for many years experienced rapid normalization of her blood pressure after acknowledging for the first time in more than 30 years that she had been raped when she was 14. She obtained further counseling from a rape counselor.

Some patients with these forms of hypertension are able to heal even without psychotherapy. Others have found psychotherapy to be helpful in processing long-repressed emotions. Trauma-informed therapists are especially helpful—you can find one by doing an online search for "trauma-informed therapist near me."

WHEN EMOTIONAL HEALING IS NOT AN OPTION

While emotional healing is the ideal outcome, many patients who have repressed trauma-related emotions might need to maintain that protective barrier of repression. For these people, getting in touch with those emotions is not an option, whether due to the severity of the trauma or turbulence in their current life… or simply because of the power of the barrier of repression.

Real-life example: David, a Holocaust survivor who was suffering from bouts of severe blood pressure elevation, insisted that he "was not affected emotionally" by that experience. The invisible—and necessary—barrier of repression was evident in his words. Fortunately, for someone like David, there is an alternative. A trial of treatment with an antidepressant to further distance the repressed emotions resulted in a complete cessation of his recurrent attacks. Two recent published studies have reported cessation of recurrent paroxysms in 80 percent to 90 percent of patients treated with an antidepressant.

OTHER CHRONIC CONDITIONS

Repressed emotions play an often-unrecognized role in other chronic medical conditions as well…

Real-life example: Robert, age 79, a retired widower and self-described optimist, came to my office for routine hypertension. He described a prior history of severe ulcerative colitis, a form of inflammatory bowel disease (IBD). Diagnosed at age eight, he had frequent diarrhea and gastrointestinal bleeding and had been hospitalized several times in his teens and 20s. He also explained that his mother had been highly critical of him as a child. The colitis ceased suddenly when he was 28, after he moved away from his mother and married. But his wife pointed out that every time his mother visited, his symptoms flared. Encouraged by his wife, Robert told his mother that if she didn't stop criticizing him, she would no longer be welcome in his home. His mother stopped criticizing, and his colitis ceased…for good!

Many studies report a significant association between IBD and childhood abuse or trauma and also confirm the beneficial effect of treatment with an antidepressant.

The connection: The gut and the brain communicate with each other via an information highway called the gut-brain axis, which is why nervousness can lead to stomach butterflies or diarrhea. This communication also may explain the link between repressed emotions and IBD.

If you have a disorder that might be linked to repressed emotions, consider exploring those emotions by yourself or with a psychotherapist. Understand that your mind did what you needed years ago to get you through a rough time. And today there is an opportunity to experience the long-repressed emotions and heal.

Stop Overthinking!

Nancy Colier, LCSW, psychotherapist, interfaith minister, public speaker, and mindfulness teacher in New York City. She is a regular blogger for *Psychology Today* and author of *Can't Stop Thinking: How to Let Go of Anxiety & Free Yourself from Obsessive Rumination* and other books. NancyColier.com

Do you ever overthink a problem to the point that you make yourself anxious and miserable? Do you obsess over inane things that you can't change? Do you ruminate, dead set on finding a solution to a mistake or a problem even though you know you can't fix it?

Just as your lungs need oxygen, your mind was designed to think…and it needs activities and difficulties to chew on. It is always searching for problems to solve. The trouble comes when we get stuck in the process of thinking and keep going over the same scenarios endlessly.

Solution: We can't stop our minds from churning out thoughts, both positive and negative, but we can change our relationship to those thoughts.

SEPARATING FROM OUR THOUGHTS

Freeing ourselves from rumination requires a radical shift in perspective. We have to recognize that thinking is something we do rather than something we are. By acting as a listener, we can learn to engage only with the thoughts that are helpful.

Consider this: Our thoughts often are random and rambling—but they're not necessarily true or accurate. A thought is just as likely to be factual as it is to reiterate unfounded criticism from a relative or remind you of an embarrassing situation.

Example: Bob expected to be named president of his company, but instead he was fired. Worse yet, he hasn't been able to find another position. He can't stop ruminating over what he did wrong and faulting himself for thinking he was in line for a big promotion. His thoughts continuously remind him of how he is falling short in life.

Research indicates that 95 percent of our thoughts are negative and 90 percent are repetitive. Most self-help books will tell you to change your negative thoughts to positive ones, but the content of your thoughts doesn't really matter. What does matter is not reacting to those thoughts in a way that harms you emotionally.

Our thoughts are colored by all the things that we have experienced—or are experiencing—in our lives.

Example: Jane is unhappy with her husband and spends a lot of time ruminating about how unlikable he is and how she is justified in wanting to leave him. But she also berates herself for not having the courage to do that. Although she enjoys her job and her children, she is not really present with them because she is perpetually entangled in her thoughts.

FREE YOURSELF FROM OVERTHINKING

These three exercises, practiced regularly, will help you shift away from overthinking and from your unwanted thoughts…

EXERCISE #1: **Stop and drop.** Awareness is freedom…so three or four times a day, turn your attention to what your mind is doing. What thoughts are popping up? How do these thoughts make you feel? After a minute or so, move your attention to your body and what you are seeing, smelling, hearing, and tasting.

Important: By focusing on your body's sensations, you experience the present mo-

Antidepressants Don't Outperform Placebos for Most Users

Antidepressants significantly outperformed placebos for no more than 15 percent of users. Patients already taking antidepressants who are satisfied might continue using them, but others struggling with depression could ask their doctors about alternative treatments, such as talk therapy, exercise programs, acupuncture, and yoga, which all match antidepressants' short-term effectiveness with potentially superior long-term outcomes.

Irving Kirsch, Ph.D., associate director of Harvard Medical School's Program in Placebo Studies, author of *The Emperor's New Drugs,* and coauthor of a study of 73,388 patients published in *The BMJ.*

ment rather than being lost in the quagmire of your thoughts.

EXERCISE #2: **Nonjudgmental seeing.** Close your eyes, and take a few deep breaths. Then open your eyes, and look at your surroundings—but don't name the things that you see. Just look. When your mind conjures up labels for the objects around you, move on.

Example: If you see a book, your mind will prompt the word "book." If you see a clock, the word "clock" may surface silently in your mind. Resist the impulse to identify everything you see.

At first, you may have only a moment or two of not hearing a word or thought while looking at these objects, but with practice, it will get easier to find the space between your thoughts, a place of silence and peace akin to what people experience during meditation.

EXERCISE #3: **Who am I now?** Try going through a whole day as if you have no history or self-narrative about what kind of person you are or what you have experienced. Just focus on who you are in the present moment.

Example: Jim's mother was critical of him and could never celebrate his victories. He thought he could have achieved much more if he'd just had a more supportive parent. This exercise helped him peel away the layers of the story he told himself. It allowed him to stop being a victim and gave him a chance to fulfill his potential.

IS THINKING HELPING...OR HURTING?

When you catch yourself ruminating, stop yourself with this exercise...

Put your hand on your heart to show yourself compassion, and silently say, *Whoa, I am stuck.* Then ask yourself, *Have I gone over this enough?...Have I done everything I can to correct this problem?...Is thinking causing more suffering than relief?* If the answer to these questions is yes, then when you notice yourself thinking about the issue again, you can consciously shift your attention away from your thoughts.

Important: Sometimes you just have to accept that there is no solution, and vow to leave an issue alone to find peace. Ironically, sometimes turning away from your thoughts leads to a solution.

By refusing to engage in overthinking, you loosen your attachment to negativity and suffering...redirect your attention to the present moment...and cultivate a sense of self separate from your thoughts so they don't have control over how you feel or what you do.

Don't Let Decision Fatigue Shut You Down

Lynn Bufka, Ph.D., associate executive director, practice research and policy, American Psychological Association, Silver Spring, Maryland, and Grant Pignatiello, Ph.D., RN, instructor, Case Western Reserve University, Cleveland.

Our brains make about 35,000 decisions daily—what to eat, what to wear, which way to turn, etc. These add up, eroding our ability to make good choices—and leading to hasty decisions...or avoiding situations that require a decision.

What to do: Turn as many daily decisions as possible into daily routines.

Examples: Have a daily go-to type of outfit, such as slacks and a blouse or shirt...a basic, nutritious go-to breakfast and/or lunch...work out at the gym or take a walk at the same time. When possible, make some decisions in advance to avoid having to make them under pressure. And share some decision-making with family members or colleagues.

Life Without Pleasure

Elizabeth A. Martin, Ph.D., associate professor in the Department of Psychological Sciences at the University of California, Irvine School of Social Ecology. Dr. Martin is a licensed clinical psychologist and a fellow at the Center for the Neurobiology of Learning and Memory at the University of California, Irvine. Her research interests include psychopathology and social anhedonia.

The pursuit of pleasure drives much of human behavior. It is why we love, eat, drink, play, and create. Without pleasure, there is no quality of life. People with anhedonia, however, have a decreased interest and sensitivity to rewarding experiences. Anhedonia is a common symptom of many psychiatric and neurological diseases, and it may be an early warning sign of dementia and schizophrenia.

A SPECTRUM OF SYMPTOMS

Anhedonia exists on a spectrum from mild to extreme. On the mild end, anhedonia may be a symptom found in people who do not have a psychological or neurological disorder. People who are very shy and introverted may have pleasure in social situations in small groups or one-on-one situations but have an-

Signs of Anhedonia

- Extreme lack of motivation
- Spending most of your time alone and avoiding other people
- No stable relationships
- Lack of interest in pleasurable activities
- A noticeable change in pleasure from things you once enjoyed
- Absence of libido
- Faking emotions you don't really feel when with others

hedonia in large groups or with strangers. People with social anxiety may also have similar anhedonia symptoms.

At the other end of the spectrum are people who have an inability to seek or feel pleasure at all. For these people, anhedonia can cut off the ability to lead a normal life. Typically, people with anhedonia are not diagnosed until it interferes with their functioning or is obvious to others. *There are two types of anhedonia…*

•**Social anhedonia** is a lack of pleasure from social interaction. Physical anhedonia is lack of pleasure from physical exposures. People with social anhedonia have no interest in friendships or intimate relationships.

•**Physical anhedonia** means people do not enjoy the taste of an ice cream cone or the touch of a loved one. They have no interest or pleasure from sex. This type of anhedonia does not usually have any relationship to the condition that causes it. Most people will have some of both types, although one type may be dominant.

CONDITIONS THAT CAUSE ANHEDONIA

Anhedonia is a symptom of brain diseases that cause death of brain cells, like dementia. It can be a symptom of psychiatric disorders caused by lack of brain messengers, like serotonin in depression and dopamine in Parkinson's disease. Finally, anhedonia can be a symptom of psychological conditions like post-traumatic stress disorder and substance abuse.

Snaith-Hamilton Pleasure Scale

The self-reported questionnaire asks patients to consider 14 questions and note whether they strongly disagree, disagree, agree, or strongly agree. Either agree response is valued at 0 points and either disagree response is valued at one point. A score of 2 or less constitutes a normal score. A score of 3 or more suggests anhedonia. The test should be interpreted by a health-care provider.

QUESTIONS	STRONGLY DISAGREE	DISAGREE	AGREE	STRONGLY AGREE
1. I would enjoy my favorite television or radio program.				
2. I would enjoy being with my family or close friends.				
3. I would find pleasure in my hobbies and pastimes.				
4. I would be able to enjoy my favorite meal.				
5. I would enjoy a warm bath or refreshing shower.				
6. I would find pleasure in the scent of flowers or the smell of a fresh sea breeze or freshly baked bread.				
7. I would enjoy looking nice when I have made an effort with my appearance.				
8. I would enjoy seeing other people's smiling faces.				
9. I would enjoy a cup of tea or coffee or my favorite drink.				
10. I would find pleasure in small things, e.g. a bright sunny day, a telephone call from a friend.				
11. I would be able to enjoy a beautiful landscape or view.				
12. I would get pleasure from helping others.				
13. I would feel pleasure when I receive praise from other people.				

Source: Snaith RP, et al. A scale for the assessment of hedonic tone the Snaith-Hamilton Pleasure Scale. Br J Psychiatry. 1995;167(1), 99-103.

Anhedonia is common, and there are many pathways to get there. A recent study published in the American Medical Association's journal *JAMA Network Open* reviewed 168 studies on anhedonia that included more than 16,000 people. Some people in the studies did not have a mental health disorder and some had either active major depression, major depression in remittance, schizophrenia, substance use disorder, Parkinson's disease, or chronic pain. All the people in these studies were tested for anhedonia with a self-report questionnaire. The studies found that people with mental health disorders tested higher for anhedonia than people without a mental health disorder, including those who recovered from major depression. Of all the mental health conditions, major depression scored highest for anhedonia. *Other studies have found more links...*

•**Anhedonia is an early and primary symptom of frontotemporal dementia,** a type of dementia that occurs in younger adults.

•**Anhedonia is one of two primary symptoms of major depression,** along with sadness.

•**Social anhedonia in a young person may predict schizophrenia.**

•**Older adults with anhedonia are five times more likely to develop Alzheimer's disease.**

•**Anhedonia might be linked to bipolar disorder and autism.**

DIAGNOSIS

Anhedonia affects the frontostriatal brain region. In frontotemporal dementia, a loss of brain cells can be seen in this region on brain imaging studies. Brain imaging with functional MRI shows that anhedonia affects areas of the brain responsible for anticipation, reward, pleasure, decision making, and motivation. However, although imaging studies may show anhedonia, the gold standard for diagnosing anhedonia is self-reporting on standardized questionnaires like the Snaith-Hamilton Pleasure Scale (SHAPS; see table previous page) and a clinical interview with a mental health-care provider. SHAPS uses 14 questions to rate a person's ability to get pleasure from foods, interests, pastimes, social interaction, and pleasurable sensations.

TREATMENT

The treatment of anhedonia depends on the cause. For example, anhedonia may improve with antidepressant medication for major depression, antipsychotic medication for schizophrenia, and medication that increases dopamine for Parkinson's disease. But a person with depression and anhedonia may not respond as well to antidepressant medications. In some cases, the medications can make it worse as they interfere with libido and the ability to have an orgasm, and may cause blunted emotions. Researchers suggest that this may be caused by serotonin inhibiting the release of dopamine, which can interfere with reward, motivation, and pleasure circuitry.

Talk therapy (psychotherapy) is a treatment that helps many people with anhedonia. A common therapy, called behavioral activation, gives patients concrete tasks, such as going to parties or socializing, that they don't find appealing. When the person completes the task and finds it somewhat pleasant, it creates a positive feedback cycle and increases the brain's sensitivity to rewards.

Treatment with ketamine, an anesthesia medication, also shows promise. In one 2014 study in the *Journal of Psychopharmacology,* a single injection of ketamine reduced anhedonia within 40 minutes, and the improvement lasted for two weeks. A growing body of research suggests that this may be an effective treatment.

Dealing with a Gambling Addiction

Antonello Bonci, M.D., executive chairman and founder of GIA Miami. He previously served at the National Institutes of Health (NIH) as scientific director of the National Institute on Drug Abuse (NIDA).

When the U.S. Supreme Court overturned the federal ban on sports betting in 2018, it set the stage for an explosion of online sports betting that has swept the country. Online sports betting is convenient, always available, private, immediate, and heavily promoted. And it's now the most common cause of gambling addiction disorder, accounting for more problem gambling than all other types of gambling combined. Today, close to 50 percent of all sports wagering happens online, and a recent study found that 16 percent of online gamblers meet the criteria for gambling addiction. The COVID-19 pandemic is likely to increase problem gambling and gambling addiction due to the combination of social isolation, more time spent at home, easy access to online gambling, stress, and boredom. Past research shows that gambling increases in times of stress and anxiety.

WHO IS AT RISK

Men are more likely to become problem gamblers than women. They tend to be well-educated and successful, and they believe that skill is the key to winning rather than luck. Many men started sports betting as adolescents and teens.

Sports betting is increasing in women, but the most common female gambler is an older woman who gambles in a casino on a slot machine.

Gambling addiction tends to run in families and probably has a genetic component. Some researchers believe that inherited genes may account for about 50 percent of gambling addiction risk. Other risk factors include having a personality type that is competitive, restless, and easily bored.

Mental health disorders like post-traumatic stress disorder, personality disorders, and drug or alcohol abuse have also been linked to compulsive gambling. In one study, people with mental health disorders were 17 times more likely to develop problem gambling than gamblers without mental health issues.

CAUSES OF GAMBLING ADDICTION

Drug and alcohol addictions are called substance-abuse addictions. Gambling and sexual addiction are called behavioral addictions, but all these addictions change the brain in similar ways. Addiction causes the release of chemical messengers in the brain called dopamine and serotonin. These messengers are responsible

---

Diagnosing Gambling Addiction

The American Psychiatric Association defines gambling addiction as "persistent and recurrent problematic gambling behavior leading to clinically significant impairment or distress." *To make the diagnosis you need at least four of these symptoms over the past year...*

- A need to gamble more and with more money to get excited from gambling
- A feeling of restlessness or irritability when trying not to gamble
- Having tried and failed to stop gambling
- Thinking constantly about gambling
- Gambling when anxious or depressed
- Having a strong urge to gamble again right after a loss to get even
- Lying to hide gambling
- Risking relationships, employment, or education
- Having to ask for money to cover gambling debts.

---

for feelings of reward and euphoria. Over time, the brain becomes dependent on these messengers and craves them when they are not stimulated by the addictive behavior.

TREATMENT

Gambling addiction is a treatable disease, with several approaches supported by strong research. In most cases, a combination of psychological, pharmacological, and behavioral treatments is most effective.

Behavioral therapy includes cognitive-behavioral psychotherapy to understand cravings and harmful behaviors, and to substitute unhealthy behaviors with positive and healthy choices.

Pharmacologic approaches include medications that improve mood, such as antidepressants and mood stabilizers. Medications may also be used to treat co-occurring conditions, such as depression, anxiety, or attention deficit hyperactive disorder. Medications that block opioid receptors may help reduce compulsive gambling.

Long-term follow-up and support from a 12-step program like Gamblers Anonymous can be very helpful.

A new therapy pioneered at GIA Miami is transcranial magnetic stimulation (TMS), which has been shown to help people with compulsive gambling. TMS uses small magnetic fields to gently coordinate brain activity in the parts of the brain that control decision-making. TMS is done through the skin without any incisions and is a painless treatment. TMS is combined with behavioral and pharmacological treatment to develop a personally tailored recovery plan.

HOW TO GET HELP

A gambling addiction can have devastating consequences on your relationships, career, or education. It can empty your bank account and leave you deeply in debt. Gambling addiction also increases the risk of depression and suicide. Unfortunately, studies show that only one in 10 problem gamblers seek help. They may not recognize gambling as an addictive disease that can be treated.

If you or someone you know has four or more of the red flag symptoms for gambling addiction in the sidebar on page 116, help is available. You could talk to your health-care provider about a treatment program or go to a Gamblers Anonymous meeting. You can find a 24-Hour National Problem Gambling Helpline at (800) 522-4700 and other resources at NCP gambling.org.

Addiction to the News Affects Physical Health

Study of 1,100 adults by researchers at Texas Tech University, Lubbock, published in *Health Communications*.

In addition to stress and anxiety, 61 percent of people whose news consumption shows signs of being severely problematic reported frequently feeling fatigued and having physical pain and gastrointestinal issues...versus only 6 percent of people who did not obsessively check the news.

Reason: Constant exposure to 24-hour news puts some people into permanent high alert because the world seems dangerous and makes them feel powerless. These people watch more news hoping to find updates to lower their emotional distress. But obsessing over news interferes with their lives and causes mental and physical symptoms.

Break Your Digital Addiction

Anna Lembke, M.D., professor of psychiatry and behavioral sciences, Stanford University, California, and author of *Dopamine Nation: Finding Balance in the Age of Indulgence*. AnnaLembke.com

Are you spending far too much time scrolling through posts on Facebook and Instagram? Sending out tweets on Twitter? Watching videos on Snapchat?

Warning: These apps are designed to be addictive. They start off as fun. With every photo of a friend or funny meme, our brain is rewarded with a hit of dopamine—the brain chemical released when we do something we enjoy. And that keeps us coming back for more.

But: The more we indulge in that digital dopamine dispenser, the more unhappy, anxious, or depressed we are likely to become.

If we continue to consume our drug of choice, over days or weeks the initial pleasure response gets weaker and shorter in duration and the after-response—pain—gets stronger and longer. Over time, we end up in a chronic dopamine-deficit state where, when we're not doing our "drug," we experience the universal symptoms of withdrawal (anxiety, irritability, insomnia, depression) from any addictive substance—nothing else is enjoyable, and we need our drug not to get high but just to feel normal.

Solution: Experiment with a dopamine fast. Take a break from digital products for a set period of time...at least one day but preferably longer. This break allows the brain's dopamine reward system to reset itself and gives us an opportunity to reflect on our compulsive use.

117

What to do: Set a specific "quit" date, and let people around you and online know before and during that you will be offline and not available.

Even better: Encourage others to take the digital break with you—there's great strength in community.

During the fast, stay active doing non-screen–based activities that involve moving your body, such as exercising and being outdoors, which can help mitigate some withdrawal side effects.

Also: Write down or record your feelings as you go through the fast, so you can be mindful of what you're experiencing and share the experience with others.

Warning: Indulging in other high-dopamine rewards, such as watching TV, eating sweets, or using addictive substances, is not helpful. Replacing one reward with another can lead to cross-addiction and prevent the reward pathway from resetting itself.

When the fast is over: Make a list of what was good about taking a digital break and what was bad. Boredom and social isolation usually top the list of bad things. Topping the list of good things includes less anxiety and depression…getting more done…reduced compulsions to check our phones/be online…and increased ability to be more present and think creatively, not just react to external stimuli.

After the fast, you will be better able to reintegrate the digital world into your life again, but with a bit more wisdom.

How to Escape Anger

Gina Simmons Schneider, Ph.D., a psychotherapist, licensed marriage and family therapist, certified coach, and the author of *Frazzlebrain: Break Free from Anxiety, Anger, and Stress Using Advanced Discoveries in Neuropsychology.*

If you're like many people, you may be feeling angrier than usual. It's no surprise, as we live in uncertain times, and anxiety and stress underlie most angry outbursts.

This creates a vicious cycle: Anger can disrupt our relationships at home and work. Those relationship conflicts can make us feel more stressed. Add complex life events, like financial setbacks, and everything can soon feel out of control, making anger more likely.

CONTROL YOUR RESPONSE

The good news is that you can learn to control your response to stressful events and circumstances. You can transform from feeling frazzled to calm by aiming your thoughts and behaviors differently.

Advances in neuropsychology—how the brain interacts with feelings, behaviors, and experiences—demonstrate how your thoughts and behaviors directly impact the structure and chemistry of your brain. When you learn to steer your thoughts, behaviors, and experiences optimally, you'll feel calmer and happier.

CAUSES OF ANGER

It helps first to understand the role that a cynical attitude plays in fueling unnecessary anger. Cynicism is the belief that people are fundamentally selfish. It primes you to feel angry and threatened by most people because you assume the worst of them. You might distrust the motives of someone even when they do something nice for you. When you distrust others most of the time, you can develop chronic anger, which can become cemented into your personality.

Without knowing quite how it happens, sometimes you might find yourself feeling angry much of the time. Psychologists call this personality trait cynical hostility. Cynical hostility is a personality style that causes you to distrust and become antagonistic toward others. You might feel more guarded, suspicious, and nervous around people you don't know. Chronic anger and cynicism keep your nervous system on alert for constant threats. It's hard to relax if you remain on vigilant alert to protect and defend yourself. Cynical hostility maintains a steady drip of stress chemicals pumping through your body. Those chemicals can make it difficult for you to trust and feel safe. That lack of trust and safety keeps you frazzled for no reason.

WHAT ANGER IS TELLING YOU

Emotions exist as signals to help us survive and cope in a complex world. If we try to stuff or ignore our feelings, they often remain longer and leak out in undesirable ways. Instead, ask yourself what the emotion is trying to tell you.

For example, if you're angry at your spouse for not helping around the house, but you ignore that feeling, you might find yourself yelling at your pet for chewing up a cushion. A cynical interpretation of your emotion might lead to you think, "My spouse just wants to make me mad by never helping."

But your anger may really be telling you that you feel overworked. Once you understand that source of the feeling, you can shift your thinking to, "I need help with chores" and begin to look for solutions that address the root of the problem. Harnessed, anger can give you energy and motivation to fix a problem.

It's important to look at what you can do to solve the problem. If the only way to feel less angry requires someone else, such as your spouse, to do what you expect, then you give away the keys to your happiness. You can't make the world work according to your specifications, but you *can* control how you respond to the world around you.

HOW TO GENERATE HOPE

Anxiety, anger, and stress can feel like a three-headed monster robbing you of happiness. To fight back, question your cynical beliefs, ask what your emotions have to teach you, and summon some hopefulness.

Hope is the belief that things can be better. You can experience terrible suffering, but hopefulness helps you endure. Physically, hope helps you recover faster from the stress chemical cortisol and allows you to aim your mind in a more optimistic direction.

When you work to generate hope, you will notice that you recover faster from disappointments and hardships. As a bonus, your problem-solving skills will likely improve as well. That will help you feel much better.

To turn your mind toward more hopeful, healthier thinking, try these hope generators…

•**Be specific.** Identify your problem in specific, measurable ways rather than in a general, global way.

General: "I'm broke."

Specific: "I need to make $300 more per month to pay my bills and save some money."

When you make a general, nonspecific statement, like "I'm broke," it can leave you feeling overwhelmed. When you define a problem in specific, measurable ways, you can develop a plan so that you will then feel less frazzled, helpless, and anxious.

•**Ask for help.** Sometimes, you can feel hopeless and all alone with a problem and see no way to resolve it yourself. Hiding problems and acting tough can wear you down and keep you feeling stuck. Ask for advice or help from a trusted friend, a professional therapist, or an expert. You will feel less alone with your problem, and you could gain new ideas that might help you fix it. For example, many people worried about financial issues never seek the help of a professional advisor. Asking for help from a professional can give you hope that you can solve your financial stress.

•**Try something new.** When you try something new, you activate neural circuits that

---

Calm and in Control

Calm is not merely the absence of stress, but the powerful presence of peace. It is a state of serene awareness. You're absorbed in the present moment. You breathe deeply and slowly. Your heart rate slows, and your blood pressure lowers. Your muscles loosen and relax. You feel an easy stillness. Your mind is alert and flexible.

The English poet John Dryden wrote, "We first make our habits, and then our habits make us." When you change your angry, frazzled, habitual response to stress, space opens in your mind for calmness to emerge. A calm brain makes better long-term decisions than an angry brain. When we're angry, our main goal is to fight, run from, or escape the source of our anger. Calmness allows us to consider other options.

speed up learning and move mental energy away from hopelessness and into action. If you do the same thing repeatedly, you will probably remain stuck in the same situation. Trying something new allows you to see, experience, and think about your problem from a different perspective.

For example, if you usually try to cope with public speaking nervousness by taking deep breaths, relaxing, and vigorous preparation, but you still feel overwhelmed, do something new and different. For example, try exercising in the morning before you speak in public. It could help you release tension and feel more confident and relaxed.

•**Comfort yourself.** Self-critical thoughts can make you feel overwhelmed, stressed, and angry. You can generate more hope when you provide yourself comfort and encouragement. Try to talk to yourself as if you were caring for a close friend. Substitute realistic, hopeful statements such as: "I can handle this. I can figure out how to solve this problem. I can learn to calm down and relax. I can ask for help." To soothe and comfort yourself, use compassionate phrases like, "May I be peaceful. May I live with ease."

Fighting cynicism, questioning emotions, and generating hope can help you lessen stress, anxiety, and anger, too.

New Screening Guidelines for Anxiety Disorders

Chris Iliades, M.D., retired ear, nose, throat, head, and neck surgeon, and a regular contributor to *Bottom Line Health*.

I n October, the U.S. Preventive Services Task Force (USPSTF) issued new guidelines for anxiety screening in primary care. They now recommend anxiety disorder screening for everyone between the ages of 8 and 65. USPSTF is an independent panel of medical experts that makes recommendations for disease prevention based on the most recent evidence.

Missed Diagnosis

It's not always easy to recognize anxiety disorder. When people tell their doctors about symptoms like headache, insomnia, or fatigue, they may not even consider that anxiety may be the cause. According to the USPSTF, less than 15 percent of people diagnosed with anxiety disorder ever complain specifically about anxiety. Depression is a red flag for anxiety disorder, because these two disorders often occur together. According to USPSTF, 70 to 75 percent of people with depression also have anxiety disorder.

There are several reasons for these new guidelines. The lifetime risk of an anxiety disorder is surprisingly high, and even higher since the COVID pandemic. Anxiety affects about 40 percent of women and 26 percent of men. Only about 10 percent of people with the disorder are diagnosed in the first year. Most people live with the disorder for about 20 years before diagnosis. Studies show that screening tests work, and that treatment is very effective.

TYPES OF ANXIETY DISORDERS

Anxiety is a normal reaction to stress that everyone experiences. It may be a protective response that helps you avoid danger. But if that response becomes too deeply ingrained in your brain, you may have anxiety with any mild stress, any reminder of stress, or even stress for no apparent reason. Anxiety disorder is anxiety at a level that affects your ability to live your life normally.

The types of anxiety disorder include generalized, panic, social, and separation anxiety. There are also several anxiety disorders based on fear, called phobia-related disorders. These types have different diagnostic criteria, but there are signs and symptoms that are common to all of them, such as restlessness, fatigue, trouble concentrating, irritability, physical symptoms, insomnia, fear, and worry. Panic attacks are common in panic disorder. Physical symptoms of anxiety can include headache, muscle ache, indigestion, dizziness, or feeling a constant lump in your throat.

SCREENING FOR ANXIETY

The good news is that there are effective and readily available question-and-answer screening tests that are supported by research as effective. If a test shows a possible anxiety disorder, USPSTF recommends a mental health consultation to confirm a diagnosis. Everyone from ages 8 to 65 should be screened at least once. Because anxiety disorders tend to get better with older age, the task force did not find enough evidence to recommend routine screening for everyone over age 65, but older patients can also be screened. How often to screen is left to the discretion of the primary care provider, but people at higher risk for anxiety should be screened more frequently.

Risk factors include a shy personality since childhood, exposure to stressful life events, a history of other mental-health disorders, and a family history of depression or anxiety. It is also important for health-care providers to rule out medical causes of anxiety symptoms, such as thyroid disease.

If you think you may have some of the symptoms of anxiety disorder, you can take an online test to get more information. The results could help you talk to your health-care provider about anxiety concerns. Two short and simple tests that are recommended are the Mental Health America anxiety test (https://screening.mhanational.org/screening-tools/anxiety/) and the Anxiety and Depression Society of America test (https://adaa.org/find-help/treatment-help/self-screening).

TREATMENT

Anxiety disorder is one of the most treatable mental health disorders. Talk therapy, such as cognitive behavioral therapy and acceptance and commitment therapy, is the most effective treatment.

An anti-anxiety medication called a *benzodiazepine* can help control the symptoms of anxiety, but only psychotherapy helps a person change the way they think and act. Lifestyle changes are also an important part of treatment and include exercising, avoiding drugs and alcohol, following a healthy diet, using stress-management techniques, and adopting healthy sleep habits.

Drug-Free Relief for Anxiety

Vitamin B₆ Beats Anxiety

High-dose vitamin B_6 could reduce anxiety, a new study suggests. Volunteers who took 100 milligrams of B_6 (pyroxidine hydrochloride) once daily for a month reported a "highly significant" reduction in generalized anxiety disorder and social anxiety. Vitamin B_6 deficiency affects 16 percent of men and 32 percent of women. Supplementation should not exceed 100 mg per day. Higher doses can cause potentially irreversible sensory neuropathy.

Pharmacy Times.

Mindfulness Treats Anxiety as Well as an Antidepressant Drug

Researchers randomly assigned 276 people either to take the antidepressant escitalopram or to follow a guided mindfulness-based stress reduction program. The program included weekly in-person classes, a weekend retreat, and 45-minute daily home practice exercises. Both groups saw a 30 percent reduction in their anxiety. "Our study provides evidence for clinicians, insurers, and health-care systems to recommend, include, and provide reimbursement for mindfulness-based stress reduction as an effective treatment for anxiety disorders because mindfulness meditation currently is reimbursed by very few providers," Dr. Hoge said.

Elizabeth Hoge, M.D., director of the Anxiety Disorders Research Program and associate professor of psychiatry at Georgetown University, Washington, D.C.

DANGER OF UNTREATED ANXIETY

Untreated anxiety is dangerous for both physical and mental health. It increases the risk for heart and digestive diseases, and it weakens the immune system. People with untreated anxiety tend to have problems at home, school, and work. They have a much higher risk of substance abuse and depression. This all leads to a poor quality of life and an increased risk of suicide, especially when mixed with depression or substance abuse.

If you are concerned about anxiety symptoms, talk to your primary care provider about anxiety disorder screening. You could try one of the online anxiety disorder tests and bring that with you to show your provider. USPSTF has issued these guidelines because anxiety disorders are a common and significant threat that can be successfully screened for and treated. Starting that process now could save years of difficulty.

Don't Get Boxed In by Fear

Michael A. Tompkins, Ph.D., codirector of the San Francisco Bay Area Center for Cognitive Therapy and faculty member at Beck Institute for Cognitive Behavior Therapy. He is author of 14 books, including *Anxiety and Avoidance: A Universal Treatment for Anxiety, Panic, and Fear.* SFBACCT.com

If you have an intense fear of snakes, dogs, heights, or tight spaces, you are not alone. An estimated 10 percent to 15 percent of people have at least one phobia—a persistent anxious response that causes them to go out of their way to avoid a particular thing or situation, even though they know their fear is out of proportion to any actual danger.

Arranging your life around a phobia might not be a big problem if the thing you're afraid of is easy to dodge. But avoidance can sap confidence, limit opportunities, and reduce life satisfaction.

Examples: Someone with a fear of heights might turn down a promotion because it would require relocating from a second-floor office to one on the thirty-second floor…someone with a fear of flying may not apply for desirable jobs that involve frequent travel…someone who fears dogs may avoid working in the yard because the neighbor's dog often is outside.

Good news: Most phobias—even ones you've had your entire life—are treatable. We asked cognitive therapy expert Michael A. Tompkins, Ph.D., to explain how you can get over your deepest fears.

SPECIFIC PHOBIAS

The most common type of phobia is *specific phobia*—fear of a particular animal, object, or situation, such as spiders or flying. This type of phobia may develop after a traumatic experience—this is called traumatic conditioning.

Example: Someone who gets bitten by a dog may be conditioned to fear all dogs.

Some people become phobic as a result of observing other people's traumatic experience—this is called vicarious learning.

Examples: Seeing someone else get bitten …watching a terrifying movie…having a phobic parent who often talks about his/her own fear.

Of course, not everyone who has a traumatic experience develops a phobia. Psychologists believe that people who are prone to phobias have high emotional reactivity, a quality that may be genetic. They react to stressful events more intensely and for longer periods of time. As a result, they experience intense anxiety and quickly learn to avoid whatever triggered those highly unpleasant emotions.

Treatment: Specific phobias often can be treated in as few as one to three sessions with exposure therapy.

How it works: The therapist and the patient together identify situations that evoke the fear, then develop a ladder, or hierarchy, of anxiety-triggering situations ranging from the least to the most fear-inducing. With the therapist present to offer support, the patient confronts each step on the ladder, beginning with the one that is least anxiety-provoking. Each situation in the hierarchy is faced repeatedly until the patient's anxiety recedes. Then he confronts the next situation in the hierarchy.

Example: Someone who is afraid of dogs might first look at a photograph of a dog…then sit in the therapist's office knowing that a dog is just outside in the waiting room…then look at the dog through the waiting-room door…sit in the same room with the dog…reach out a hand toward the dog…pet the dog…let the dog sit on his lap…let the dog jump on and off his lap.

You can try exposure therapy on your own, but persisting through the discomfort at each phase can be difficult without professional support.

To find a therapist who specializes in treating phobias: Consult the Association for Behavioral and Cognitive Therapies website (ABCT.org).

AGORAPHOBIA

Specific phobias are different in some ways from another common phobia—agoraphobia. In popular culture, agoraphobia is oversimplified and defined as fear of leaving the house. But agoraphobia can be a form of specific phobia (situational specific phobia) or a feature of panic disorder with agoraphobia. A diagnosis of panic disorder with agoraphobia must include a panic attack. People can develop agoraphobia, however, as a specific situational phobia through traumatic conditioning.

Example: Someone who is actually trapped in an environment for a period of time.

The initial panic attack usually isn't caused by the environment itself. Typically, the first panic attack is a bit of a perfect storm scenario. First, the person tends to be a bit of a worrier...second, the person is experiencing a period of chronic stress...third, the person is in a situation and becomes aware of intense body sensations associated with high physiologic arousal and then makes a catastrophic misappraisal of physical symptoms, such as *I'm dying* or *I'm going crazy*...and then the person has the panic attack, a sudden rush of fear or terror. The cause may be unknown, or the incident could stem from other stressors going on in the person's life. But after the attack, the feeling of panic is connected to the site of the attack. The fear may then spread to similar environments—from shopping malls to any atrium-like space...or from bridges to freeways to even neighborhood streets. The person's zone of comfort becomes smaller and smaller, and in extreme cases, she may fear going any distance from home.

Treatment: Exposure therapy helps a client deal with the environmental triggers, but the panic attacks need to be addressed as well. Cognitive behavioral therapy (CBT) has an excellent success rate in treating panic disorder. CBT for agoraphobia includes the important element of *interoceptive exposure*—a series of exercises that trigger the physical sensations that the patient fears and that were associated with the panic attack so the patient can learn to tolerate those sensations in a safe environment.

Example: The therapist might ask the client to spin in a circle to create the sensation of dizziness...breathe through a straw to create shortness of breath. As the client gets better at accepting these uncomfortable sensations, she learns that these feared physical sensations aren't dangerous and becomes increasingly confident when approaching situations she used to avoid.

Along with interoceptive exposure, the individual and therapist build a situational hierarchy of situations or activities that evoke the feared physical response.

Example: Someone who fears feelings of suffocation might have a ladder that includes wearing a mask, sitting in a hot room, etc.

CAN MEDICATION HELP?

Benzodiazepines such as *alprazolam* (Xanax) and *clonazepam* (Klonopin) are not recommended for the treatment of a phobia or any anxiety disorder. They may help people who are experiencing high levels of stress and anxiety due to a stressor or perhaps even a panic attack, but the use of this type of medication is temporary until the stressor subsides.

Example: A doctor might prescribe a benzodiazepine to someone who has lost his job and is stressed and overwhelmed and experiencing occasional panic attacks. However, ongoing prescription of benzodiazepines for anxiety disorders is not recommended. Long-term use can lead to dependence, and recent research suggests that benzodiazepines negatively influence the brain centers where learning occurs, which could potentially interfere with the effectiveness of exposure therapy. Benzodiazepines are not recommended for people over 60, because the drugs can impair balance and memory.

Safer: Antidepressants in the SSRI category, such as *fluoxetine* (Prozac), may be helpful in reducing emotional reactivity and don't interfere with learning.

Borderline Personality Disorder

Jerold Kreisman, M.D., psychiatrist, associate clinical professor at St. Louis University, and author of *I Hate You, Don't Leave Me, Sometimes I Act Crazy*, and *Talking to a Loved One with Borderline Personality Disorder*. He has been designated a Distinguished Life Fellow of the American Psychiatric Association.

People with borderline personality disorder (BPD) experience intense, unstable emotions, stormy relationships, deep insecurity, and a lack of a strong identity. They often have an intense fear of abandonment but are triggered and angered by seemingly insignificant things, making it difficult to maintain relationships.

To learn what separates a "difficult" personality from a personality disorder, we spoke with Jerold J. Kreisman, M.D., a psychiatrist, BPD expert, and author of *Talking to a Loved One with Borderline Personality Disorder.*

What are some common characteristics of BPD?

Some of the defining characteristics of BPD are a history of unstable relationships and a problem with abandonment. You may have a partner who is clingy, who is very insecure about the relationship, or whose attitude about the relationship is very changeable.

For example, for someone with BPD, people in their lives may be idealized one moment but, after a minor disappointment (you didn't call back early enough, you couldn't give me a ride), that person is suddenly demonized. It can change immediately.

Another trait that makes BPD recognizable is that there's a chameleon effect. There isn't a strong consistent sense of identity. Someone with BPD is a Democrat when they're with Democrats and a Republican when they're with Republicans, but when it's 2 a.m. and they're alone, they don't know what they believe or who they are.

What is the difference between a personality disorder and a mood disorder?

BPD is often confused with bipolar disorder because people with both conditions have tremendous mood changes, as well as impul-

BPD Diagnostic Criteria

To be diagnosed with BPD, a person must have at least five of the following nine criteria…

1. Frantic efforts to avoid real or imagined abandonment

2. A pattern of unstable and intense interpersonal relationships characterized by alternating between extremes of idealization and devaluation

3. Markedly and persistently unstable self-image or sense of self

4. Impulsivity in at least two areas that are potentially self-damaging (such as sex, spending, reckless driving, substance abuse, and binge eating)

5. Chronic feelings of emptiness

6. Recurrent suicidal behavior, gestures, threats, or self-mutilating behavior

7. Inappropriate, intense anger or difficulty controlling anger

8. Transient, stress-related paranoid ideation or severe dissociative symptoms

9. Periods of intense irritability, anxiety, or dissatisfaction with life, usually lasting a few hours and only rarely more than a few days.

Realistically, these syndromes are on a spectrum. If you have three or four of these, you're not defined as having BPD. Many people have borderline characteristics, but the difference is when it interferes with your life.

When relationships are continuously disturbed, when jobs are threatened, when anger management is out of hand, or when substances are abused, then you cross the line into pathology and should seek treatment.

sivity and difficulty dealing with interpersonal relationships.

The difference is that in mood disorders, the mood changes often last for extended periods. In bipolar disorder, for example, people go through high or low moods that last for days or even weeks. Importantly, there are periods between those extremes when the person's moods are fairly stable.

In people with BPD, however, mood changes are usually stimulated by some environmental stimuli and they change on a dime. A person with BPD could be walking down the street and get a compliment that makes them feel really good and positive. But if they then hear a derogatory remark, they can suddenly become depressed, angry, or even suicidal.

This tendency is an ongoing thing. They don't have extended periods where their moods remain stable.

What treatment is available for people with BPD?

There are no medications specifically available for BPD yet, but there is a European company with a drug in phase 3 studies.

Medications can, however, help comorbid conditions.

BPD rarely stands alone: It often accompanies another disorder, such as depression, anxiety, or substance abuse. There is a role for medication for many of those accompanying symptoms.

The primary treatment for BPD is therapy. Over the years, several treatment approaches have been developed that are manualized, which means you can "go by the book"…

•**Dialectic behavioral therapy** is a form of cognitive therapy that teaches group skills, such as what to do when you feel a sense of abandonment, when you get angry, or when you feel lost and empty.

•**Mentalization-based therapy** teaches people how to think through what they are feeling underneath the problematic emotions and to empathize more with the person on the other end of the relationship.

•**Transference focus therapy** is more psychodynamic and analytic. It looks into past relationships and the therapeutic relationship to understand and improve current relationships.

•**Schema-focused therapy** also has to do with past experiences growing up.

The problem with a lot of these formalized treatment approaches is that they usually require a lot of training for a therapist and they're not readily available. Overall, mental health treatment isn't readily available in this country. There's a terrible shortage of professionals.

So the best approach may be another manualized program called Good Psychiatric Management. It's more informal and it focuses on

---

Men, Women, and BPD

Bipolar disorder is likely equally represented in men and women, but three out of four people diagnosed with BPD are women. I think it's a gender bias because so many of the symptoms are more culturally attributable to women. If you see a man who is impulsive, reckless, drinking too much, involved with drugs, and changeable, he may be diagnosed with an antisocial personality disorder. But a woman with the same symptoms may be seen as being histrionic and borderline. When there is an emotional breakup between a man and woman, the blame will often be on the more expressive woman. In our society, there is often a common assumption that everyone's first wife was borderline.

There's a cultural element. We're talking about a disorder in which one of the main features is a changeable sense of identity. A woman's identity changes a lot more than a man's. When a couple has a child, traditionally, the man goes to work and his role remains largely the same. But for the woman who has the baby, takes time off work, and becomes the primary caretaker, the roles change a lot more. I think that lends itself more to some of the anxieties and characteristics that might be incorrectly associated with borderline syndrome.

—Jerold Kreisman, M.D.

---

understanding BPD and addressing a person's symptoms.

What is the prognosis for people with BPD?

In the past, BPD was stigmatized. Patients had a reputation for being demanding and difficult. Further, there was a belief that "this is your personality: You're never going to get better."

But research shows otherwise. Studies have shown that, over time, BPD tends to even out. The good news is that more than 90 percent of people get better over time—even without treatment. And those same studies have provided insights that can make treatment more effective

Beat the Mid-Winter Blues

Jamison Starbuck, ND, naturopathic physician in family practice in Missoula, Montana, and producer of *Dr. Starbuck's Health Tips for Kids*, a weekly program on Montana Public Radio, MTPR.org. She is a past president of the American Association of Naturopathic Physicians and a contributing editor to *The Alternative Advisor: The Complete Guide to Natural Therapies and Alternative Treatments*.

If winter finds you a bit down in the dumps, you are not alone.

Studies show that more than 5 percent of the U.S. population suffers from seasonal affective disorder (SAD), a winter condition with symptoms of fatigue, irritability, indifference, sleep disorders, weight gain, suicidal thoughts, and generalized depression. It's more common in northern latitudes, though southern dwellers are not immune. That's because SAD is caused by winter's diminished light, not by low temperatures.

Having practiced medicine in Montana for close to three decades, I've seen lots of patients with SAD, and I know that natural medicine can really help. However, people with severe symptoms or a preexisting mental health diagnosis should consult their doctor before using any new medicine, including natural medicine, to treat SAD.

Here are my tried-and-true recommendations for conquering the winter blues. You don't have to use all of them and can combine the ones you like best. Getting outside is essential. If possible, that should top your list.

•**Spend time outside in the morning.** Melatonin is a sleep-inducing, mood-improving hormone that our bodies make in the evening in response to early morning sunlight entering our eyes. Go outside in the morning as often as you can. If you can exercise outdoors, do. But even sitting outside, facing the sun without sunglasses, for 20 minutes a day will bring benefit.

•**Melatonin.** If you can't get outside, melatonin is available as a supplement. For SAD, I generally recommend a liquid, sublingual dose of 1 to 2 milligrams (mg) at bedtime.

•**Vitamin D deficiency is linked to mood disorders and depression.** Like melatonin, vitamin D is produced in the human body in response to sunlight on our skin. If you can arrange a long holiday at the equator in mid-winter, you may store enough vitamin D to get you through until spring. But if that's not possible, consider vitamin D supplementation. For most of my patients, 2,000 international units (IU) daily, taken with a meal, is an effective dosage for SAD.

•**Ginkgo biloba is a plant medicine that promotes circulation in small blood vessels, such as those in our brains.** I've found that a daily dose of 80 mg of ginkgo biloba, available in capsules, helps reduce SAD symptoms of listlessness, foggy thinking, and depression.

Note: If you have a circulatory disorder or are on cardiac or blood-thinning medication, speak with your doctor before starting ginkgo.

•**Lemon balm is another of my favorite plant medicines for SAD.** A member of the mint family, lemon balm has been consumed in tea form as a nervine herb (soothing to the nervous system) since the Middle Ages. Because lemon balm can also help with indigestion, restless legs, and insomnia, take it in the evening, an hour or more after dinner. You can find lemon balm in loose- or bag-tea form. Use one bag or one-half teaspoon loose tea per 8 ounces water. Steep for 6 minutes and drink the tea an hour away from food. Lemon balm has a pleasant taste, though it can be combined with mint or sweetened with honey if desired.

Seasonal Depression Can Strike Even in Warm Weather

Christine Crawford, M.D., associate medical director, National Alliance on Mental Illness, Arlington, Virginia. NAMI.org

Seasonal affective disorder (SAD) typically is associated with the shorter days of winter.

But summer's long days and short nights can disrupt sleep/wake cycles as well.

Other summer stressors that affect mood: Summertime pollen, which can cause agitation and irritability…social pressure to find summertime enjoyable and relaxing…and pressure to have a well-toned body.

Self-defense: Set limits according to your comfort level, not the expectations of others.

Examples: Skip a planned brunch or beach trip if you need to sleep in. Seek treatment for insomnia. If you find yourself struggling, reach out to people you trust and/or for professional help if necessary.

Extreme Heat Worsens Mental Health

Boston University School of Medicine.

A study found that there are a higher number of emergency room visits for mental health conditions, including substance use, anxiety, stress disorders, and mood disorders, on very hot days. Researchers defined extreme heat as temperatures above the 95th percentile of temperature distributions by county. Heat affected men and women of all age groups equally.

The Science of Grief: Five Important Findings

Mary-Frances O'Connor, Ph.D., associate professor of psychology at University of Arizona and director of that school's Grief, Loss and Social Stress Lab. She is author of *The Grieving Brain: The Surprising Science of How We Learn from Love and Loss.* MaryFrancesOConnor.com

---

If you've endured the loss of a loved one, you don't need anyone to explain what grief feels like. But why does grief hurt so much…why is it often hard to come to terms with loss…and what are the best ways to cope?

Psychologists and neuroscientists have made progress unraveling the secrets of grief and grieving. In fact, prolonged grief has been added to the *Diagnostic and Statistical Manual of Mental Disorders. Five findings are worth knowing if you have recently endured the death of a loved one…*

•**It's normal to expect a recently deceased loved one to walk through the door even though you know he/she is gone.** Grieving people who experience this disconnect sometimes worry that they're losing their grip on reality, but recent studies suggest this is simply a symptom of how the brain works.

In a 2013 study, Norwegian neuro-scientists monitored rats' neural activity as the rodents encountered a LEGO tower in the same spot every day for 20 days. The neuroscientists then removed the LEGOs and discovered that neurons in the rats' brains fired when they neared the spot where the tower used to stand. The rats' brains reacted to something they *expected* to encounter even though it was obviously gone. It took days for the rats' brains to update to the missing tower. If it takes days to adjust to missing LEGOs, it's only natural that it can take months to adjust to the loss of a loved one.

Further research suggests that it's especially difficult to adjust to the loss of a loved one because this forces the brain to reconcile two powerful but divergent sources of information. The memory reports that the loved one has died…but the bond between you and the deceased loved one continues to exist in your brain. This bond is very real to the brain, and there's reason to believe it operates completely separately from memory.

In one compelling experiment, researchers at the University of Iowa showed that a patient gravitated toward the caretakers who treated him best. That wouldn't be surprising, except that this patient had suffered a brain injury that made it impossible for him to form new memories—his memory couldn't tell him how his caretakers treated him. If the relationship bonds formed in the brain operate independently from episodic memory, as this research suggests, it makes perfect sense that these bonds would not automatically update to reflect that our loved one has died, even though our memories assure us this is true.

Coping strategy: When you can bear it, spend some time in the places that you used to visit with your deceased loved one. This might be painful, but it can help update your brain to the reality that he/she is gone. Until that update occurs, accept that you might have a strange sense that your loved one is both gone and yet somehow still in existence.

Also be aware that this could trigger unexpected feelings of anger toward the deceased—if part of your brain believes your loved one is still around, you might get angry that he hasn't called or returned home. This anger does not mean you harbored latent anger toward the deceased or that you need to reevaluate the relationship—it's a symptom of your brain's divergent messages.

•**Your *grief* might recur for many years…but your *grieving* means your grief will likely ebb over time without ever completely going away.** A man whose wife got home from work at 6:00 pm every day for years hears a sound at that time, and for a moment, he imagines that his wife is coming through the door. Suddenly the truth hits him—his wife died, and she is never coming home again. The whipsaw of emotion triggers a wave of grief.

A woman who lost her husband felt lost for a few months but slowly began to feel reconnected to her life. One day, she realizes that the anniversary of the day her husband died is fast approaching, and she's plunged into grief again.

Grief has a habit of returning unexpectedly—but grief is not the same as grieving. Grief is a moment in time, a wave crashing on shore when something brings a lost loved one to mind, then retreating back into the ocean. Grieving is the long-term process of coping with a loss. And while it's common to experience moments of grief in the years following a loss, only a modest percentage of people suffer from extended problems related to grieving.

A project by researchers at University of Michigan followed 1,500 older married adults, starting when their spouses were alive and continuing after one spouse in each couple died. They found that while moments of grief are common after the death of a spouse, the trajectory of grieving turns toward adaptation for the majority of widows and widowers. Most never fall into depression…and only perhaps 10 percent endure severe grieving that continues to dominate the mind without improvement, a condition sometimes called "prolonged grief."

Coping strategy: If a year or more has passed and the loss and grief still dominate your life, visit Columbia University's web page about prolonged grief to locate a therapist (on ProlongedGrief.Columbia.edu, click the "For the Public" tab).

But: Wait at least one year following a loss to seek this help—until then, it can be difficult to determine whether or not someone is experiencing prolonged grief. Don't let moments of grief convince you that you're not healing.

•**Neurochemicals deepen our suffering when we lose a loved one.** Prairie voles live very different lives than humans, but these little rodents mate for life and form close bonds with their one-and-only. A neuroscientist at Germany's University of Regensburg investigated what happens inside the brains of prairie voles that are kept away from their partners.

Answer: The voles' brains were flooded with a neurochemical similar to the human stress hormone *cortisol,* and the stress continued until these rodents were reunited with their mates. Humans are subjected to comparable neurochemical encouragements to return to our loved ones, and these stress-inducing neurochemicals are released even when it's impossible to reunite.

One more prairie vole trait worth noting: When voles reunite with their mates, they comfort each other with grooming. Human partners provide comfort for their mates at stressful times, too. This points to an additional challenge when we lose a life partner—not only are we flooded with stress-causing neurochemicals, we no longer have the person we depended on to help us through stressful times.

Coping strategy: Engage in activities that reduce cortisol production and increase neurochemicals that produce positive feelings, such as *dopamine* and *oxytocin*—exercise, yoga, anything else that makes you feel relaxed.

•**Working hard to overcome grieving isn't the best way to overcome grieving.** A study conducted by social psychologists at California State University Channel Islands and University of Arizona asked participants their opinion of four potential strategies for dealing with the loss of a loved one—journaling about grief…sharing stories about the deceased with other people who cared about him/her…going to a party and having fun…and watching a favorite movie. Most participants believed the first two options were most likely to be effective. They were wrong. There's a widely held belief that the way to overcome grief is to work our way through it by confronting negative emotions. Doing things that bring us joy may seem like it's shirking this necessary work, but engaging in activities that increase positive emotions can be more effective at reducing sadness than confronting negative feelings. Among other benefits, positive emotions have the power to change a grieving person's cognitive state, improving creative thinking and broadening attention.

Coping strategy: The takeaway from this is not that sharing stories about a loss or journaling is bad, but that activities that bring happiness tend to be more beneficial. If going to a party doesn't bring you joy, do it anyway… again and again. A new activity might not bring happiness until we repeat it enough that the brain accepts it as a habit.

•**Sleep medication slows the recovery process.** Insomnia is a common side effect of grief—ruminating over a loss when the lights go out keeps grieving people awake…as does elevated levels of the stress hormones *cortisol* and *adrenaline*. Well-meaning doctors often prescribe sleep medications to grieving patients—but they probably shouldn't. A study by researchers at Imperial College School of Medicine found that sleeping pills don't make people feel less grief, and, counterintuitively, they actually make bereaved people sleep worse in the long term. These medications might bring sleep on the nights they're taken, but they prevent people from learning how to sleep without medication.

Coping strategy: Force yourself to get up from bed on schedule each morning, even if

grieving kept you from sleeping the prior night. Enforcing the morning part of a sleep routine encourages the evening and nighttime routine to eventually fall back into place, too. If that fails, seek help from a sleep medicine practitioner.

Looking Stressed Makes You Look Likeable

Study of 131 people by researchers at Nottingham Trent University, U.K., published in *Evolution and Human Behavior.*

When study participants rated videos of people performing a stressful task, they rated people who showed more nonverbal signs of stress—such as fidgeting or nail biting—as more likeable.

Possible explanation: Signs of stress could have had an evolutionary advantage—possibly making the stressed person seem more honest in his/her reactions…and it could have increased the likelihood that other humans would treat the stressed person with kindness.

How to Beat Burnout

Monique Valcour, Ph.D., executive coach based in France who writes about topics including burnout regularly for *Harvard Business Review.* She previously has been a management professor at Boston College and France's EDHEC Business School. MoniqueValcour.com

In 2019, the World Health Organization updated its definition of burnout, classifying the consequences of chronic workplace stress as a legitimate syndrome. A 2021 survey by Indeed.com found that 52 percent of employees felt burned out as the pandemic wound down, versus 43 percent before it began.

Are you feeling burned out? *Here are strategies to take away the burn…*

•**Identify what depletes you**—specific circumstances—then reduce your exposure to them. When people experience burnout, they often feel that their schedules are crammed full—but only certain aspects of their lives might be producing most of the stress.

What to do: Track your activities and interactions. For each block of time during the day, note what you worked on...who you dealt with...how well this time helped you achieve your goals...and how drained or joyous it made you feel on a one-to-10 scale. After a week or two, review your notes to determine which of your activities are productive and directed toward your goals and which are more stressful than useful. Search for ways to avoid stressful, unproductive activities—could these be delegated to others, handled differently, or eliminated entirely?

•**Coordinate with colleagues.** Is burnout caused by workplace factors...or by how one employee copes with workplace factors? The individual employee side of burnout gets most of the attention, but research suggests that the organizational component likely is the larger of the two.

What that means: A significant percentage of your colleagues likely are feeling burned out as well—but they might not be talking about it.

What to do: Brainstorm with colleagues about solutions for the issues causing the group to feel burned out. Frame this session as seeking efficacy/productivity strategies.

Examples: A group of colleagues might resolve to schedule meetings only during certain blocks of time each week...or to cease work communication between 6 pm and 8 am.

•**Deepen your engagement with free-time activities.** Engaging in relaxing activities outside the workplace can help control job-related stress. But when people are under that stress, they often feel too tired to do anything with their evenings and weekends...and even when they do, some portion of their attention remains focused on work responsibilities.

What to do: Prioritize self-care activities even when work is stressful. If you're working at home, create an intentional step or two to signify the end of each workday.

Example: Shut your laptop, then walk around the block to replicate a commute home. Experiment with "mindfulness" practices during your free time—spend 10 minutes

focusing your thoughts on things for which you're grateful and/or focusing on your breathing...and when engaging in enjoyable off-hours activities, strive to pay close attention to these experiences on a moment-to-moment basis.

How to Bust That Stress

Debra Kissen, Ph.D., clinical director of Light On Anxiety CBT Treatment Center in the greater Chicago area. She is author of *Overcoming Parental Anxiety.* LightonAnxiety.com

The holidays are over...and yet you are still feeling stressed. You probably already know some potential remedies—exercise...listen to soothing music...meditate. But those strategies don't work for everyone, and they're not practical in every situation. *Here are six lesser-known possibilities backed by academic research...*

•**Improve your seated posture.** According to researchers at New Zealand's University of Auckland, sitting upright with your shoulders back reduces fears and fosters self-esteem and a more positive mood. Why? When we sit hunched over, the mind receives the message that we're curled into a ball trying to protect our vital organs from attack.

•**Do a crossword puzzle...or a Sudoku... or play chess.** A UC Berkeley psychologist found that mentally challenging activities are more effective anxiety-reducers than passive distractions such as watching TV.

•**Do something for someone else.** Not surprisingly, researchers at University of Miami School of Medicine found that people's anxiety decreased when they received three massages a week for three weeks. But the study also found that people experienced even greater anxiety declines when they gave three massages a week for three weeks. Other studies have found that donating money to people in need is a better mood booster than splurging on oneself.

•**Chew gum.** Researchers at Australia's Swinburne University found that gum chewing reduces stress—probably because chewing

Magic Mushrooms for Mental Health and Addiction

Psilocybin May Treat Depression

Two doses of psilocybin, the active ingredient in hallucinogenic "magic mushrooms," provided substantial depression relief for at least one year.

Caution: Psilocybin treatment should be done only through mental health professionals—taking such drugs on your own is illegal and dangerous.

"Magic Mushrooms" Could Help Heavy Drinkers

Patients with alcohol use disorder who received two doses of the mushroom hallucinogen psilocybin plus talk therapy drank heavily only 22 days of the following 32 weeks...versus 53 days for patients receiving placebos and talk therapy. Supervised therapeutic use of psilocybin has been legalized in Oregon and could spread to other states.

Joseph Feuerstein, M.D., integrative medicine consultant and assistant professor of clinical medicine at Columbia University, New York City, commenting on a study in *JAMA Psychiatry*.

burns off anxious energy when other options aren't available. If gum chewing isn't for you, squeeze a ball of putty or play with a fidget spinner.

•**Cool your fears with cold water.** A 2021 study by researchers at England's University of Chichester found that a 20-minute dip in 56°F water significantly improved participants' mood, lowering tension, anger, and depression while boosting self-esteem. Another 2021 study by an international team of researchers at Australia's Swinburne University and Canada's Queen's University found that immersing one's face in a bowl of cold water can reduce feelings of panic. This might be because cold slows the heart rate...or because the cold jolts the stressed brain away from its ruminations, like hitting a reset button. If sitting in a cold bath or plunging your face into cold water isn't practical, try running cold water over your wrist or hold an ice cube against it.

•**Lean into your anxieties.** If diversion attempts fail, try the opposite—allow your mind to roll around in the "crumminess" of your situation. Stop trying to convince yourself that your problem is no big deal, and let yourself dive into the fact that it truly stinks. Numerous studies have shown that increasing exposure to a source of anxiety can slowly reduce its power. A stressed brain can be like a young child throwing a tantrum. Sometimes the best option is to get the child to a private place and let the tantrum happen. Soon the child will yell himself out and be ready to move on.

Spironolactone May Help Alcohol Use Disorder

Lorenzo Leggio, M.D., Ph.D., senior investigator, Translational Addiction Medicine Branch, Joint National Institute on Drug Abuse/National Institute on Alcohol Abuse and Alcoholism, National Institutes of Health.

In mouse and rat models of excessive alcohol drinking, increasing doses of spironolactone—a diuretic used to treat conditions like heart problems and high blood pressure—decreased alcohol consumption. In a parallel study, researchers examined health records of people from the U.S. Veterans Affairs healthcare system and found a significant association between spironolactone treatment for heart problems or high blood pressure and reduction in self-reported alcohol consumption. Spironolactone blocks mineralocorticoid receptors. Preclinical research suggests that higher mineralocorticoid receptor signaling contributes to increased alcohol consumption. There are three medications approved for alcohol use disorder in the United States, but new medications are needed to provide a broader spectrum of treatment options.

Bird-Watching Lifts Mental Spirits

Seeing or hearing birds improves mental well-being. A recent study used a smartphone application to collect people's real-time reports of mental well-being, their reports of seeing or hearing birdsong, and information on existing diagnoses of mental health conditions. Bird exposure was associated with improvements in mental well-being in both healthy people and those with depression.

Kings College London.

Folic Acid May Reduce Suicide

JAMA Psychiatry.

An observational study suggests that taking the synthetic form of vitamin B$_9$ is associated with a 44 percent reduction in suicide events. Every additional month of treatment was associated with an additional 5 percent reduction. Previous research has shown that folate may enhance the effects of antidepressants, and that folate deficiency can predict poorer response to antidepressant medications. Folate may also help prevent strokes and reduce age-related hearing loss in adults.

Kanna Boosts Brain Health

Joseph Feuerstein, M.D., integrative physician and assistant professor of clinical medicine, Columbia University, New York City.

Kanna (*Sceletium tortuosum*) is a succulent plant used in Africa for hundreds of years for brain health. Claims that kanna helps with mood balance, executive function, cognitive ability, and resilience to stress now are supported by scientific studies.

Example: The alkaloid compounds in kanna increase the brain's access to serotonin (the "good-mood" neurotransmitter)…reduce physiological responses to stress…improve brain performance…and promote calmness or "alert serenity."

Caution: Although kanna is available in teas, extracts, tablets, and caplets, it can cause "serotonin syndrome"—a buildup of potentially life-threatening levels of serotonin—and interacts with antidepressants, such as SSRIs and MAOIs.

Safest: Take kanna only under the guidance of a doctor trained in integrative medicine… don't exceed 25 milligrams daily or use for longer than six weeks.

When Someone Else's Chewing Bothers You

Jennifer Brout, PsyD, certified school psychologist, founder, Misophonia and Emotional Regulation Program, Duke University, Durham, North Carolina, and director, International Misophonia Research Network, writing in *Psychology Today.* MisophoniaInternational.com

Misophonia is intolerance for certain repetitive sounds, such as chewing, sniffling, typing, or even breathing—regardless of how loud or soft the sounds are. Research has found that the repetitive sounds trigger the fight-or-flight response in people with misophonia because their brains misinterpret the sounds as a threat.

How to cope if you have misophonia: Since background noise can mask some repetitive sounds, try using a fan or music to prevent or stop being triggered by the sound. Regular exercise can help relieve stress so you're more able to stay calm when you hear the sound. Keeping to a regular sleep schedule also can help—fatigue seems to make misophonia worse. Take breaks from triggering situations when you need to let your system calm down.

CHAPTER 8

Family Health Matters

Helping Your Spouse Get Healthy

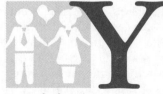

Your spouse is a package deal—you get all the great as well as what you consider the not-so-great. Perhaps you are concerned about your partner's eating and exercising habits, smoking, drinking, sleep, doctor visits, even subtler things such as getting out more, making friends, and avoiding depression. It is a common cause of strife in a marriage or relationship—when one partner feels that his/her lifestyle is healthier than the other's and tries to motivate the less health-conscious partner to improve.

Whatever your reasons, you'll certainly fail if nagging is your only approach. *We asked marriage and family therapist Michele Weiner-Davis for her strategies to help a spouse to adopt healthier behaviors…*

•**Don't complain—request.** When most of us want our partners to behave differently, we complain. "I can't believe you're still smoking cigarettes. You know how harmful it is for your health. It's a disgusting habit." That is a complaint, prompting your spouse to immediately go on the defensive.

Strategy: Make a request for change. "I know smoking has been a big part of your life, but it would mean the world to me if you would consider cutting back." A request for change is speaking about the future, while a complaint addresses what has happened in the past—something that can't be undone. There's no guarantee that your request will be honored, but it stands a better chance than mere complaint.

•**Find "the hook."** I recently counseled a woman who was concerned about her husband's drinking. She didn't think he was an alcoholic, but she feared for his brain health,

Michele Weiner-Davis, MSW, licensed clinical social worker, marriage and family therapist, Boulder, Colorado, and author of *Getting Through to the Man You Love: The No-Nonsense, No-Nagging Guide for Women.* DivorceBusting.com since dementia ran in his family. She complained, pointed him toward studies linking alcohol to brain health, asked him to change for her—but nothing prompted him to change. Finally, she realized there was one thing that might motivate him—he was an incredibly doting grandfather. She asked him how he felt about the possibility that he might not be around to enjoy his grandkids…that he might not be present for them mentally…that they might never know the real him.

Result: He cut back his drinking. This woman had found what I call "the hook."

Strategy: Ask yourself what motivates your partner. You can be completely honest and sincere about your own needs and preferences, but if you haven't hit upon the thing that your spouse truly cares about, you won't get him to change. Present the problem using the hook.

• **Use positive reinforcement.** Humans respond better to positive reactions than negative ones, yet many of us can't vocalize our approval of incremental progress. Instead, we focus on the fact that the problem still exists—"Sure, you went for a walk one evening, but one walk per week just isn't going to cut it." That is a surefire way to kill anyone's motivation.

Strategy: When you notice any small sign of change—even if it's far from where you want it to be—bring on the fanfare. Positively acknowledge, out loud, every small step toward the ultimate goal. "I was really glad to see that you took a walk Wednesday evening, honey. That's awesome."

• **Lead by example.** Maybe you can eat dessert every night without gaining weight. Lucky you—but if you're asking your partner to go without, you've got to model the behavior.

Strategy: Start living the healthier lifestyle yourself. Buy healthier food, serve low-calorie meals, join a gym, take a daily walk or run—and ask your partner to join you. Present it as a fun thing for you to do together.

• **Try "The Opposite."** In a famous episode of *Seinfeld*, luckless George Costanza gets fed up with his unsuccessful efforts with women. He decides that since everything he has tried has met with failure, he'll do the opposite of

what his instincts tell him. And of course, that's what finally works (at least for a while—he is, after all, George Costanza).

While that is, of course, fiction (and comedy, at that), there's some truth in it. When people try to get their spouses to change, they often follow a predictable pattern. First, they state how they'd like things to be. When nothing changes, they try again, this time with feeling. When there's still no result, they escalate and get angry. I call this method "more of the same only louder."

Result: You build more resistance to your ideas with every round.

Strategy: Instead of doing the same thing over and over and expecting a different result, try something completely different.

Real-life example: A woman I was counseling was concerned about her husband, a truck driver who had been injured on the job and became depressed. He withdrew from the family, spent all day in bed, drew disability benefits, and refused to look for work that wouldn't aggravate his injury. Her life with him came to a standstill. She tried everything to motivate him to start living again, but he grew increasingly angry at her failure to appreciate the extent of his injury.

My advice: Immediately stop asking him to change. Instead, I suggested she bring home some brochures from assisted-living facilities and nursing homes and leave them where he would see them. Then she was to have a conversation with him in which she said, "I have an apology to make. I guess I didn't fully understand your disability and how hard it must be for you, and I realize I've been pushing you too hard. I understand now, and I promise I won't do it anymore. I'm going to get on with my life, and I want you to just rest and take it easy." It was like a lightning bolt—he instantly got up and started moving again, integrating himself back into the family life.

• **Accept what you cannot change.** Not everyone thinks that just because you're married to someone, you have a say in how that person lives his life and what he does with his body. And different people have different standards for healthy living. Are you perfect? If you'd married an ultramarathoner, would you want him harping on you for not exercising enough? If you'd married a bodybuilder, would you want him griping about the hot fudge sundae you ate on Labor Day?

Strategy: Consider the dynamic within your marriage. You and your spouse may have the kind of relationship in which it's fine to have preferences about the other's lifestyle choices. And if you want your spouse to do better, try the steps above. But after a certain point, you simply may have to accept that backing off is your only option. In fact, research shows that even among happily married couples, a full two-thirds of what they argue about is completely unresolvable. No matter how spectacular your partner is, there will be some things you have to learn to live with.

Sleeping with Your Partner Is Good for You

Study by researchers at University of Arizona, Tucson, published in *Sleep*.

Compared with sleeping alone, sleeping with a romantic partner was associated with longer and deeper sleep, less fatigue, better mood, lower stress, and greater relationship satisfaction.

But: Having children sleep in your bed had the opposite effect—more stress and sleep disruption.

The Science of a Successful Marriage

W. Bradford Wilcox, Ph.D., director of the National Marriage Project at University of Virginia, Charlottesville, and senior fellow at the Institute for Family Studies. Virginia.edu

Putting something as ethereal as love under the microscope may seem cold, but it's effective. Simply by observing couples' interactions, marriage scientists are able to predict their likelihood of divorce with 90 percent accuracy. But it's important to remember that most of these findings are associations, not direct causal links. Still, aiming for the habits associated with happy marriages makes sense.

We asked sociologist W. Bradford Wilcox, director of the National Marriage Project, to explain the science behind successful unions...

•**Couples with joint checking accounts are happier.** In this age of individualism, couples are frequently advised to maintain separate accounts so each spouse feels free and independent. But when researchers at Northwestern University assigned newly married people to maintain joint or separate accounts, those with joint accounts were more likely to be flourishing in their marriages.

The finding is probably only partly about money. A joint checking account exemplifies what I call the "we before me" mentality in marriage—the idea that you and your partner are a team, taking on the world as one unit.

•**Marrying early is a bad idea—but so is marrying late.** It's no surprise that teen marriages are at high risk for divorce. For every additional year of age before a person marries, the couple's divorce risk falls by 11 percent, according to our research at the Institute for Family Studies. But interestingly, after age 32, the opposite starts to happen—divorce risk climbs by 5 percent for each additional year.

It's easy to explain why too-early marriages fail. In our late teens and early 20s, we have lots of growing and changing to do. By our late 20s, we're more stable and have some life experience under our belts and a decent start on a career.

But what happens after age 32? Nicholas Wolfinger, Ph.D., on whose research this finding is based, admits that there's no clear reason why divorce rates increase for those who marry later in their 30s, but he speculates that those who've waited that long may have grown too comfortable as singles to be as suited for long-haul marriage.

•**Cohabit with caution.** Americans are delaying marriage for longer, partly thanks to the lack of stigma around cohabitation. Today, more than 70 percent of couples live together before marriage (up from only 5 percent in the 1960s). Premarital cohabitation makes intuitive sense—why not make sure you and your partner are truly compatible before committing? But my own research and that of others have found that cohabiting comes with some caveats.

Couples who cohabit before marriage have an increased risk for divorce over the next 15 years. In fact, cohabitation boosts divorce risk by about 15 percent. And there's an exception to the rule of thumb about the inadvisability of early marriage—religious couples who marry in their early 20s without first cohabiting have lower divorce rates than cohabiting couples who marry in their late 20s. Religion may add spiritual or psychological stability to a marriage through shared values and a strong support group.

•**Novelty-seeking couples are happier.** Date nights, of course, are good for a marriage because they're a time to focus on one another. Many couples faithfully drop the kids with a sitter to pursue their go-to activity once a month or so—very often dinner and a movie. But as crucial as such routine rendezvous are, doing new and exciting things together is what really causes relationship satisfaction to surge.

Researcher Arthur Aron, professor of psychology at State University of New York at Stony Brook, asked 53 married couples to engage in date-night activities that were deemed either "pleasant" or "exciting." Before-and-after assessments of the couples' marital satisfaction showed that exciting activities—think escape room, indoor skydiving, surfing lessons—renewed couples' excitement about their partners more than did pleasant activities, such as dinner, drinks, and a movie.

Why? Using the language of social scientists, Aron and colleagues wrote, "Habituation [is] an obstacle to relationship maintenance." Put in plain speech, when things get stale, we start taking our partners for granted.

Additional research went further, however, showing that spouses get an immediate burst of renewed attraction toward their partners when they try something new and challenging together—even a seven-minute activity, as long as it's "novel and arousing." Beyond just staving off boredom, shared activities outside the comfort zone make us feel freer and more fulfilled as individuals, and that excitement

and novelty open us up psychologically to those old honeymoon vibes.

By the way, if you're scheduling date nights once a month, you may want to up the ante. A study done by the National Marriage Project found that both husbands and wives are three times more likely to be very happy in their marriages if they have a date night once a week. That may be a tall order, but the implication is clear—more time spent alone together predicts a lower risk for divorce.

•**Tiny gestures matter.** For their book *The Normal Bar: The Surprising Secrets of Happy Couples*, Chrisanna Northrup, M.D., and Pepper Schwartz, Ph.D., studied thousands of couples to isolate the variables associated with happy, lasting marriages. At the top of the list were factors humbling in their simplicity—physical and verbal expressions of affection, cuddling on the couch, a peck on the cheek in passing, a love note or warming your spouse's feet under the blankets at night.

Any of these gestures is trivial by itself, but researchers agree that the accumulation of these expressions of love is what makes people feel they have a true partner. Whether consciously or not, we're constantly looking for reassurances of our spouse's commitment. Whenever we find evidence of it, the bond grows stronger.

Text messaging lends itself perfectly to these gestures of affection. Researchers at Brigham Young University found that, among 276 young adults in committed relationships, texting to express affection—even just a simple love emoji—was associated with a stronger sense of attachment to their partners. When you receive a text from your spouse during the workday—no matter what it actually says—the subtext is clearly, *I'm at work, but I'm thinking about you.*

•**There is a magic number for handling conflict.** We all know that married life isn't a bed of roses, and that conflicts will arise. How we handle those conflicts matters—a lot.

Renowned marriage scientist John Gottman, Ph.D., analyzed discussions between thousands of couples. He found that during conflicts, couples who remained respectful and positive were more likely to stay with their partners in the years ahead. But it wasn't simply a matter of countering every negative interaction with a positive one…or of making sure to have more positive than negative exchanges. Instead, successful couples had, at minimum, five positive exchanges for every negative exchange. Fewer than that put them into fragile territory.

You're not expected to keep track of how many positive versus negative interactions you have, but marriages are susceptible to both virtuous and vicious cycles. Being empathic, engaged, and affectionate creates a virtuous cycle that predicts both quality and stability of marriage. Getting bogged down in defensiveness and contempt creates a vicious cycle that can threaten the marriage.

•**Be vigilant.** It's alarming how quickly a previously happy union can crash-land in divorce court. You can be in a seemingly good spot in your marriage, but if you're not making a regular effort to maintain the quality of your married life, you can end up in trouble.

Reframing Dementia as "Deeply Forgetful"

Stephen G. Post, Ph.D., author of *Dignity for Deeply Forgetful People: How Caregivers Can Meet the Challenges of Alzheimer's Disease.* He is founding director of the Center for Medical Humanities, Compassionate Care and Bioethics at Stony Brook University Renaissance School of Medicine, Stony Brook, New York. Stony BrookMedicine.edu

---

Watching a loved one with Alzheimer's disease (AD) or another form of dementia struggle to remember and communicate can be deeply upsetting… and frustrating and exhausting if you are his/her caregiver. People with dementia often are branded "empty"…"a shell of their former self"… or even "dead inside."

Stephen G. Post, Ph.D., is a medical ethicist who has worked with this population for decades and also helped care for his own cherished family member with AD. He believes that these labels not only are inaccurate but stigmatizing and destructive. After all, we all age, and we all forget things. Individuals with dementia

continue to experience awe and know love. They are human beings who simply happen to be further along on the continuum of human forgetfulness than most of us.

In fact, "we" are not all that different from "them"…unless we decide to value independence, intellect, and the ability to reason over other vital human characteristics such as consciousness, creativity, and the appreciation experienced when in the presence of others.

"DEEPLY FORGETFUL PEOPLE"

When it comes to describing people with various medical conditions, words matter. As seen with the move toward putting the person before his/her disability—"a woman who uses a wheelchair" versus "wheelchair-bound woman" or "a boy with autism" versus "autistic boy"—prioritizes who the person is, as opposed to the condition. Similarly, we have moved away from stigmatizing, judgmental labels such as "crippled" or "crazy."

So it makes sense to look at the 55 million people worldwide living with this condition in a new light. The term "deeply forgetful" is intended to help us notice and remember their dignity and the fact that they deserve care and love. The deeply forgetful may struggle to remember and communicate, but these limitations don't strip them of their personalities, their artistic creativity, and more.

Using respectful language also helps imbue caretakers with a layer of mindfulness that can encourage patience during trying encounters. More than that, it benefits the deeply forgetful person—no matter how advanced their dementia may be, people almost always respond better to health-care providers and caretakers who express respect and use kind language.

4 WAYS TO CONNECT

To date, there have been no great scientific breakthroughs in terms of eliminating Alzheimer's or most of the other diseases that cause dementia. If pharmaceutical solutions remain out of reach, we need to get creative about how we treat and care for this massive and ever-growing population. *The techniques below all encompass the "deeply forgetful" ideology, reminding us that these individuals should not be devalued or discounted…*

•**Play music.** The region of the brain involved in appreciating music is believed to be spared from AD and other dementias. This is why many deeply forgetful people light up when they hear music they identify from earlier in life.

Exciting findings: In 2020, researchers at the Betty Irene Moore School of Nursing at UC Davis found that nursing home residents with dementia who participated in a personalized music program called "Music & Memory" needed less antipsychotic and antianxiety medication…displayed fewer distressed or aggressive behaviors…experienced less pain and depressive symptoms…and fell less frequently. Other research has linked personalized music interventions with improved swallowing in people with advanced dementia, which may reduce the need for a feeding tube.

Try it: For 15 minutes a day, play for your loved one music that she enjoyed years ago. If faith and religion have historically been important to her, try a hymn. If your loved one used to sing "You Are My Sunshine" while putting you to bed every night, try that. Watching this person respond will remind you that she is "still there" beneath the surface…she just needed an alternative way to connect with you.

Resource: The Music & Memory nonprofit organization (MusicAndMemory.org) can help you use music in the care of a deeply forgetful person.

•**Expose them to art.** Deeply forgetful individuals are capable of artistic creativity and appreciation. The famous Dutch-American artist Willem de Kooning painted for more than a decade after he was diagnosed with AD, and art therapy is considered a nonpharmacologic treatment for the deeply forgetful, improving self-esteem and providing a means of expression.

Fact: Deeply forgetful people "have a preserved capability to paint, with and without instructions, even those in the later stages" of dementia, according to a study at the University of Gothenburg, Sweden, published in *SAGE*

Open. Some deeply forgetful people may experience a newfound burst of creativity. Language abilities may be lost, but new painting or sculptural skills may emerge…even in those with no previous artistic experience.

Try it: Many memory-care centers offer art-therapy programs or host art exhibits for residents. If those aren't available, try showing your loved one a coffee-table book of art…a book of interesting photos of celebrities from his younger years…or a book of well-known landmarks such as the Lincoln Memorial or Taj Mahal. You also can read to your loved one his favorite poetry. (Robert Frost's "The Road Not Taken" tends to work well because it's widely recognized.) Notice his body language, and ask questions about anything that seems to evoke a response.

If your deeply forgetful loved one is able to travel, try a day trip to a museum. Many of them—from The Met and The Smithsonian to The Nasher Museum of Art at Duke University and the Milwaukee Public Museum—offer programs specially curated for the deeply forgetful and their families or care partners.

•**Be open to surprises.** One of my students told me about the caretaking relationship between his mother and his grandfather. Hours before his grandfather died due to complications from dementia, he experienced a period of lucidity. He looked at his grown daughter and reminisced about the old times, such as walking her to school. Then he told her how proud he was of her.

Sometimes called *rementia* or *paradoxical lucidity*, these bouts of awareness and other improvements can happen at any time…and often do, especially after positive stimulations such as personalized music, poetry reading, art or social engagement, or in the morning after a good night's rest. The deeply forgetful person may have a lot to say, or it may be an emotional look or squeeze of the hand. Veterans may stand at attention and sing along when "You're a Grand Old Flag" is played. These moments are what I call "surprises," evidence that even though dementia is progressive and incurable, anyone can experience improvements, even if they're short-lived.

•Adopt a dementia support dog.

You don't need a specially trained service dog to reap the benefits, though you can get one. Sometimes called "dementia assistance dogs" or "dementia service dogs," these animals have undergone training to learn how to help their humans manage daily living, including providing balance support…fetching medication…and maintaining an eating and sleeping routine. You can learn more at 4 Paws for Ability (4PawsForAbility.org). But generally speaking, any loving, well-behaved dog can ease loneliness and anxiety and enhance mood. No currently available drug compares with what a dog can offer—for the deeply forgetful and for their caregivers, whose burdens can be somewhat lessened. Work has been done at the University of Southern Maine going back two decades on the effects of animal-assisted therapy on agitated behaviors and social interactions of older adults with dementia. And, at UCLA Health, research in animal-assisted therapy indicates that even robotic cats and stuffed animals can be beneficial in moderating agitation.

Overcome Loved Ones' Fear of Home-Safety Tech

Stephen Golant, Ph.D., gerontologist and professor at University of Florida, Gainesville. He is a fellow in the Gerontological Society of America, a leading national speaker and writer, and author of *Aging in the Right Place*. UFL.edu

Technology that could help seniors live independently for longer is rapidly reaching the market—but its intended users often are less than enthused. Seniors' resistance to "gerontechnology"—wristwatches that alert loved ones when the wearer falls… home-monitoring sensor systems that send alerts when the resident doesn't leave his/her bedroom…and other tech products—may surprise younger generations. After all, living at home for as long as possible is a common goal of older Americans, so surely, they should embrace technology that can help them do so safely, right? But gerontech's would-be bene-ficiaries may have valid concerns about this tech. *Here's how to address those concerns…*

CONCERN: Constant monitoring makes it difficult to relax at home. Home is supposed to be where we're free from the scrutiny of others, but gerontech could undermine that.

Example: A system that alerts loved ones when a parent is too ill to get out of bed also could trigger a warning when the parent simply decides to sleep in. *What to do…*

•Ask your parents to decide which loved ones will receive the alerts and how those recipients should respond. A parent might select the least panicky family member and request that family members send text messages, not call, when alerts seem unlikely to be true emergencies. In some systems, notifications can be customized so that different family members receive messages at different times of the day and can be enabled or disabled according to the older person's needs.

•Discuss together the degree of monitoring—systems that offer extensive oversight might seem invasive. Monitoring systems that rely on cameras rather than ambient sensors should be avoided. Also discuss whether the parent can occasionally turn off the system for privacy.

CONCERN: Data could be misused by marketers or scammers. Confirm that the company has privacy rules in place before purchasing any product or service. Information shouldn't be sold to third parties, for example—and the company should have a track record of protecting customers' data from hackers.

CONCERN: High-tech monitoring might mean less human interaction. Reassure parents that loved ones' calls and visits won't become less frequent.

CONCERN: Safety tech can promote overconfidence and tech dependance. A monitoring system that summons help if a parent falls might embolden him to climb a ladder to change a lightbulb…or make an adult child less likely to rush to that parent's house when he doesn't answer his phone. Stress that parents should request assistance with potentially risky chores…and parents should agree not to use tech monitoring as an excuse to be less vigilant themselves.

CONCERN: Tech surveillance could speed parents' transition to senior-care

facilities. When a family starts receiving alerts that the parent has fallen or forgotten to close an outer door, family members may become convinced that the parent needs to move into a senior-care facility.

Exploring Senior Living Options

Lisa Sanders, director of media relations for Leading Age, the professional association that represents not-for-profit senior living communities in the United States.

The senior housing sector is made of more than nursing homes: It offers a continuum of services that can provide everything from a little help with housekeeping to 24/7 medical care. By familiarizing yourself with the many options, you can begin to plan what may work best for you or a loved one.

ADULT DAY PROGRAMS

Many people prize staying in their own homes as they age, and a variety of senior services can help address the medical and psychosocial needs that can make that challenging. In adult day programs, for example, seniors who need assistance spend an average of eight to 12 hours in a community setting, where they have access to health, social, functional, and therapeutic activities. They may receive help with transportation to activities and appointments as well as assistance with activities of daily living (ADLs), such as eating, bathing, and dressing.

Coverage: These programs may be paid for by Medicaid, some Medicare Advantage plans (but not traditional Medicare), and private funds.

Cost: The national average for adult day care is $80 per day, according to the 2021 Genworth Cost of Care Survey, but prices vary widely by location. For example, if a person attends five days per week, the monthly cost averages $620 in Alabama but $2,900 in Alaska.

PACE

Programs for All-Inclusive Care of the Elderly, which are available in 30 states, offer preventive, acute, and long-term services to

Tips for Hiring a Home Care Aide

Persuade your loved one—people who need care often are resistant. Enlisting a doctor to make the case or referring to the aide as a housekeeper might help. *Don't wait*—labor shortages can cause delays, so start your search as soon as you've identified the need. *Vet the aide carefully*—ask the agency how aides are screened. Make sure they're licensed, bonded and insured. *Check whether changes will need to be made to the insurance policy of the person being cared for by the aide*—for instance, adding the aide to the car insurance policy if he/she will be driving your loved one's vehicle. *Look for aides whose personality traits and interests* match those of your loved one. *Ease into it*—stick around for at least part of the first few sessions to help train the aide on your loved one's specific needs, then gradually ease off your presence.

Christina Irving, client services director, Family Caregiver Alliance (Caregiver.org), San Francisco, and Connie McKenzie, president, Aging Life Care Association (AgingLifeCare.org), Jupiter, Florida.

Medicaid-eligible seniors who can safely live in their communities. (About 5 percent of PACE participants live in nursing homes.) Programs are available in Alabama, Arkansas, California, Colorado, Delaware, Florida, Iowa, Indiana, Kansas, Louisiana, Massachusetts, Maryland, Michigan, North Carolina, North Dakota, Nebraska, New Jersey, New Mexico, New York, Ohio, Oklahoma, Oregon, Pennsylvania, Rhode Island, South Carolina, Tennessee, Texas, Virginia, Washington, and Wisconsin.

Coverage: PACE programs are covered fully for people who are enrolled in both Medicaid and Medicare. People who are not eligible for Medicaid can pay privately.

Cost: $0 for Medicaid-eligible seniors; $4,000 to $5,000 per month if paying privately.

HOME HEALTH SERVICES

When a person transitions from a hospital to home, a physician may order a range of services, such as nursing care, wound care, and occupational and physical therapy. People may also use companion care services that include help with meal preparation, shopping, transportation, laundry, dressing, and bathing.

Coverage: Medicare covers medically necessary services that have been prescribed by a physician, but not companion care services. Medicaid coverage depends upon the state.

Cost: Without Medicare or Medicaid coverage, the average cost of home health care is $5,148 a month. Nonmedical care averages $4,957 a month, with a low of $3,623 in Louisiana and a high of $6,547 in Washington, according to Genworth.

HOSPICE

People with a terminal illness and an expected life span of less than six months can receive hospice services at home usually at no charge. These services include care that is focused on reducing pain and suffering, while attending to patients' emotional and spiritual needs.

Coverage: Medicare covers most or all of the cost of hospice. Medicaid coverage depends upon the state.

Cost: $0

AFFORDABLE HOUSING FOR LOW-INCOME OLDER ADULTS

There are also a variety of options for people who want or need to move to a new setting. Affordable senior housing allows older adults with low incomes to live independently in cost-controlled apartments. In about half of these communities, professional service coordinators can help residents locate local services and support. These programs are funded by the Department of Housing and Urban Development (HUD), the U.S. Department of Agriculture's Rural Housing Service, and the Low-Income Housing Tax Credit program. These programs are extremely limited, however, and there are far more applicants than available homes.

Coverage: Limited availability through federal programs.

Cost: Resident rents vary by federal program. In most HUD programs, called Section 202, for example, residents pay about 30 percent of their incomes for rent.

ASSISTED LIVING

People who need a little more assistance with activities of daily living and medical care, but don't require a nursing home, may choose an assisted living facility. There, they have the privacy of living in their own apartment or suite, but also have access to medical care, medication management, meals, help with personal care, housekeeping, and recreational activities. Assisted living facilities are regulated by the state, not the federal government, so there can be significant differences in cost, services, and quality of care between states.

Coverage: Most assisted living is private pay. Some states offer assisted living coverage through Medicaid waivers, but demand outstrips supply.

Cost: The national median cost of assisted living facilities in 2021 was $4,500 per month with a range from $3,000 per month in Missouri to $6,978 in Washington, D.C.

NURSING HOMES

Nursing homes provide the highest level of medical care around-the-clock. Unlike assisted living facilities, nursing homes are federally regulated, so the care and services provided are more consistent state-to-state. You can review information on all Medicare-approved nursing homes through Medicare's Nursing Home Compare website (Medicare.gov/care-compare/).

Coverage: Most, but not all, nursing homes accept Medicaid. Medicare does not cover long-term nursing home care, but it may cover short-term stays in skilled nursing facilities for people who need rehabilitation care. Most nursing home care, then, is paid for privately.

Cost: The average cost is $7,900 per month for a shared room and $9,034 for a private room, but prices vary by state. Texas has an average cost of $5,125 compared with $13,764 in Connecticut.

LIFE PLAN COMMUNITIES

LPCs cover the spectrum of care, so people can transition to higher or lower levels as needed. An LPC will often have independent living, assisted living, memory care, and nursing

Better Way to Check Out Nursing Homes

Two new sites—Data.CMS.gov and Medicare.gov/care-compare—now allow prospective users to look up ownership information on 15,000 nursing homes certified by Medicare and Medicaid. The data will include whether the home is part of a larger chain or consulting firm. The Medicare.gov site, which has a five-star rating system, also evaluates a home's health inspections, staffing, and quality measures. Releasing this information to the public is intended to help consumers make more informed decisions about a facility—and also allows the government to find out whether for-profit chains are building stakes in the nursing-home industry, possibly reducing competitiveness, which could lead to more expensive care.

USAToday.com

home residential areas, and some offer home-based care services.

Coverage: Most LPCs are private pay. Some require that you agree to apply for Medicaid if you run out of funding, and you may have some medical bills processed through Medicare.

Cost: Most LPCs have two costs to consider: entrance fees and monthly fees. An entrance fee could be as low as $20,000 if you will be renting your home or hundreds of thousands of dollars if you are buying it. The monthly fees also vary widely and depend upon what they cover. As the level of medical care that you need rises, so do the fees.

The costs also vary depending on your contract type...

•**Extensive contracts provide a lifetime guarantee of housing and all the care that you need.**

•**Modified contracts are cheaper, but they limit care coverage.** When you exceed that care, you will be charged for additional services.

•**Fee-for-service contracts allow you to pay only for the services that you use.** While these may cost the least initially, it is best to budget for unexpected and additional expenses, since health care and other needs can change as you age but can lead to surprise bills.

When investigating communities, be sure to ask about their policies if you spend all of your assets and still require care.

How to Reconcile with Your Estranged Son or Daughter

Joshua Coleman, Ph.D., psychologist in private practice in the San Francisco Bay area and author of *When Parents Hurt: Compassionate Strategies When You and Your Grown Child Don't Get Along* and, most recently, *Rules of Estrangement: Why Adult Children Cut Ties and How to Heal the Conflict.* DrJoshuaColeman.com

Some parents are suffering from broken hearts that they could have never imagined or prepared for—because an adult child has cut them off. Phone calls and text messages go unanswered...they haven't seen their grandkids in years.

These parents don't understand how this could have happened or why their parenting mistakes were egregious enough to cause such an ugly rift. Their anguish often turns to intense resentment and shame. After all, no one who provided ample love and devotion deserves to be treated this way by their own child.

Joshua Coleman, Ph.D., who specializes in helping estranged families, says the situation is far more common than you would think. In one survey of the dynamics of 566 families by researchers at Purdue, Cornell and Iowa State Universities, 11 percent had a child estranged from a parent.

Coleman himself knows the pain of this situation—he was estranged from his own daughter for several years following his divorce and remarriage. But he was eventually able to find a way back into her life.

We spoke to Dr. Coleman about the strategies he has developed that have helped hundreds of his patients reconcile with their adult children…

What causes a child to stop communicating with a parent?

As a child enters adulthood, longstanding resentments and conflicts over everything—from emotional abuse to clashes of personality or values to traumatic family events—can intensify. The child may be furious at the parent for being controlling, judgmental, untrustworthy and/or impeding his/her personal growth and development. I have found that healing this estrangement requires the parents to adopt a very different mindset than they may be used to.

Keep in mind that there are many other pathways to estrangement beyond parental mistakes or abuses.

Example: The adult child may be mentally ill or have addictions and thus be unable to navigate the slings and arrows of parent/adult-child conflict. He may have been the victim of parental alienation when, after the parents' divorce, one parent turned him against the now-estranged parent. The parent may have married someone who said, "Choose them or me—you can't have both." Finally, the child may know no other way to feel separate from the parent than to be estranged.

Two big misperceptions about reconciliation…

MISPERCEPTION #1: The process will be based on fairness. Parents assume that they and the child can hash out each other's shortcomings and what wrongs were committed and then both agree to make concessions in the future and move forward. But that's not how it works.

Estranged children have all the power in the relationship because the parent is the one who wants back into their lives and must regain their trust. To reconcile, you will have to listen to all the child's complaints without criticism or defensiveness…alter your behavior in ways he/she defines…and agree to his boundaries, regarding contact, visits, etc.

What's more, this process can take years until you are on solid and secure enough ground with your child to request a more equitable

relationship. I know this sounds one-sided. But if you cannot accept it, you just wind up reinforcing the reasons the child has cut off contact with you.

MISPERCEPTION #2: Explaining or rationalizing your past behavior will help make things right. Trying to convince your child that her negative sentiments about you are wrong and you were justified in how you acted will never get her back.

Reason: Her emotions constitute the absolute truth of the matter for her, regardless of how differently you may see things.

Example: You say, "I was a single parent trying to raise you, and your father made life impossible for me after the divorce." Focusing on your own experiences and blaming others just reinforces that you aren't interested in acknowledging the child's emotions and perspective or in really taking responsibility for your mistakes.

How do I begin the process of reconciliation if my child isn't even speaking to me?

E-mail him a letter of amends. The goal of the letter is to build credibility and trust by having the courage and self-awareness to apologize for any specific hurts/mistakes that your child has mentioned. You want to communicate your willingness and desire to learn more and see past events from his perspective…to show respect for his choices…and to let him know you are interested in reconnecting when he is ready.

Example of a letter of amends: "I'm so sorry for the ways that I let you down as a parent. I know that I was harsh in many ways, and that was hurtful to you. I could understand why that might make it harder to spend time with me. It is true that I was preoccupied in many ways when you were young and that it prevented me from being as involved with you as would have been good for you. I'm glad that you let me know how you feel about that, and I hope there are ways that I can make it up to you in the future."

Wait at least six to eight weeks for a reply. If you hear nothing, send a follow-up e-mail that says, "Just following up to see if you've had a chance to read my letter. I'm sure I left out some details that would have been good to address, but I just wanted to try to get the conversation started. Let me know if you have any thoughts or reactions, positive or negative. "

If a letter of amends works and my child seems willing to talk, what's the next step?

Let the child take the lead on what contact with you looks like. *Whether it's e-mail, a Zoom call, or a face-to-face meeting, focus on two strategies…*

• **Empathize without retaliating.** Your child needs the space and time to talk to you about why the estrangement was necessary. You will probably hear lots of negative sentiments about you, so you need to tolerate any pain, sorrow, and guilt that evokes. Your job is to acknowledge what the child is feeling and show curiosity about understanding her perspective more deeply.

Example: Your daughter says, "You were always gone when I was growing up." You reply, "I was gone a lot, and that was really painful and unfair to you. I was focused on my career and making money instead of on spending time with you."

• **Own up to your parenting mistakes without any hedging or excuses.** It's powerfully healing to an adult child when she sees that her parent actually gets it.

What if my child raises issues that are highly exaggerated or just not true? Am I supposed to apologize and take responsibility for everything?

The short answer is…yes. Strive to find at least a kernel of truth in your child's complaints that you can work with. Even if it's just saying, "Clearly I have blind spots, and I don't have a better understanding of why you are doing this. But I know you wouldn't have done it if it wasn't the healthiest thing for you." This allows your adult child to feel that you are really forming an alliance with him—even if the alliance is against you! It also establishes some credibility with the child that you are sincerely interested in understanding how he came to feel the way he does.

What if nothing works, and my child just refuses to have any more contact?

You always have the option of taking a break from your efforts if it's too painful or you feel the estrangement is compromising your life. Leave a message for your child that says, "I accept your decision. I'm sorry things are in the state they are right now, but I love you. I will continue to love you and will be available for contact, whatever that might mean, when you are ready."

If you decide to take a break, I recommend waiting at least a year before trying again. This may feel like you are giving up. But an extended period of no-contact actually can be productive. It proves to the child that you can respect her boundaries and choices with no pressure. It also allows her to work on feeling less triggered and to develop a new perspective on her own. And it lets you focus on self-healing. Should your child seek contact in the future, you want to be able to greet her as a more peaceful, whole person, not someone who is embittered or a martyr.

After a year of no contact with your adult child, reach out again, perhaps on an occasion like a birthday or holiday. Write another letter of amends with the subject line, "It was clear you needed time. I wanted to check in."

Help Your Adult Children Through Tough Times

Richard Horowitz, EdD, partner at the coaching and training company Growing Great Relationships, LLC, Palm Harbor, Florida, and author of *Family Centered Parenting*. GrowingGreatRelationships.com

---

If it hasn't happened to you, then it's probably happened to a friend—an adult child either fails to launch or gets hit so hard by life that he/she comes knocking for help. Maybe he has suffered through a divorce, flunked out of school, lost a spouse, had an unwanted child, gotten fired, developed a drug or alcohol problem, run afoul of the law, or fallen victim to mental health issues. As a parent, you want more than anything to help your offspring become happy and problem-free. While no two situations are exactly alike, here are some guiding principles to help you navigate these crises.

•**Keep the relationship in focus.** When there's a threat to our children's well-being, we're desperate to make it go away. If we feel unable to help, we often take out that frustration on our children—especially when the problem stems from the child's own bad decisions. Mixed in is a sense of failure—*Is this really how I raised my child?*—and disappointment and even grief for the loss of a once-imagined future.

Take a deep breath, and look at the big picture. The most important thing—long before this problem came along and long after it passes—has been and forever will be the relationship you have with your child. Whatever help you do or don't give, your top priority should be preserving the rapport you've spent a lifetime developing. With that as your guide, you'll increase your odds of hitting on the right strategy for helping.

A big part of your role has always been to teach and model responsibility, resilience, and autonomy. When a child enters adulthood, that aspect of the relationship should taper off and be replaced by trust and friendship. Ask yourself if you've done your part in letting your child be an adult. If not, that might have contributed to this crisis, and establishing an adult-to-adult dynamic probably will be part of the solution.

•**Seek some understanding.** Yes, our younger generations generally have a resiliency problem. They find it difficult to act independently and figure their own way out of tough situations. That may be partly because of the way we've raised them. Ours is the generation of helicopter parenting and adult-monitored recreational activities. Sometime in recent years, it became commonplace for parents to edit their kids' university term papers and intervene when they got bad grades—even in college! So it is difficult for children who were raised that way to suddenly start fending for themselves.

Reality: Today's young adults face economic challenges that we never faced. Between 1987 and 2017, tuition at public universities increased by 213 percent adjusted for inflation.

Rent prices increased 12.5 percent faster than inflation. Median home prices increased by 60 percent over the last 44 years, while median incomes for people ages 25 to 34 have barely increased. In 2020, more than half of American 18-to-29-year-olds were living with their parents, the highest percentage since the Great Depression, and the pandemic made it worse. When your child says she can't make ends meet, a lecture about how well you were doing at her age won't help.

Listen to the problem without interrupting. Ask questions only to help understand. State what you've heard the problem to be—"It sounds like you're saying your boyfriend has decided it's over, and since the apartment is in his name and your bank account is empty, you have nowhere to go. If I don't have that right, please correct me."

You may be thinking all kinds of things—*I knew that guy was a bum! I told you to save for a rainy day!*—but this is not the time to say them.

Remember: The most important thing is the relationship. Make your child feel heard and supported. Share your opinions later.

•**Make a specific plan.** Once you're sure you understand all aspects of the problem, it's time to formulate a solution. It might be as simple as reflecting on the situation and deciding you're unwilling or unable to help. It might require some prolonged discussion with your own spouse and/or co-parent(s). Brainstorm some possible plans. When you have some ideas to propose, set up a meeting with all interested parties and float your possible solutions. If necessary, construct a mutually agreed-upon contract specifying those solutions.

Whatever you and your child agree on, make sure everybody agrees to what's expected of them.

Example: "We're going to cover your car payments while you're in rehab and for two months afterward. It won't be our responsibility after that or if you quit rehab."

If you're lending your child money, make sure he knows your expectations about being repaid. Saying "whenever you can pay me back" is a bad idea if your goal is to recoup your money or instill accountability. Set up a repayment plan, clarifying the first-payment date…due dates for monthly installments…interest rate…and term of the loan.

When an adult child is going to live under your roof, you might have a longer list of expectations. Negotiate those before you come to an agreement.

Example: You might want to impose a midnight curfew for your peace of mind, but your child might push back by insisting that she doesn't need one. Talk it out, and compromise as necessary.

Set a move-out date as well as deadlines for steps such as finding a job, getting transportation and so on. Talk about what will happen if those deadlines aren't met. Will the child need to find other accommodations? Will she have to provide a reason for falling short?

Tell your child how much she will be expected to contribute toward the mortgage and other monthly bills. To prevent future friction, you even can set expectations around sharing food, space, and other things.

Examples: The top shelf of the refrigerator is Dad's…Mom gets to park inside the garage. A long list might seem nit-picky or demanding, so make sure your child understands that you're trying to ensure a successful arrangement—and ask her what expectations she has of you, which also are negotiable.

Make sure your boundaries and expectations are as clear and measurable as possible.

Example: If an adult child will be moving back into the home, some parents might insist, "While you're living in my house, you must not be disrespectful toward me." But because "being disrespectful" is vague, enforcement will be a challenge. Instead, talk through your definition of disrespect—eye-rolling, name-calling, or whatever it is that makes you feel undermined.

●**Stay involved.** To make any plan work, you need to stay on top of how things are going. It's your right, as someone who has been approached for help, to get periodic progress updates. If you've just helped your child out of financial trouble, check in to see if he is starting to save. If you've bailed him out of jail, find out if he is making his court dates. If you're shelter-ing your child until he lands a job, find out how many interviews he has had each week.

It's not your job to micromanage any of this. Offer to help where you can and where you want to, but don't overburden yourself or steal your child's opportunity for personal growth.

Example: Instead of, "You haven't gotten any interviews yet? Let me see your résumé," try, "Let me know if you'd like a second look at your résumé. I have a friend who does that for a living."

By staying involved in a positive and unobtrusive way, you help your child be accountable…you acquire information that you need to be an effective support…and you signal to your child that you love him and have his back.

●**Get help.** Some problems almost always require professional help—mental illness, substance abuse, legal woes. Even for some less drastic problems, you might seek a professional. If your kid has destroyed her finances, part of your bailout plan might include credit counseling or hiring a financial planner. For a spiritual crisis, a pastor or rabbi might provide better counsel than you could.

Get help for yourself as well. Resentment can build when the empty-nester years that you've been looking forward to become as much of a self-sacrificial grind as the years that preceded them. Find a confidante—a friend, a counselor—and make good use of that person as a sounding board.

●**Help…but don't enable.** Too many young adults learn to manipulate their parents—even unconsciously—into providing for them endlessly. If you give unconditionally, not only will you never be free of that burden, your child will be deprived of the gift of autonomy. Any kind of bailout plan should include a good portion of tough love and steps for the child to take to extricate herself from the situation. Be open-minded…sympathetic…supportive—but also be on the lookout for manipulative behavior or a spirit of entitlement on the part of your child. That may be a signal that it's time to re-evaluate your role.

Screen Time Can Be Good for Infants and Toddlers

Study by researchers at Université Paris Nanterre and Sorbonne Université, both in Paris, France, and University of Portsmouth, U.K., published in *Frontiers in Psychology*.

There is widespread concern about the amount of time children age three and under watch TV, computer, smartphone, and other screens and how it affects their cognitive development.

Recent finding: Screen time can be beneficial for young children's cognitive development if what is shown on the screen is appropriate for the child's age…viewing is supervised by an adult…and screens are viewed as a foreground activity rather than in the background while the child is doing other things. Negative effects are more likely when screen content is not age-appropriate—for instance, when narrative is weak, pacing and editing are fast, and stimuli are too different from reality.

Third-Hand Smoke Is Still Pervasive

Study of 504 children, age 11 and younger, by researchers at San Diego State University and University of Cincinnati, Ohio, published in *JAMA Network Open*.

Third-hand smoke affects nearly all children—even in nonsmoking homes. Third-hand smoke is the residue of tobacco smoke left in dust and on surfaces after someone smokes or vapes. Smoking bans, including in homes and cars, are not preventing kids from being exposed to third-hand smoke. More than 97 percent of children studied had nicotine residue on their hands, including 95 percent of those who lived in nonsmoking homes.

Self-defense: Avoid taking children to indoor spaces that were used by smokers.

Homemade Baby Formula Can Be Dangerous

Steven Abrams, M.D., pediatric professor, The University of Texas at Austin. UTexas.edu

The American Academy of Pediatrics strongly advises against making your own baby formula. Even before shortages, there were recipes circulating on the Internet, but these homemade formulas are not safe and have resulted in hospitalizations and even death.

Important: Cow and plant-based milks do not have the same nutritional profile as breast milk—for instance, cow's milk has too much protein, while coconut and almond milks lack adequate protein and calcium for infants.

Baby formula options: Parents can ask their doctors for formula samples…and they can look for a local breast milk bank, such as Human Milk Banking Association of North America (HMBANA.org).

How to Spot Hepatitis in Children

Alexander Weymann, M.D., director, Liver Center, Nationwide Children's Hospital, Columbus, Ohio.

The sudden increase in acute hepatitis (liver inflammation) among otherwise healthy children under age 10 has prompted the CDC to issue an alert to health-care providers.

Symptoms to watch for: Fever, fatigue, joint/muscle pain, loss of appetite, nausea, diarrhea, vomiting, abdominal pain and/or tenderness, dark urine, pale or clay-colored stool and especially jaundice (yellowing of the skin or eyes), a hallmark of the illness. Symptoms may come on suddenly and in any combination. *Adenovirus*, which spreads through respiratory droplets and touching contaminated surfaces, is suspected to be causing the outbreak.

Prevention: Wash hands often…avoid touching the face and mouth as much as possible. Hepatitis can be mild, but severe cases can lead to liver failure and even require a liver transplant.

How to Find a Vet for Your Best Friend

Nancy Kerns, editor of Whole Dog Journal, a publication that has been providing dog-related guidance for 24 years. Whole-Dog-Journal.com

Ask local pet-sector professionals, such as the owners of pet-supply stores, kennels, and pet-grooming businesses, which local veterinary practices they trust most. You also can ask friends and neighbors who have pets for their opinions, but individual pet owners can share only their own experiences, while pet pros have a broader sense of vets' reputations.

Also ask these people why they trust the vets they recommend—it's a great sign if you hear things like, "The practice has a wonderful way with animals"…"You can tell how much they care"…and/or "They take the time to answer my questions."

Nutritious Treats for Dogs and Cats

Nancy Kerns, editor-in-chief of *Whole Dog Journal,* a guide to natural health care and training. Whole-Dog-Journal.com

To our pets, food means love, security, and reinforcement…and delicious treats can be a great tool for training our furry friends.

But: Selecting healthy treats can be challenging. *Here's how to buy the right ones to keep your companion happy and healthy…*

•**Consider the appeal.** Treats are simply high-value foods. Try different types to see which ones excite your pet. Their appeal can center around meatiness, fattiness, sweetness, and novelty.

•**Remember it's food—and should be healthy.** Use the same criteria that guide your food purchases. In fact, regular dinner kibble works as a treat, especially when intermixed with sexier fare, such as bits of roasted chicken and feta cheese. Nutritionally, treats shouldn't be radically different from your pets' daily diet. And for training purposes, they should be small—pea-sized—so rewards can be frequent.

•**Think "kitchen foods" first.** The healthiest choices are not packaged but single-ingredient, unadulterated items from your kitchen.

Examples: Cooked meat—lower-fat, white-meat chicken, especially…eggs—bits of scrambled or hard-boiled…fish—for both cats and dogs…cheese—start with pea-sized amounts and see how it affects your pet's digestion… fruit—most dogs love chunks of watermelon, apple slices, and strawberries…vegetables— carrots, zucchini, and broccoli.

Use fatty foods sparingly, mixed in with low-fat treats for training. Cats lack taste-bud receptors for sweetness, but dogs love sweets. Most pets respond to variety, so try a "trail mix" of goodies.

•**Don't scrimp.** You get what you pay for. Inexpensive foods don't contain good-quality ingredients.

Also: Don't be lured by cute presentation and packaging.

•**Read the ingredients.** Never buy treats without studying their contents. Start by ruling out artificial colors, flavors, and preservatives. Avoid such preservatives as BHA, BHT, and ethoxyquin. ("Mixed tocopherols"—vitamin E—is an acceptable natural preservative.) The longer the ingredients list, the more likely it is that a treat contains junk.

By-products and food fragments are signs of low quality. If you don't recognize an ingredient, don't buy the product.

After eliminating the bad stuff, look for the good—whole meats, grains, fruits, and vegetables. Organic ingredients are best. Look for specificity regarding meats—species of origin and body part. Pets love treats that combine both muscle and organ meats.

Where to buy treats: Grocery stores mainly stock junk foods, so don't buy there. You'll fare better by supporting local artisans, buy-

Leaving a Cat Home Alone...

Rule of thumb: If you will be away for more than 24 hours, get a sitter. Left on her own for too long, a cat can become destructive or eliminate outside of the litterbox.

Reminder: Even if you have a sitter come in to check daily, your cat still will be alone most of the time.

When leaving your cat alone: Keep shades open in at least a few rooms so your cat can enjoy some natural light...keep the heat/air-conditioning at comfortable levels... leave a TV or radio playing if that's something you normally do...block doors so the cat can't accidentally get shut inside a room...remove the cat's collar...for especially active cats, unplug unneeded lights and appliances...and take breakable objects off countertops.

Pamela J. Perry, DVM, Ph.D., behavior resident, Cornell University College of Veterinary Medicine, Ithaca, New York. Vet.Cornell.edu

ing from an independent pet-supply store or ordering from a reliable online supplier such as Chewy.com.

Cannabis Poisonings in Pets Have Been Rising Since 2018

Survey of 222 veterinarians in the U.S. and Canada by researchers at Ontario Veterinary College, University of Guelf, Ontario, Canada, published in *PLOS One.*

Dogs are most likely to ingest cannabis, usually through edibles or discarded joint butts. Edibles also contain other substances that are toxic to dogs and cats, including chocolate, grapes, raisins, citrus, and aspartame.

Symptoms of poisoning: Disorientation, distress, anxiety, lack of muscle coordination, and involuntary urination. Most pets recover, but a few pets have died.

Warning: The products' childproof containers are not pet-proof—dogs and cats can chew through the plastic.

Happy Dogs Wag Their Tails This Way

Whole Dog Journal. Whole-Dog-Journal.com

Happy dogs wag their tails to the right. Right-side motion is controlled by the left side of the brain, which is associated with positive feelings—so a happy dog typically wags to the right. The right side of the brain—which controls movement on the left side of the body—is associated with negative feelings, so a dog that is fearful likely will wag to the left.

Is Your Pet's Skin Problem Really an Allergy?

Natalie Marks, DVM, CVJ, veterinarian and assistant medical director at VCA Blum Animal Hospital in Chicago. VCAHospitals.com/Blum

Patchy fur and itchy red skin often are the first and most obvious clues that a dog or cat has an allergy. Unfortunately, those clues frequently are misinterpreted, mistreated, or ignored, leaving the pet to suffer unnecessarily. *Here's when to suspect that your pet has an allergy and what you can do about it...*

FOOD ALLERGY

Dog signs: The skin of both of the dog's ears and its rear end are itchy and/or red. The dog's rear-end discomfort might result in frequent "scooting" across lawns or carpets.

Cat signs: Excessive scratching that leads to red and/or balding areas, especially on the head and/or neck. A food allergy also might make a cat vomit and/or overgroom, though this is only one of many potential explanations for these symptoms. In fact, vomiting and frequent grooming are so common in cats that they often are thought to be "normal." However, there usually is an underlying reason for this, and often it is allergies.

Rule of thumb: There's cause for concern if the cat vomits several times or more per week...or when grooming becomes so common that patches of the cat's fur are rendered short and stubbly.

What to do: If a food or treat was introduced to the pet's diet within 72 hours of the onset of symptoms, stop providing this and see if the symptoms clear. If that is the cause, you should see improvement in five to seven days.

If the food is not the cause, take the pet to a vet to confirm that a food allergy is to blame and that there isn't a secondary infection in the ears and rear. Also discuss diet modifications. Options might include a "novel diet"—with limited ingredients and a new protein, such as bison, venison, pork, or rabbit, not commonly found in commercial pet foods...or a "hydrolyzed diet," which breaks the proteins down enough that the dog or cat's body doesn't recognize them or attack them, causing the allergic response.

Misinformation alert: You might have heard that the best way to solve a dog's food allergy is to feed it a grain-free diet. In truth, grains such as corn are not common causes of food allergies among dogs. And when given to the animal long term, grain-free diets are associated with heart failure in many dogs.

FLEA ALLERGY DERMATITIS (FAD)

Dog and cat signs: Extreme itchiness and discomfort—the pet is so distressed that it can't eat or nap without scratching. Areas of thinning fur and inflamed, red, scabby skin develop, especially around the base of the tail or elsewhere near the pet's hindquarters, rear legs or belly. Among cats, overgrooming is a common symptom as well...and the areas of thinning fur and red skin also might appear on the head and neck.

A flea allergy could be the problem even if you don't see any fleas on the pet. When a dog or cat is allergic to flea saliva, even a single flea bite days earlier can cause discomfort.

What to do: A vet can prescribe drugs such as corticosteroids to relieve the animal's severe discomfort. Flea-preventive medications and lawn treatments can reduce the odds of future flea bites.

Best: Use pet-friendly flea treatments to treat carpeting, flooring, bedding, and lawns. They all are different so follow instructions on the product label.

Related: If a pet is scratching at a single spot because of what appears to be a single bug bite, an ongoing allergy likely isn't to blame. Apply a light layer of 1 percent hydrocortisone cream two or three times daily to this spot to ease the itchiness. If the pet can lick the spot, apply Aquaphor instead—it's less likely to cause digestive distress or other issues when small amounts are ingested.

ENVIRONMENTAL ALLERGY

Dog signs: The inside and flap of one ear—not both ears—is red and itchy. The animal's eyelids also might be swollen and red.

Cat signs: Itchy, flaking skin on the head and face or potentially elsewhere. Scratching or overgrooming might lead to hair loss, stubbly hair patches, and/or hairballs. Other potential symptoms among cats include watery eyes, runny nose, sneezing, respiratory congestion, vomiting, and/or ear infections.

What to do: Reducing exposure to the allergen could lessen the symptoms—keep the pet indoors as much as possible if pollen or other outdoor allergies are suspected based on seasonality...and clean the house thoroughly if dust-mite allergies are a possibility. Routine weekly bathing can remove allergens from the pet's skin and fur. A vet can prescribe medications to reduce the pet's allergy symptoms including itchiness.

Misinformation alert: It used to be common to give pets suffering from environmental allergies over-the-counter antihistamines primarily intended for humans, such as Benadryl. Recent research suggests that these provide little or no benefit for pets—they appear only to offer relief because they make pets so sleepy that they temporarily scratch less.

CHAPTER 9

Food, Diet, and Fitness

Are You Addicted to Processed Foods?

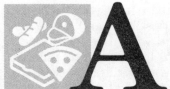**A**merica's obesity epidemic usually is blamed on poor dietary decisions, but a growing body of evidence suggests that the root cause is our addiction to processed foods—hot dogs, soda, sugary breakfast cereals, potato chips, etc.—and that affects how we should go about trying to lose weight. Some people have a hard time believing that we can become addicted to food, but consider the facts...

Brain scans of obese people indulging in processed foods reveal the same neural activity seen in drug, alcohol and other addicts—deactivation of brain regions related to inhibition and reasoning, coupled with hyperactivity of rewards pathways. Overeaters' relationship with processed foods mirrors the American Psychological Association's 11 symptoms of substance dependance listed in the fifth edition of the *Diagnostic and Statistical Manual of Mental Disorders*. Experiments have shown that sugar—a primary ingredient in many processed foods—has an effect on rodent brains similar to that of morphine.

While the research is less extensive, experiments suggest that other common processed-food ingredients might have a similar effect, including gluten and flour products, excessive amounts of salt, nonsugar sweeteners and trans fats.

Convinced yet? *Here's a six-step plan to help you determine if you or someone you love might be addicted to processed food and what to do about it...*

1. Determine if your eating habits fit the symptoms of addiction. The following selected statements are based on the American

Joan Ifland, Ph.D., food addiction specialist and fellow of the American College of Nutrition. Based in Seattle, she is coeditor of the textbook *Processed Food Addiction: Foundations, Assessment, and Recovery*. ProcessedFoodAddiction.com

Psychological Association's symptoms of addiction. If even just two or three apply to you, you might be addicted to processed foods… and the more that apply, the more serious that addiction.

I regularly eat more than intended. Maybe you think, I'll have one and then eat the bag of chips…or I'm not stopping for fast food, then you stop anyway.

I have tried to cut back without success. You diet but regain the weight.

I have spent a lot of time getting food, eating, and recovering from eating. Food has an outsized place in your schedule.

I experience cravings or urges to eat processed food. It's normal to feel a bit hungry as dinner nears if you missed lunch…but yearning for processed foods throughout the day isn't normal.

My eating makes it hard to fulfill my roles at home, work, school, etc. Indulging in a vice even though it's making it difficult to complete your obligations is a sign of addiction.

I have relationship problems because of my eating. Has someone you care about begged you to eat less?

I eat for reasons other than hunger, such as boredom, fatigue, loneliness, anger, or depression.

2. Learn to identify addictive foods. When people are watching what they eat, they tend to scan ingredients lists and track calories.

Problem: There are far too many troublesome ingredients with long chemical names to remember and avoid them all.

What to do: Rather than worry about each ingredient and calorie, group foods into addictive and nonaddictive, and then avoid the former.

How to determine which foods are addictive: If a food looks like it did immediately after being removed from nature, it's probably unprocessed and nonaddictive. But if it looks like it's been created in a factory or lab, it's probably processed and addictive. That means items from the produce, butcher, and seafood sections of the supermarket usually are safe choices, while anything found in boxes or cans in other aisles usually isn't. And yes—this includes packaged processed foods that are marketed as "diet foods." They might have low calorie counts but almost inevitably contain addictive ingredients.

Surprising: Dairy products such as milk and cheese seem healthy and natural, but they contain *casomorphin,* a naturally occurring peptide that studies suggest is addictive. After all, milk is meant to help baby mammals rapidly pack on pounds—it's not something nature intended adults to consume.

3. Remove processed foods from your life. Some people can go cold turkey and eliminate processed foods overnight. But most people prefer slow, steady modifications.

What to do: Remove one processed food from your diet each day. Start by eliminating processed foods that you consume only occasionally and won't miss much—starting small can create a sense of progress toward a larger goal without feeling overwhelming.

4. Make it difficult to make eating mistakes. If you constantly convince yourself not to eat processed food, you're likely to fail. Instead, arrange your life so temptations are less common, particularly during the first few months. *What to do…*

Restrict availability: Processed foods should not be where you can easily reach them. Completely remove them from your home and workplace if that's possible—and when you remove an item from your diet, also remove it from your kitchen. Unfortunately, this isn't always an option—you might share your living space or workspace with someone who doesn't want to do without these foods. If so, at least keep these items out of your reach and out of sight.

Examples: Perhaps the people who share your living space would be willing to store their processed foods in a separate closet or locked box in the kitchen…or perhaps your co-workers could exclude you from group e-mails announcing when snacks are available in the break room.

Avoid activities and places linked in your mind to processed-food consumption: If you always eat a hot dog when you visit a local park, avoid that park…if you shovel unhealthy food into your mouth when you sit

Eat Fruit—Be Happy!

Fruit Boosts Mental Health

According to a recent study, people who ate fruit most often scored highest for mental well-being and had the lowest scores for depression. On the other hand, the more frequently people ate savory snack foods such as chips, which are low in nutrients, the more likely they were to report low mental well-being and frequent "everyday mental lapses"—for instance, forgetting why they'd walked into a room, where they'd left an object or trying to remember the name of an acquaintance.

Note: The benefit was specific to frequency of eating fruit, not quantity of fruit eaten...and to fruits, not vegetables.

Reason: Nutrients in vegetables, which also are known to benefit mood and cognition, often are lost during cooking...and most vegetables are eaten cooked. Fruit, on the other hand, usually is eaten raw.

Study of 428 adults by researchers at Aston University, Birmingham, U.K., published in *British Journal of Nutrition.*

Three Cheers for Watermelon!

Watermelon supports cardiovascular and metabolic health. Watermelon's beneficial nutrients include essential vitamins, minerals, antioxidants and amino acids—including citrulline and arginine, which help control blood pressure, lipids (fats), and glucose. Researchers are looking into how much watermelon has the most beneficial effect.

Study by researchers at Illinois Institute of Technology, Chicago, published in *Current Atherosclerosis Reports.*

in front of the TV, take up a hobby that keeps your hands busy.

5. Cultivate negative mental responses to processed food. When tempted to eat processed food, don't tell yourself that you can't have a food you want. Instead, tell yourself why you don't want it.

Examples: Think, I don't want that—it makes me feel unhealthy or I don't want that—

it's ruining my life. These negative mental responses might not feel accurate at first, but they will gain power as your rational frontal lobe begins to regain control from your brain's rewards pathways.

6. Spend time with people who eat unprocessed foods. Humans are likely to behave the way we see the people around us behaving—our brains contain cells called mirror neurons that respond to the actions we see performed by others as though these were our own actions.

Result: It is much harder to overcome food addiction when we spend time around people who eat unhealthy processed foods and easier when we spend time with people who eat right. Seek out healthy eating support groups in your area or online.

Resistant Starch: The Good Carbs

Michael Greger, M.D., physician who specializes in clinical nutrition and is a founding member and fellow of the American College of Lifestyle Medicine. Dr. Greger writes at NutritionFacts.org and is the author of several bestselling books, including *How Not to Die, The How Not to Die Cookbook, How Not to Diet,* and *How to Survive a Pandemic.*

If you think starches will make you fat and play havoc with your blood sugar, you're not alone. Starchy foods have a bad reputation. But that reputation is undeserved for foods high in a particular kind of starch. We're talking about resistant starch, a kind of fiber most abundant in beans and other legumes. It's also found in whole grains, vegetables, seeds, green bananas, and nuts such as cashews and almonds.

BODY BENEFITS

Resistant starch gets its name because it resists fast digestion. The enzymes in our small intestines don't break down these carbohydrates easily, which prevents a quick rise in blood sugar. It also means that more of these starches make it into our colons, where they act as prebiotics: substances that provide food for helpful bacteria.

When helpful gut bacteria are well fed, they multiply, creating a healthier microbiome. That's the community of bacteria that lives in every person's digestive tract. When we eat lots of resistant starch, we get more bacteria that make certain short-chained fatty acids, such as butyrate. These fatty acids are absorbed into our bloodstreams, where they travel through the body and even to the brain. Benefits may include improved immune function, lower inflammation, and positive effects on mental health, metabolism, and body fat.

Eating more fiber, including resistant starch, also directly improves digestive health, creating softer, bulkier stools, and reducing colon cancer risk.

HOW TO GET MORE

The emerging science has led to a vast array of supplements that claim to supply resistant starch in pills and powders, but studies have shown no benefits from these products. And there's no reason to think that a supplement could work as well as whole foods. After all, when you eat a bean or a nut or a vegetable, you get not just resistant starch, but all kinds of fiber, plus vitamins and minerals.

Here are some ways to get more resistant starch…

•**Eat more beans and other legumes,** such as lentils, chickpeas, and split peas. Aim for three servings a day. A quarter-cup of hummus, a half-cup of cooked beans, or a cup of peas is a serving.

•**Stick to whole grains.** Whole-grain bread has more resistant starch than refined white bread. Grains such as oats, quinoa, and barley are great sources.

•**Eat more intact grains, beans, nuts, and seeds.** While it's fine to eat bean dip and hummus, when you have whole beans or chickpeas on a salad, more resistant starch gets to your colon. A traditional muesli, made with raw oats, seeds, and nuts, is full of intact food for your gut.

•**Eat starchy foods with berries,** which block enzymes that digest starches. A little raspberry jam on your toast, blueberries on your

---

Dr. Greger's BROL Bowl

Ingredients…
½ cup hulled barley
½ cup rye berries
½ cup oat groats
½ cup dried black lentils
4 cups water
Directions…
Mix all ingredients and cook in an electric pressure cooker for 30 minutes. Add toppings as desired. For a sweet breakfast bowl, try frozen dark cherries, cocoa powder, dates, and walnuts.

Nutritional Information Per Cup: *calories* 280; *carbohydrate* 55 g; *fat* 2 g; *cholesterol* 0 mg; *fiber* 15 g; *protein* 13 g; *sodium* 12 mg.

---

cereal, or strawberries on your pancakes will leave more food for gut bacteria.

•**Get more resistant starch from potatoes, pasta, and rice by cooling them after cooking them.** The temperature shift causes some of the starch to recrystallize into resistant starch. That can make cold pasta or potato salads a little healthier than their hot counterparts.

Cereal Fiber Lowers Inflammation Better Than Vegetable Fiber

Columbia University's Mailman School of Public Health.

Researchers report that cereal fiber, but not fruit or vegetable fiber, is consistently associated with lower inflammation and cardiovascular disease incidence in older people. Cereal fiber is found in bran, whole-wheat bread and pasta, brown rice, seeds, barley, and other whole grains. The researchers don't know why cereal fiber showed more benefits, but suggest that other nutrients in foods rich in cereal fiber may play a role.

Fiber and Constipation

Anish Sheth, M.D., gastroenterologist at Princeton Medical Group and an attending physician at the University Medical Center of Princeton at Plainsboro, New Jersey.

Getting more fiber from plant foods (especially pears, apples and sweet potatoes—all with skins on—and cooked greens) will usually increase the frequency and comfort of bowel movements, but not for everyone. A form of constipation known as slow-transit constipation (STC) occurs when the intestinal muscles contract less often and with less force than normal. Some patients with STC improve when they get more fiber, but others will still need laxatives or other treatments. If you have constipation that hasn't responded to dietary changes, ask your doctor whether you might have STC.

It's also important to take medication into account. Many prescription and over-the-counter drugs and supplements can cause constipation as a side effect. Psychiatric medications, including tricyclic antidepressants, such as *imipramine* (Tofranil) and *amitriptyline* (Elavil), are notorious for causing constipation. If a new medication is causing constipation, ask your doctor if you can get by with a lower dose or switch to a different drug.

Eating prunes can help, too. Prunes are high in fiber, but the main benefit comes from sorbitol, a sugar that draws water into the intestine. Two servings of prunes (about 10 fruits) contain 12 g of sorbitol and 8 ounces of juice has about 15 g. If you don't like prunes, consider trying rhubarb, artichokes, and/or peaches—all of which promote regular bowel movements.

Drinking more water and getting more exercise help keep stools soft and intestinal muscles active, too.

Buckwheat: The Wheat and Gluten-Free Superfood

Janet Bond Brill, Ph.D., RDN, FAND, registered dietitian nutritionist, a fellow of the Academy of Nutrition and Dietetics, and a nationally recognized nutrition, health and fitness expert who specializes in cardiovascular disease prevention. Based in Hellertown, Pennsylvania, Dr. Brill is author of *Intermittent Fasting for Dummies, Blood Pressure DOWN, Cholesterol DOWN*, and *Prevent a Second Heart Attack*. DrJanet.com

Buckwheat is a *pseudocereal*, the name for seeds from nongrass plants commonly consumed in the same way as grains. (Quinoa is also a pseudocereal.) Buckwheat is the seed of the *Fagopyrum esculentum* plant, which is related to rhubarb and sorrel. A grain and a seed are similar, but not identical. A grain is the small edible fruit harvested from grassy crops. A seed is an ovule that contains an embryonic plant. Both seeds and grains are highly nutritious and should be eaten in their whole, unprocessed forms.

Buckwheat is considered an "ancient grain," meaning a plant that has been cultivated for centuries, even millennia. Other examples of ancient grains include quinoa, barley, rye, and millet. All types of ancient grains are whole grains, and, for that reason alone, they deserve consideration as a part of your healthy diet. A large body of scientific evidence illustrates the spectacular health benefits of consuming whole grains daily.

Buckwheat has no relation to wheat and is gluten-free. Gluten is a protein found in wheat and some other cereals, but it is not found in seeds. Buckwheat groats (the hearty, hulled seed of the buckwheat plant) can be eaten roasted or in products such as buckwheat flour and kasha. Buckwheat is the primary ingredient in Japanese soba noodles. (If you're avoiding gluten, check the label. Many brands include some wheat flour as well.) Buckwheat is exceptionally rich in fiber, which most Americans don't get enough of.

Experience its toasty, nutty flavor and a soft, chewy texture with this fiber-packed recipe…

KASHA VARNISHKES

Ingredients…

4 cups uncooked bow tie pasta
2 large white onions, chopped
1 cup sliced fresh mushrooms
2 tbsp. extra virgin olive oil
1 cup roasted whole-grain buckwheat groats (kasha)
1 large egg, at room temperature and beaten lightly
2 cups low-sodium chicken broth, heated
½ tsp. salt
Dash pepper
Minced fresh parsley

Directions…

Cook pasta according to package directions. In the meantime, sauté onions and mushrooms in oil in a large skillet until lightly browned, 7 to 9 minutes. Remove from pan and set aside.

Combine buckwheat groats and egg in a small bowl and add to the same skillet. Cook and stir over high heat for two to four minutes or until the buckwheat is browned, separating grains. Add the hot broth, salt, and pepper.

Bring to a boil. Add the onion mixture. Reduce heat, cover, and simmer for 10 to 12 minutes or until the liquid is absorbed. Drain the pasta, add to pan, and heat through. Sprinkle with parsley.

Yield: Makes 8 servings

Nutrition per serving (¾ cup): 270 calories, 6 g fat, 28 mg cholesterol, 408 mg sodium, 47 g total carbohydrate, 4 g sugars, 4 g fiber, 9 g protein.

How to Eat Meat Responsibly

David L. Katz, M.D., board-certified specialist in preventive medicine/public health, author of several best-sellers, including *How to Eat: All Your Food and Diet Questions Answered*, and founder/CEO of Diet ID, a digital tool that enables doctors to assess patients' nutrition profiles. DavidKatzMD.com

It's no secret that red meat, especially processed red meat, is not healthy when it makes up the lion's share of your calories.

What is only recently getting attention, however, is how bad red meat is for the planet. Global demand for beef is a leading driver of the loss of the Amazon rainforest. The rainforest is being eliminated through burning, clear-cutting, and other methods to create more grazing land for cattle. And the methane gas produced by cattle and the fossil fuels used in gas-guzzling farm machinery contribute to climate change.

We spoke with preventive medicine and public health specialist David L. Katz, M.D., who started the nonprofit TrueHealthInitiative.org, which is running the #NoBeefWeek campaign to encourage people to give up beef for one week and get motivated to reduce meat consumption over time.

No matter how much red meat you currently eat, doing it "responsibly" means eating it less frequently and making important choices when you do…

Where the meat comes from: Meat tends to be healthier for you when it comes from well-fed, active animals—grass-fed, pasture-raised beef and lamb, and pastured pigs (pigs can't feed only on grass). A Google search will turn up many farms offering humanely raised meat that can be shipped right to your door.

Type of meat: It's difficult to tell if one type of red meat is better for you than another—most nutrition studies aren't specific enough to draw firm conclusions. But it's always smart to look for cuts that are lean, with minimal or no marbling, to limit your consumption of saturated fat. While saturated fat is not "bad" per se, problems start when there's an imbalance between the amount of saturated fat you consume and other foods, such as vegetables, fruits, and whole grains, which help counter the inflammation linked to red meat.

Portion size: Four to six ounces is reasonable for most of us (a tall, muscular, physically active man may want more). Think of meat as the garnish rather than the main attraction on your plate…make better use of inexpensive legumes…and experiment with ethnic cuisines that place little emphasis on meat.

Frequency: To empower you to eat less meat, consider Suzy Amis-Cameron's *The OMD Plan*, which encourages at least one plant-based meal a day (OMDForThePlanet.com)... and *Mark Bittman's VB6* (MarkBittman.com), which stands for eating only vegan before 6 pm each day.

What about fake meat? We don't yet know whether plant-based meat alternatives are healthier for you, but I recommend it for people who would be eating meat otherwise. We do know that they're healthier for the planet. Yes, they're processed, but so is the meat used to make burgers at fast-food chains and even the ground beef sold at supermarkets.

Surprising Sources of Vegetable Protein

Roseanne Rust, RDN, registered licensed dietitian/nutritionist and freelance nutrition writer. RustNutrition.com

Eating meat or legumes such as navy and pinto beans aren't the only ways to meet your protein requirement. The following plant-based foods may not be familiar as protein sources, but they pack a protein punch. *Spinach:* 6 grams (g) of protein per cup. *Peas:* 4g in one-half cup. *Average-sized baked potato:* 3g. *Broccoli:* 3g per cup. *One medium ear of corn:* 3g.

Helpful formula for proper protein intake: Multiply your body weight in pounds by 0.36. The result is the number of grams of protein you need daily, at a bare minimum.

Example: Someone who weighs 150 pounds needs 54 grams of protein per day.

Protein from Meat Alternatives Is Harder to Digest

Study by researchers at The Ohio State University, Columbus, published in *Journal of Agricultural and Food Chemistry.*

A recent study revealed that when compared with cooked chicken breast protein, hu-

man gut cells absorb 2 percent less protein from a plant-based meat alternative, indicating that protein from meat alternatives may be less available to the body. While the study did not determine if the difference is significant enough to be a dietary concern, including protein from both animal and plant sources in your diet will help ensure that you are getting adequate amounts.

Ode to Chocolate: Food of Love and Health

Janet Bond Brill, Ph.D., RDN, FAND, registered dietitian nutritionist, a fellow of the Academy of Nutrition and Dietetics, and a nationally recognized nutrition, health, and fitness expert who specializes in cardiovascular disease prevention. Based in Hellertown, Pennsylvania, Dr. Brill is author of *Intermittent Fasting for Dummies, Blood Pressure DOWN, Cholesterol DOWN,* and *Prevent a Second Heart Attack.* DrJanet.com

Isn't it incredible news that everyone's favorite indulgent treat can help improve our heart health? All chocolate is not created equally, though, and some types are better than others. *Here are key concepts that you should know...*

•**Choose dark.** Dark chocolate has a much higher percentage of cocoa than milk chocolate, and it's the cocoa that contains most of the flavonoids—plant substances that provide your body with a host of health benefits. Flavonoids work as potent antioxidants to protect us from free-radical damage, the process that accelerates aging and promotes chronic illnesses, such as heart disease and cancer. The darker the chocolate, the higher the percentage of cocoa, and the more flavonoids it will contain. A large amount of cocoa can make the food taste bitter, so try different products to see what appeals to you.

Dark chocolate, while very good for health, is not a low-calorie diet food. Chocolate products are often loaded with calories, fat, and sugar, which is why if you choose to eat a chocolate confection, I suggest you make it no more than 1 ounce of at least 70 percent dark chocolate per day. The American Heart Asso-

157

ciation includes sugar on its blacklist of ingredients—joining the ranks of saturated fat, trans fat, dietary cholesterol, and sodium—foods that consumers need to limit for better heart health. Also watch out for imposters like white chocolate, which has no antioxidants, and hot chocolate mixes, which have negligible antioxidants. Instead, make your own sinfully delicious hot chocolate with dark cocoa powder, low-fat milk or light soy milk, and a touch of sweetener and keep your heart and your soul healthy and happy.

Dr. Janet's Decadent European Hot Chocolate

Ingredients…

1½ cups 1 percent milk

½ cup soy creamer

1 packet Splenda, stevia, or the sweetener of your choice

1 teaspoon instant coffee

4 oz. 72 percent chocolate. (I use ½ bar of Trader Joe's Pound Plus 72 percent chocolate bar)

Fat-free whipped cream

Directions…

In a medium-sized saucepan over medium heat, whisk together milk, creamer, sweetener, and instant coffee until small bubbles form around the edges. Do not boil. Chop the chocolate bar into small pieces and add to saucepan. Stir the mixture for about five minutes to melt or until desired consistency is reached. Serve in an espresso cup and top with fat-free whipped cream.

Tip: Serve in espresso cups for a one-quarter cup serving size. This recipe is very rich and satisfying even at a small serving size.

Yield: 8 servings (3.2 ounces, ¼ cup serving size)

Nutrition per serving: *Calories:* 230; *Total fat:* 15g; *Saturated fat:* 1g; *Cholesterol:* 1mg; *Sodium:* 35mg; *Carbohydrates:* 18g; *Fiber:* 0g; *Sugar:* <1g; *Protein:* 4g.

Lighten Up Southern Comfort Foods for Better Health

Harvard Health Letter.

Researchers have linked a traditional American Southern diet with a higher risk of cardiovascular disease, owing to ample servings of meat and fried fare. But plenty of beloved Southern dishes are based on heart-healthy vegetables, beans, and whole grains. With a few quick swaps, you can build a complete, and completely satisfying, meal by combining some meat-free sides.

•**Greens.** Stir-fry collard greens, kale, cabbage, or chard in olive oil with garlic, a splash of vinegar, and red pepper flakes.

•**Beans.** Saute diced onion and garlic in olive oil, and then add rinsed black-eyed peas or pinto beans. Simmer for a few minutes.

•**Corn bread.** Use whole-grain cornmeal and skip the white flour or sugar. Use vegetable oil instead of bacon drippings.

•**Sweet potatoes.** Toss one-inch cubes in olive oil and roast at 425 degrees for 20 to 30 minutes.

Bust Dangerous Belly Fat

Kimberly Gomer, RD, director of nutrition at Body Beautiful Miami in Florida, and former director of nutrition at the Pritikin Longevity Center & Spa. Body BeautifulMiami.com

There are two main types of fat storage. *Subcutaneous fat* is stored right under your skin, and *visceral fat*, the so-called "belly fat," is stored deep in your body, packed between abdominal organs like the stomach, liver, kidney, and intestines.

Visceral fat is downright deadly. One reason is that fat cells inside the abdomen secrete high levels of an inflammatory molecule called interleukin-6, according to researchers at Washington University in St. Louis. And higher levels of inflammation are linked to nearly ev-

Lifestyle Tips for Losing Belly Fat

To lose belly fat, diet is crucial, but it's not the whole story. Scientific research shows you need a healthy lifestyle, including regular exercise, stress management, and at least seven hours of sleep per night.

•**Stress management.** A study from researchers at Yale University shows that normal-weight women with negative moods and higher levels of life stress had higher levels of the stress hormone cortisol and more abdominal fat. When you feel stressed, take a few deep breaths for a quick calming effect.

•**Regular exercise.** Even small amounts of exercise reduce the inflammatory components of belly fat, according to research from the University of Illinois. Other studies show that aerobic exercise, like brisk walking, resistance training, and high-intensity interval training, can all help reduce belly fat.

•**Sufficient sleep.** A study from the Mayo Clinic, published in the *Journal of the American College of Cardiology* in March 2022, showed that lack of sufficient sleep increased belly fat by about 10 percent.

•**Mindful eating.** Researchers from Brown University found that people with less "dispositional mindfulness"—being aware of and paying attention to current feelings and thoughts—had an average of an extra pound of belly fat. Mindfulness, say the researchers, helps a person eat healthier and exercise regularly. When you eat, don't look at your smartphone or the TV. Pay attention to your meal instead.

ery chronic health problem, including insulin resistance (prediabetes) and type 2 diabetes, high blood pressure, heart disease, cancer, chronic obstructive pulmonary disease, and Alzheimer's disease.

Do you have excess belly fat? To find out, put a tape measure around the largest part of your waist. You have excess belly fat if you're a woman with a waist measuring 35" or more, or a man with a waist measuring 40" or more.

EXTRA BELLY FAT, EXTRA RISK

Scientific research shows that if you have excess belly fat—just that one risk factor—you might be at extra risk for a host of ailments…

•**Heart failure.** In a study published in *Circulation*, every additional ten centimeter (3.9 inch) increase in waist circumference was linked to a 29 percent higher risk of heart failure.

•**Cancer.** In a study of nearly 6,000 older women, those with more belly fat had a 68 percent higher risk of lung cancer and a 34 percent higher risk of gastrointestinal cancers.

•**Cognitive decline.** A study in the *British Journal of Nutrition* showed that older people with more belly fat had a greater level of cognitive decline.

•**Dementia.** If you have excess belly fat in your 40s, you're 2.3 times more likely to have dementia in your 70s, according to a study published in *Neurology.*

•**Chronic obstructive pulmonary disease (COPD).** In a 10-year study, researchers found that people with excess belly fat had a 72 percent increased risk of developing COPD.

•**Asthma.** People with more belly fat are 1.4 times more likely to develop asthma, according to the European Lung Foundation.

•**Premature death.** In a 14-year study from the Mayo Clinic, normal-weight individuals with excess belly fat had double the risk of dying from any cause.

Bottom line: If you want good health and long life, lose excess belly fat.

HORMONAL IMBALANCES

Belly fat tends to accumulate because of imbalances in several hormones…

•**Insulin,** which ushers blood sugar out of the bloodstream and into the cells.

•**Estrogen.** Menopause and its falling levels of estrogen trigger the accumulation of belly fat.

•**Ghrelin and leptin.** These hormones control appetite and satiety (feeling full after eating).

•**Cortisol,** a hormone generated during times of stress.

Sample Meal Plan

There is no one-size-fits-all approach to meal plans, but a day's worth of meals should look something like this...

- **Breakfast.** Eat an omelet loaded with veggies such as onions, peppers, tomatoes, and avocado. If you're not sensitive to dairy, add a little cheese. Have a chicken sausage on the side. You could also add a serving of yogurt and berries (blueberries, raspberries, strawberries, etc.).
- **Lunch.** Eat a vegetable salad (dressed with olive oil) or vegetable soup. Include a protein, such as salmon, and a small amount of carbohydrates, such as a serving of sweet potato or squash.
- **Dinner.** This meal should also be protein-centered, featuring a serving of meat, poultry, or fish. For carbohydrates, include a serving of roasted vegetables or a root vegetable such as butternut squash.

It takes healthy eating, regular exercise, stress management, and sufficient sleep to re-balance those hormones.

DIETARY CHANGES

Dietary changes will get you to about 70 percent of your goal. (See sidebar for the other 30 percent.)

- **Cut refined carbohydrates.** Cut back on (or eliminate) sugary processed foods and refined carbohydrates such as white bread and white pasta.
- **Cut vegetable oils.** Eliminate pro-inflammatory, hormone-disrupting vegetable oils, including soybean, canola, sunflower, corn, cottonseed, vegetable, safflower, and peanut oils. (These may also be lurking in packaged foods.) Instead, favor anti-inflammatory olive and avocado oils. Use olive oil on salads and avocado oil (which has a high burning point) for cooking.
- **Emphasize protein, vegetables, and good fats.** Keep carbohydrates to a minimum and focus on complex carbs (like vegetables) over simple carbs (like white bread). This ap-

proach will balance blood sugar and hormonal production and regulate appetite.

- **Eat three meals a day and limit between-meal snacking.** Include dairy if you're not sensitive to it. For those who prefer less or no meat, protein-rich beans are a good alternative.
- **Drink plenty of water and other non-caloric beverages, such as coffee or tea.** Limit diet soda to no more than one serving per day.
- **When you eat out,** choose a protein-centered entrée such as steak, chicken, or fish, and ask for it grilled, which helps you avoid unwanted oils.

5 Big Myths About Weight Loss

Samantha Cassetty, MS, RD, nationally recognized food, nutrition, and wellness expert with a private nutrition counseling practice in New York City. She is a contributor to *The New York Times* best sellers *7 Years Younger* and *7 Years Younger: The Anti-Aging Breakthrough Diet*, and coauthor of *Sugar Shock*. Samantha Cassetty.com

We all know that there are no magic bullets when it comes to weight loss. The truth is, it requires substantial mental and physical effort. We asked weight-loss expert Samantha Cassetty, MS, RD, to dispel some commonly held myths about dieting that could be preventing you from reaching your healthy weight...

MYTH #1: **Losing weight is just a matter of calories in and calories out.** For many years, experts believed that all calories were alike—but that just isn't true.

Fact: Some calories work harder for you—and promote better nutritional outcomes—than others.

Example: The 150 calories in one can of regular soda will not have the same effects on your body and appetite as 150 calories of broccoli, salmon, nuts, or quinoa.

MYTH #2: **You have to drastically restrict what and when you eat to lose weight.** Some misguided diet plans focus on certain nutrients, such as protein and fat, at the expense of healthy carbohydrates. Other diets let you eat only certain foods that you might not find palatable or only at certain times of the day. These plans are tough to follow for a long enough time to lose weight.

Fact: The best diet plan contains a healthy balance of protein, carbs, and fat, and emphasizes good-for-you foods. But it also lets you indulge, at least occasionally, in the foods that you really enjoy.

Examples: Bread and highly processed snacks often are cited as foods to restrict. That's because you tend to eat them quickly…they stimulate your appetite…and they don't leave you feeling full.

Better: Prioritize healthy fruits and vegetables in your diet…beneficial fats such as olive oil, avocados, nuts, and seeds…and good-for-you proteins including low-fat dairy products, eggs, fish and seafood, and lean poultry.

If you like big portions: Go for water-rich foods that you can eat more of.

Example: A cup of grapes takes up more room on your plate than a small box of raisins, so the portion looks and feels more satisfying. Fresh and frozen fruits and veggies and broth-based soups are examples of water-rich foods.

MYTH #3: Any diet plan will work—if you just do it. This is partly true. Any plan that has you eating fewer calories than you burn can lead to weight loss. In this way, you even could lose weight eating fast food—but it's highly unlikely that you'll keep the weight off long-term because you won't have changed the unhealthy behaviors that led you to gain weight in the first place, and you won't be getting the nutrients your body needs to function well.

Fact: You will achieve sustained weight loss only if you're ready to commit to a new way of eating and living. You have to find a healthy eating plan that plays into your individual preferences and lifestyle. *Healthy plans to consider…*

•**Weight Watchers (WW) and Noom** are based on solid research and focus on both the physical and mental aspects of the weight-loss journey while helping you adopt a healthy lifestyle.

•**The Mediterranean diet** emphasizes whole and plant-based foods such as olive oil and nuts and minimizes added sugars and red meat.

Note: Olive oil and nuts are high in calories, but eating controlled portion sizes will make you feel full for a long time. These tasty foods also are good sources of nutrients. One study conducted by the University of Barcelona and other institutions in Spain even found that regular consumption of nuts and olive oil can reduce belly fat over a five-year period.

Not ideal: Prepackaged diet plans such as *Jenny Craig* and *Nutrisystem*. There is some research to back up the benefits of kickstarting weight loss with one of these diets, but they are unlikely to keep the weight off permanently because they don't give you the behavioral tools to make necessary changes in your eating habits.

Worst: The low-carb, high-fat ketogenic diet has been named the least healthy diet plan of 2022 by *U.S. News & World Report* in its annual diet ranking because it is so restrictive. Although there are some data to support ketogenic diets, they don't provide balanced nutrition.

Even worse: Some people take them to an extreme and gorge on bacon and other heavily processed foods. If you follow a ketogenic diet, you miss out on the many benefits of carbs, including the fiber in whole grains, which supports your gut bacteria and the health of your immune and digestive systems. Several research studies show that eating whole grains in moderation every day actually can assist with weight loss rather than stymie it.

Easy ways to eat more whole grains: Choose brown rice over white rice…whole-grain pasta over white pasta…whole-grain bread over white bread…low-sugar whole-grain cereals over sugary processed cereals.

MYTH #4: Willpower is the key to sustained weight loss. This sets you up to feel like a failure if you can't control your impulse to eat. Your brain perceives certain foods—cookies, candy, cake, potato chips, frozen pizza, and other processed foods—as highly rewarding, so they become more enticing, especially when you are tired or stressed out and your willpower is at its weakest. Processed foods require minimal or no preparation, so it is easy to overindulge in them without thinking about it.

Fact: Willpower comes and goes, and the more decisions you have to make—especially during times of stress—the more your willpower gets used up, causing you to make unhealthy decisions. Rather than relying on willpower, take a behavioral/psychological approach to weight loss, and plan what you are going to eat in a variety of potentially problematic settings.

Examples: What are you going to have for dinner if a meeting runs late? Which snacks are you going to have to satisfy your hunger pangs? A 2018 report from the U.S. Preventive Services Task Force confirms that people lose more weight by making behavior changes like these than with typical cut-your-calorie diets.

MYTH #5: Your doctor is the best source of weight-loss advice.

Fact: Most doctors don't have the training, tools, or time to help their patients lose weight. A 2018 survey of 141 U.S. medical schools conducted by researchers from the Cleveland Clinic and Northwestern University found that programs spend only about 10 hours educating doctors-to-be about obesity, nutrition, and behavioral-change techniques for weight loss.

Some doctors are not even good role models themselves. Although physicians are less likely to be obese than non-health-care professionals, nearly 48 percent of doctors say they are trying to lose weight, according to the *2021 Medscape Physician Lifestyle and Happiness Report*. When doctors are overweight, it impacts how they counsel patients about weight loss and whether patients follow their advice.

Better: Turn to a registered dietitian or a group such as WW or Noom to help you stay accountable to your goals. Expect that you will have ups and downs, plateaus and challenges during your weight-loss journey. Start anew each day…when you overeat…and when you make poor food choices.

Is Time-Restricted Eating Right for You?

Krista Varady, Ph.D., professor of kinesiology and nutrition at the University of Illinois, Chicago. She has published more than 100 scientific papers on intermittent fasting, including time-restricted eating, and is the author of *The Every Other Day Diet*.

Every year, 45 million American adults go on a diet. That's not surprising when you consider that 180 million American adults—70 percent of us—are overweight or obese. But no matter which diet you choose—high-protein or high-fiber, low-carb or low-fat, keto or paleo, vegan or carnivore—it's likely that dieting itself, with all its demands and deprivations, will be a difficult ordeal. It's equally likely that when you go off your diet, you'll slowly but surely regain all the weight you lost. It's estimated that only one in 20 people who lose weight on a diet maintain weight loss long-term.

RESTRICTING TIME, NOT FOOD

The good news: Research my colleagues and I have conducted at the University of Illinois shows that there's a way to lose weight that doesn't involve dieting. This unique approach to weight loss is called time-restricted eating (TRE). Rather than restricting the *foods* you can eat, you restrict the *times* you can eat. On a daily basis, you eat all your food within a limited window of time—for example, between noon and 8 p.m. There are no special foods to emphasize, no "bad" foods to eliminate, and no calories to count. You just eat during fewer hours.

With TRE, you consume fewer calories because you spend less time during the day eating. Research shows that an eating window of eight hours accomplishes a daily reduction of 300 to 500 calories. This research is summarized in a scientific paper in the May 2022 issue of *Nature Reviews/Endocrinology*.

LESS WEIGHT, BETTER HEALTH

Studies show that, along with weight loss, TRE produces many health benefits in people who are overweight and obese…

Preventing Age-Related Weight Gain

After studying thousands of people on a time-restricted diet, it's clear that this approach could help prevent age-related weight gain, the slow but sure addition of extra pounds with aging, at the rate of about one to two pounds per year, usually starting around the age of 50. Some people try to prevent that "weight creep" by counting calories—an approach that almost never succeeds. But time-restricted eating is an easy—almost effortless—way to restrict calories and keep pounds at bay.

• **Less body fat,** which generates inflammatory compounds that raise the risk for chronic disease

• **Lower levels of fasting insulin.** High levels of this glucose-regulating hormone are a risk factor for type 2 diabetes.

• **Less insulin resistance,** another risk factor for type 2 diabetes

• **Balanced levels of blood sugar,** which helps prevent or normalize type 2 diabetes

• **Lower blood pressure.** High blood pressure is a risk factor for heart attack and stroke.

• **Lower triglycerides,** a heart-harming blood fat

• **Lower levels of 8-isoprostane,** a biomarker of chronic inflammation.

Importantly, TRE does a *better* job of reducing insulin resistance than calorie restriction. That's probably because not eating for a stretch of time helps the body know when to release insulin to regulate blood sugar and helps make cells more insulin sensitive.

In fact, in a study being readied for publication, my colleagues and I compared TRE to a calorie-restricted diet in people who had type 2 diabetes for at least 15 years. We found that calorie restriction was ineffective for weight loss and blood sugar control. It hardly worked at all. But TRE helped people with diabetes lose an average of 8 percent of their body weight—one of the most successful studies on weight loss in diabetes ever conducted. Some

of the study participants were able to get off their diabetes medication, and some achieved full remission from type 2 diabetes, with A1c levels in the normal range.

TIPS FOR TRE

Scientific research shows that people who successfully lose weight on a time-restricted diet adopt these simple habits…

• **Eat between noon and 8 p.m.** You can do TRE *any* time that works for you, but in informal surveys, 95 percent of people who have made a lifestyle of time-restricted eating have chosen noon to 8 p.m. as their eating window. Many study participants tend to dislike a time-restricted eating period of 10 a.m. to 6 p.m., because it's likely they'll miss the evening meal—the most social meal of the day. Don't worry about skipping breakfast, which is sometimes touted as the "the most important meal of the day." A recent study in *BMJ* analyzed 13 studies on breakfast and weight loss, involving more than 1,400 people, and found there was no health risk in skipping breakfast—and a slight advantage in losing weight.

• **You can lose weight eating almost any foods.** In my research, we often provided weekly nutritional counseling to study participants, guiding them to increase their intake of fruits, vegetables, and other whole foods. It almost never worked. It is very hard to change dietary patterns, most of which are learned in childhood.

TRE can accomplish *weight loss* without changing the foods you eat. However, for overall health, it's still important to try to eat more fruits, vegetables, and whole grains, and less processed foods, sugars, and saturated fats.

• **Feel free to skip a day.** Skipping TRE one day a week—for example, Saturday, so you can do more socializing—is fine. It won't affect your ability to shed pounds and keep them off.

• **Stay hydrated.** It's important to stay well-hydrated during the fasting period. Try to drink at least 68 ounces (2 liters) of water every day (along with any other beverages you drink).

• **Drink no more than two diet sodas daily.** Some research indicates that drinking diet soda increases cravings for sugary foods and imbalances insulin. For that reason, limit your

Weight Maintenance and TRE

Most people who lose weight regain it—making *maintenance* of weight loss the Holy Grail for weight loss researchers. In a one-year study conducted by researchers at the University of Illinois, participants who lost 6 percent of their body weight after six months on a time-restricted diet maintained that weight loss over the following six months. Why? Because time-restricted eating is an easy habit to maintain—a long-term solution for losing weight and keeping it off.

intake of diet sodas to no more than two per day.

•**Coffee and tea.** Add no more than 1 teaspoon of sugar and 1 teaspoon of cream (or milk or half-and-half) to any cup of coffee or tea. Limit coffee and/or tea to no more than four cups per day.

•**Alcohol is permitted.** During your eating window, men can safely have two drinks, and women can have one. (A drink is 12 ounces of beer, 5 ounces of wine, or 1.5 ounces of distilled spirits.)

•**If you have a history of eating disorders, don't engage in TRE.** TRE doesn't cause eating disorders. But in people with a history of eating disorders, such as binge-eating disorder, TRE might trigger the problem. Also, TRE is contraindicated for pregnant or lactating women and for children under the age of 12, since the safety of TRE for these groups hasn't been scientifically evaluated.

The Secret to Portion Control

Lisa R. Young, Ph.D., RDN, adjunct professor of nutrition at New York University and author of *The Portion Teller Plan* and *Finally Full, Finally Slim.*

A recent International Food Information Council survey found that nearly half of Americans cannot correctly distinguish serving size—a standard unit of measure upon which nutrition labels are based, such as one cup or two tablespoons—from portion size, which is the amount of food you are served or choose to eat. Your favorite cereal may list a serving as three-quarters of a cup, but if you pour yourself two cups for breakfast, your portion is actually more than double the serving size.

One of the problems lies in the fact that our notion of a proper serving has been distorted beyond recognition by super-sized fries and 1,000-calorie smoothies. When a restaurant server brings us an enormous plate of pasta, we consider it to be an individual *serving* when, in fact, what we've been given is a *portion*. They're not the same thing.

Very generally speaking, most people should aim for the following serving quantities and sizes…

•**Grains.** Eat four to six servings per day. One serving is one-half cup of cooked rice, pasta, or oatmeal; one slice of bread; or one cup of ready-to-eat cereal flakes.

Hint: One cup looks like the amount of space taken up by a closed fist.

•**Protein.** Aim for two to three servings per day. One serving is three ounces of cooked fish, poultry, or lean meat; two eggs or four egg whites; one cup of cooked beans; one-half ounce of unsalted nuts or seeds; or one cup of tofu.

Hint: Three ounces looks like the amount of space taken by an open palm (not including the fingers or thumb).

•**Dairy.** Eat or drink two to three servings per day. One serving is one cup of low-fat or fat-free milk or yogurt; or one-third cup of shredded cheese.

Hint: A cup is 8 ounces, not a full drinking glass, some of which can hold 16 ounces or more.

•**Fruits and vegetables.** With fruits and vegetables, there's really no reason to worry about serving sizes or portions. They're packed with nutrients as well as fiber, which helps keep you fuller longer. The more produce you eat, the less room you'll have for junk food.

Note: This doesn't include fruit juice or dried or canned fruit, all of which are somewhat processed, high in sugar, calorie-dense, and easy to overeat.

As for those tasty, addictive ultra-processed sweets and treats, there's still room for them at the table, but be choosy and rein in the portions.

***Portion Hack #1:* Buy big bags, and then portion them out at home.**

It's human nature to eat more out of a large bag than a single-serving one. But single-serving packages of food, whether it's ultra-processed (like chips or candy) or healthy (almonds or baby carrots), cost more, so people tend to go for the bulk sizes.

That's fine, just portion the snacks out once you get home, keeping serving sizes in mind. Check the nutrition label and make sure it lists a single serving size. Most candies and chips will specify how many pieces per serving (for example, 12 peanut M&Ms or 17 pretzel twists). If you're still hungry, supplement your snack with a fruit or veggie.

***Portion Hack #2:* Scoop cereal.**

It can be all too easy to pour out several cups of cereal for breakfast, especially if you're in a rush and aren't being mindful. What you assume is one cup is usually closer to three. In a *Consumer Reports* test, people were asked to pour out the amount of cereal they'd typically eat for breakfast. Ninety-two percent of participants poured themselves more than the recommended serving size.

Some cereals, such as granola and muesli, are quite dense and high in calories. They can easily contain close to 300 calories for a two-thirds-cup serving. Two cups of your favorite granola could easily have more calories and sugar than a chocolate-covered ice-cream bar.

Keep measuring cups and scoops handy and aim for one cup of cereal flakes or two-thirds of a cup of chunkier cereal.

***Portion hack #3:* Use small bowls.**

In that same *Consumer Reports* test, people were given bowls in three different sizes: 12, 18, and 28 ounces. When using a 12-ounce bowl, study participants tended to pour themselves 24 to 92 percent more cereal than would be in a single serving. When using an 18-ounce bowl, it was 43 to 114 percent more.

Larger dishes make portions seem smaller. Select smaller bowls and dishes and whatever you're eating will appear to be more plentiful, which helps make you feel more satisfied.

You can also use this to your advantage to load up on vegetables and salad. In a 2019 study at Australia's Deakin University, people were given either a small or a large bag of baby carrots. Those presented with the bigger bag ate more carrots. Large portions of veggies will encourage you to eat more: the best-case portion distortion scenario.

Look at Labels, Not Just Names

Kellogg's Smart Start cereal sounds healthy, right? But a quick look at the nutrition label shows that it has the same amount of sugar in each serving as Cap'n Crunch: 4.5 teaspoons. Don't trust the name and always check the nutritional information label.

Consumer Reports.

Low-Protein Breakfasts Lead to Higher Calorie Intake

University of Sydney.

The Protein Leverage Hypothesis argues that the body craves protein over any other type of food. Because modern diets consist of highly processed and refined foods, which are low in protein, people eat more overall in an attempt to satisfy their protein demand. Researchers from the University of Sydney analyzed data from 9,341 adults and reported that those who ate less protein at breakfast (or whenever you eat your first meal) ate more calories, fat, sugar, salt, and less grains, vegetables/legumes, fruit, dairy, and meats for the rest of the day. People who received the recommended amount of protein, on the other hand, ate less throughout the day.

Get Rid of Your Bad Health Habits…for Good

Katy Milkman, Ph.D., James G. Diann Endowed Professor at The Wharton School of The University of Pennsylvania, author of *How to Change: The Science of Getting from Where You Are to Where You Want to Be* and host of the podcast *Choiceology.* KatyMilkman.com

Who hasn't lost 10 pounds only to gain back 15…or started working out every day only to fall back to once a week? Changing unhealthful habits is important—40 percent of premature deaths are linked to small things we can change. But the things we rely on to accomplish change—from journaling to willpower—often fall short. *Behavior scientist Katy Milkman, Ph.D., recommends these new research-based tools to get past the obstacles…*

•**Pick a meaningful "reset" day to start.** A symbolic day will have a "clean slate" effect—the start of a season…a holiday…the first day of the next month…or simply the very next Monday.

•**Build instant gratification into your plan.** *Add elements of fun to turn reaching the goal into a game…*

•Temptation bundling. Restrict an indulgence to when you're doing a virtuous activity. *Example:* Watch your favorite TV show only when you're exercising.

•Gamification. Look for a goal-oriented app that rewards daily achievements with badges or stars.

•**Deploy "commitment devices."** Set up binding deadlines with penalties if you miss them. *Examples…*

•Cash commitments. Set a goal…ask someone to track your progress…and give him/her a set amount of money that you'll forfeit to a charity if you don't stick to your plan.

•Psychological price tag. Tell friends about your goal, and post it on social media. You will feel uncomfortable if you don't reach it after having shared it with others.

•**Engineer new-habit reminders.** The more things we juggle, the harder it is to keep track of our intentions. It's easy to ignore the earlier bedtime you set for yourself when you're working on an important project. *What to do:* Set a go-to-sleep alarm on your phone.

•**Link the new habit to something you already do.** Floss right after brushing your teeth…link eating fruit with your morning coffee. The more you repeat a new task, the more habitual it becomes.

•**Be very detailed.** Break big goals into manageable chunks, and write down the steps you'll take to accomplish each chunk. If you are trying to lose 20 pounds, drill down to how you will lose one pound this week—how many fewer calories you will eat and where will you cut them out. Create a daily checklist to tick off each action.

•**Put actions on autopilot.** Create automatic deposits into your retirement account with every paycheck. Use an online grocery-delivery service to stock up on healthy foods.

•**Factor in flexibility.** Acknowledge that you might sometimes miss a workout or eat a high-calorie meal. Doing this will allow you to pick up where you left off and avoid letting a small slip turn into a major slide.

•**"Copy and paste."** Look to your circle of friends for people who were successful at what you want to achieve. Copy the strategies that fit your style.

Stick to Your Health Goals

Barry A. Franklin, Ph.D., Director of Preventive Cardiology & Cardiac Rehabilitation at Beaumont Health, and author of *GPS for Success: Skills, Strategies, and Secrets of Superachievers.* DrBarryFranklin.com

Here's a comprehensive six-point plan that can help you set goals—at any time of year—and achieve them.

STEP ONE: WRITE IT

•**Write down your goal.** "If it's not on paper, it's vapor," quipped Sir John Hargrave. Recognize that your subconscious mind is a powerful magnet for bringing goals into your life. Writing them down is the first step to making them a reality.

STEP TWO: PLAN IT

•**Develop a written, detailed plan to achieve your goal.** "A goal without a plan is just a wish," said writer Antoine de Saint-Exupéry.

•**Break down major goals into smaller manageable tasks.** Then use daily to-do lists to bring aspirations, desires, and goals into your life. For example, if your goal is to exercise more, break it into small, measurable tasks, such as taking a walk for 20 minutes each day or taking two 10-minute-long walks. Plan the time that will work best for you and mark it on your calendar. Think about possible conflicts and plan ahead so they don't derail you. For example, if you normally walk outside, but the weather forecast calls for rain, walk through the local mall instead. The more detailed your plan, the greater your likelihood of success.

STEP THREE: GET STARTED

•**Start the journey today.** Taking action helps you overcome inertia, which allows you to develop momentum. That makes it much easier to keep going and get the job done. Lao-Tzu said, "A journey of a thousand miles begins with a single step." If you don't start your journey, it's impossible to reach your goal.

STEP FOUR: TAKE ACTION EVERY DAY

Daily action toward your goal is the most powerful secret of success. It's better to spend one hour per day every day on a task to get you to your goal than it is to spend five hours on the weekend.

STEP FIVE: PERSIST

Most people try to meet a goal for a little while, but when the results come too slowly, they quit and look for something easier. They don't realize that if they had hung on a bit longer, they could have achieved their goals and reaped the rewards.

STEP SIX: BELIEVE

Radiate happiness, optimism, and gratitude for what you've already achieved in life. People who believe that good things invariably happen to them exhibit behaviors that attract the resources and circumstances they need to achieve their goals. Instead of viewing temporary setbacks with self-doubt, look at them as opportunities in disguise.

Get Back on Track

I've counseled countless people who had followed a healthy eating and exercise plan for a while, then attended a celebratory function and deviated for a day or two. All too often, they give up the entire plan because they mistakenly reason that all is lost. To avoid this pitfall, buy a half-gallon jar and display it prominently in your home. Put a penny in the jar for each day you work toward your goal. If you fall off the wagon for a day, remove a penny—but don't empty out all the precious pennies that you've earned to that point. The next day, get right back on track. When the jar is full, you'll be well on your way to achieving your goal. Cash in the pennies and buy yourself something special.

Time of Day You Burn the Most Calories

Study by researchers at Brigham and Women's Hospital, Boston, published in *Current Biology*.

Because of natural circadian rhythms, our bodies burn 10 percent more calories when at rest in the late afternoon and early evening than in the morning. And they burn the fewest resting calories during our "biological night"—when our body temperature falls. This finding may help explain why people with irregular sleep schedules are more likely to gain weight.

New Guideline for Calculating Healthy Weight

Recommendations from National Institute for Health and Care Excellence, which publishes guidelines based on evidence-based recommendations, London, U.K. NICE.org.uk

Body mass index (BMI), which uses height-to-weight ratio to calculate obesity-related health risks—such as high blood pressure, diabetes, heart disease, and stroke—does not take into account central adiposity (weight around the waist). New guidelines recommend that in addition to BMI, the height-to-waist ratio also should be taken into account—with a healthy ratio being a waist size that is less than half of height.

Note: Height-to-waist ratios are applicable for both sexes and all ethnic groups but are not appropriate for people with BMI over 35, pregnant women, or children under age two.

Exercise Preserves Muscle Better Than Protein

Study of 22 older women led by researchers at McMaster University, Hamilton, Ontario, Canada, published in *The Journal of Nutrition*.

The average American diet provides at least the recommended amount of protein (0.38 grams per pound of body weight)…but consuming higher amounts has not been shown to maintain muscle.

Recent finding: More protein synthesis occurred when participants increased their amount of daily walking than was associated with consuming extra protein through dairy and alternative dairy products.

Stretch to Feel Your Best

Michelle Leachman, professional education services program manager at the American Council on Exercise, San Diego, California.

Waking up with stiff, achy muscles and joints? Taking a few minutes to stretch can help you warm up your body and get your day off to a good start. *After taking a few deep breaths and drinking a cup of water, you might start with these moves…*

OVERHEAD TRICEPS STRETCH

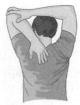

Stand with your feet hip-width apart. Roll your shoulders down and back. Reach your left arm up, bend it at the elbow, and let your hand drop to the middle of your back. Reach your right hand up and place your fingers on your left arm, near your elbow. Apply light pressure to deepen the stretch. Hold for 15 to 30 seconds. Repeat two to four times with each arm.

KNEELING HIP-FLEXOR STRETCH

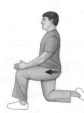

From a kneeling position, place your right knee on the floor, directly under your hip, and place your left foot forward, with your knee over your ankle. Place both hands gently on your left thigh. Keep a tall, straight spine, brace your abdominal muscles, and pull your shoulders down and back without arching your back. Lean forward into your right hip, keeping your left knee pressed down. Hold for 30 to 45 seconds and repeat two to five times on each side.

SHOULDER STABILITY STRETCH

Lie flat on your back with your knees bent and your feet on the floor. Place your arms out to the side, bent at the elbows, with your palms facing up. Stiffen your abdominal muscles and pull your shoulders back and down. Exhale

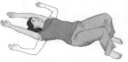

and slowly extend your arms above your head without shrugging your shoulders or arching your

Stretching Tips

•**Avoid holding your breath.** Instead, maintain smooth, steady breathing.

•**Don't bounce or jerk.** That can cause injury.

•**Stretch to the point of tension,** but don't stretch to the point of pain.

•**Take advantage of warmth.** If you miss the chance to stretch after exercise, when your muscles are warm, do some stretches after a hot bath or shower.

•**Accept that flexibility varies from person to person and even muscle to muscle.** A stretch that is easy for your workout partner may be hard for you. And you may find you are more flexible in one part of your body than another. If you keep working on your flexibility, hard moves should get easier.

back. Keep reaching until your thumbs touch the floor behind your head or to the point of tension. Hold for 15 to 30 seconds; then relax and return to the starting position. Repeat two to four times.

WORKOUT STRETCHES

There's a lot of confusion about whether it's best to stretch before or after exercise. In general, stretching after exercise, when your muscles are warmed up, is most effective. Stretching before some kinds of exercise can hurt performance. For example, serious weightlifters shouldn't stretch before lifting, because elongating muscles beforehand might interfere with the muscle-building process. However, there is a role for light stretching before some kinds of exercise. Brief static stretches, in which you stretch out a muscle and hold your position, can be helpful before exercises such as yoga or Pilates that involve more prolonged stretching. And dynamic stretching, in which you move your body fluidly through a stretch, can be part of your warm-up for activities such as running or dancing. A dynamic stretch might be something as simple as crossing your arms, one at a time, over your chest, while gently swinging your hips. Here are a few simple static stretches you might want to try after your main workout. *Try holding each for 10 to 30 seconds...*

HAMSTRING STRETCH

This stretch focuses on the back of the thigh and relieves tension in the back. Sit with your legs stretched out in front of you, or bend one leg and straighten the other. Straighten your back, and gently fold your upper body forward.

RECLINING FIGURE-4 STRETCH

This stretch focuses on the outer hip and gluteal muscles. It can relieve lower back tension. Lie on your back, with both knees bent and your feet flat on the floor. Cross your right foot over your left thigh and bring your legs toward your torso. Avoid straining. Instead, allow gravity to bring your legs closer to your body to deepen the stretch. Hold, and then repeat on the other side.

You can find more stretches at the American Council on Exercise's exercise library at: https://www.acefitness.org/resources/everyone/exercise-library/

Healthy Hot Weather Exercise

Jonathan Su, DPT, CSCS, TSAC-F, C-IAYT, physical therapist, yoga therapist, and former U.S. Army officer based in the San Francisco Bay area. Dr. Su is author of *6-Minute Fitness at 60+* and *6-Minute Core Strength*. https://sixminutefitness.com/about/

When consistently warm weather arrives, millions of Americans are out jogging, running, hiking, and biking. But summer exercise comes with some risks. Here's how to maintain your healthy habits while keeping yourself safe.

DEHYDRATION

Working up a sweat is great for health, but rising temperatures can set you up for dehydration. Older adults are especially prone because, as we age, we have a diminished ability to regulate temperature, recognize thirst, and store water. (The last has to do with age-related loss of muscle mass, as muscle helps hold on to water.) Older adults are also more likely to take medications that increase dehydration risk, like diuretics (for high blood pressure and heart failure) and antacids. Dehydration can cause dizziness, muscle cramps, balance issues, and can even land you in the hospital.

Stay safe: Most people assume that feeling thirsty is the first sign that they need to start hydrating, but by the time you feel thirsty, you're already on your way to becoming dehydrated. ***Prepare for outdoor exercise by prehydrating:*** increasing water intake for one or two days before the workout. This gives your body the chance to fully soak up all that hydration.

While exercising, sip water every 15 minutes. Plain water works well, or try electrolyte-enhanced water. Electrolytes are minerals (usually sodium, potassium, or magnesium) that help regulate hydration, blood pressure, and muscle contraction. Unsweetened coconut water is naturally rich in electrolytes and lower in sugar than many commercial sports drinks, so it may be a better choice, especially for people with diabetes.

If your urine is dark yellow or amber, it's an indicator you need more water. Pale yellow is ideal.

OVERHEATING

When your body is too hot for an extended period of time, it can overheat, just like your car. Peoples ages 65 and older are more likely to experience heat-related health complications than the general population, potentially even requiring hospitalization. *Overheating, also called hyperthermia, can lead to several dangerous conditions…*

- **Heat syncope can cause dizziness or fainting.** (If you take beta-blockers, you are especially susceptible to this condition.)

- **Heat exhaustion can manifest as weakness,** dizziness, thirst, nausea, poor coordination, excessive sweating, rapid heart rate, or clammy skin.

- **Heat stroke is an emergency requiring immediate medical care.** Signs include loss of consciousness; confusion, aggressiveness, or otherwise odd behavior; weak pulse; and not sweating despite extreme heat.

Stay safe: If possible, avoid exercising outdoors between 10 a.m. and 3 p.m., the hottest parts of the day. Check the heat index, a measure of how hot it feels once humidity is factored in, before heading out. (Humidity intensifies heat and prevents sweat from evaporating, hampering the body's natural cooling mechanism.) Exercise indoors if the heat index surpasses 90. Stay hydrated and wear light-colored, sweat-wicking materials and a hat that also covers the back of your neck. (Lighter colors absorb less heat.) If you feel faint, rest in a cool, ideally air-conditioned, area, with your legs elevated above your heart, and hydrate.

FALLING

Hiking is a wonderfully healthy activity for both body and mind, but it comes with the risks of tripping over rocks or branches, losing your footing while climbing up or down hills, and falling. Heavy backpacks can compromise balance. Nearly half of all mountain hiking accidents are caused by falls.

Falls happen on paved surfaces, too. In fact, many of my patients between ages 50 and 65 have fallen when walking on sidewalks or stepping off of curbs, usually because they were using their phone or otherwise not paying attention. This sort of distracted walking also changes your gait and speed.

Stay safe: Pay attention to your surroundings while hiking, running, speed-walking, or engaging in your favorite outdoor activity. Scan the ground for trip hazards, such as rocks, twigs, and holes. Avoid multitasking (such as texting while walking, jogging, or biking). If you are wearing a backpack, make sure there's not too much weight in the top half, which can throw you off-kilter.

Nordic-style walking poles, also called trekking poles, offer an additional layer of insur-

More Fitness Safety Tips

●**Always carry identification,** a bit of cash, and your phone with you in case of an emergency.

●**Tell a family member or friend where you're headed and when you plan to return.**

●**Brightly colored clothes in the daytime** and reflective materials and/or a flashlight at night will help drivers see you.

●**Wear proper shoes for your activity.** Avoid shoes with worn treads, which can be too slippery.

●**Try to avoid talking on the phone or listening to loud music;** both can make it difficult to hear approaching cars or bikers. (If you hear someone say, "On your left," it means a bike is coming up behind you and will pass on your left side.)

●**Choose routes with places to sit in case you want to stop and rest.**

●**Walk facing oncoming traffic,** but bike in the direction of traffic.

●**Always cross at intersections or crosswalks, with the crossing signal.** Don't assume a driver sees you when you're crossing. If possible, make eye contact with drivers as they approach.

●**If you are facing bad weather,** consider walking around malls or stores.

Source: The National Institute on Aging.

Toxic Combo: Sitting and Screen Time

Sara K. Rosenkranz, Ph.D., an associate professor in the Department of Kinesiology and Nutrition Sciences at the School of Integrated Health Studies, University of Nevada, Las Vegas, and Emily Mailey, Ph.D., an associate professor in the Department of Kinesiology, and director of the Physical Activity Intervention Research Lab, at Kansas State University.

Studies show that sitting *and* watching a screen, such as a TV, computer, smartphone, or video game, is worse for you than just sitting. Scientists aren't sure why. One reason may be that bouts of sitting tend to be more prolonged when you're watching a screen. Another possible factor is that screen time means you're likely to be sitting *and* mindlessly eating unhealthy foods such as chips and sweets.

Stepping Up Your Health Is Easier Than You Think

Kaberi Dasgupta, M.D., professor of medicine at McGill University, in Montreal, Canada, and director of the Centre for Outcomes Research and Evaluation at the Research Institute of the McGill University Health Centre. Dr. Dasgupta is the author of more than a dozen scientific studies on steps and health.

You and your doctor already use many "metrics" or measurements to monitor, protect, and improve your health: your weight, blood pressure, cholesterol, and blood sugar. But there's another metric that is just as informative about your health and well-being that you and your doctor probably don't track, but should: the number of *steps* you take every day.

Steps are an objective and accurate measure of how much you walk every day. And physical activities like walking (or the lack thereof) play a key role in your health and longevity. Two recent scientific studies show the crucial link between daily steps—and staying alive.

RISK OF DEATH HALVED

In a study published in September 2021 in *JAMA Network Open*, scientists from the Uni-

ance. Held like ski poles, they improve balance and stability while also working the upper body, which doesn't normally happen while hiking or walking. Look for ones with removable rubber tips that can be used on paved surfaces and then removed for hiking. Poles can be especially helpful for arthritis sufferers, offsetting the pressure on hips and knees. YMCAs often offer pole-walking classes.

Wear appropriate footwear, such as hiking sneakers or boots that provide traction and ankle support. Also, remember to pace yourself. When we're fatigued, we tend to not properly pick up our feet, which can lead to stumbles.

versity of Massachusetts Amherst tracked the daily steps of more than 2,000 middle-aged people. After 15 years, those who walked an average of at least 7,000 steps per day had an astounding 50 percent lower risk of premature death from any cause, compared with people who walked fewer than 7,000 daily steps.

That result may surprise you because taking 10,000 steps per day is routinely recommended for optimal health, but there is little scientific evidence to support that recommendation. That result may also hearten you and motivate you because 7,000 steps a day is much easier to achieve than 10,000.

In another study, published in *Lancet Public Health* in March 2022, an international team of researchers analyzed data from 47,000 people across 15 studies on daily step count and mortality. They found a much lower risk of "all-cause mortality" (death from any cause) in people over age 60 who regularly took 6,000 to 8,000 steps a day, compared with people who walked less.

MANY BENEFITS

Walking 7,000 steps a day doesn't just keep you alive; it also keeps you healthy...

•**Studies show that it can lower high blood pressure,** the number-one risk factor for heart attack and stroke.

•**It lowers your risk of developing and dying from heart disease.**

•**It improves insulin sensitivity,** the main risk factor for developing diabetes. (Insulin is the hormone that ushers blood sugar out of the bloodstream and into cells.)

•**It lowers A1C**—a measurement of long-term blood sugar levels—suggesting that it helps prevent or control type 2 diabetes.

•**It helps prevents overweight** and helps you maintain weight loss after you've shed pounds. Maintaining a normal weight reduces the risk of osteoarthritis and chronic pain because there's less strain on the knees and hips.

•**Walking 7,000 steps a day is also linked to better mood**—particularly less depression and anxiety.

•**It also helps build bone density,** strengthen lungs, and deepen sleep.

SMALL INCREASES, BIG BENEFITS

You don't even need to reach 7,000 steps a day to see significant benefits to your health. Research from McGill University in Canada shows that taking just 1,200 additional steps per day can decrease your risk of heart attack, stroke, heart failure, and dying from heart disease. It also can lower blood sugar, insulin, and insulin resistance, helping you prevent or control diabetes. It can even decrease your risk of all-cause mortality. These improvements are less than what you would achieve by walking 7,000 steps a day, but they're still significantly protective.

The benefits of increasing your step count by 1,200 a day are greatest in people who currently take the fewest steps. For example, if you're already walking 9,000 steps a day, increasing to 10,200 won't make that big of a difference in your health. But if your steps per day are currently 4,000—a common level for people who aren't physically active—getting to 5,200 can dramatically improve your health.

COUNTING YOUR STEPS

Counting your daily steps is easier than ever. There are many step-counting apps you can download to your phone, or you can buy a pedometer, a device you wear on your waist or put in your pocket that measures steps. Devices such as Fitbit and other smartwatches can track your daily steps along with other metrics, such as heart rate and blood oxygen level.

Find the app or device that fits your budget and lifestyle. However, don't spend less than $15 to $20 on a pedometer—devices less expensive than that aren't likely to be accurate. *Next, make a plan to get the optimal number of steps...*

***STEP 1:* Figure out how many steps you're walking every day.** To do that, use your step-counting device to track your steps every day for three days. If your device doesn't store daily steps, use a written log, noting your daily step total at bedtime. Make sure to note the daily total before midnight, when your pedometer may automatically reset your step count to zero. Your total number of steps divided by three is your daily average.

Boost Your Motivation

There are several reasons why monitoring daily steps is uniquely motivating in helping you achieve your goal for regular physical activity.

Tracking steps is ideal for goal-setting and goal-reaching: A step count tells you where you are right now, helps you know where you want to go, and lets you know whether or not you got there—and adjust accordingly.

The device you use to count your steps also gives you *instant feedback*—you can periodically check it throughout the day to see how you're doing, making it much more likely you'll achieve your daily goal.

The device also measures your physical activity all day, not just when you're exercising. It's motivating when everything you do—short of sitting—counts as physical activity.

Bottom line: Research shows that people who have a steps-per-day walking goal and wear a step-counting device tend to get more steps than people who have a minutes-per-day goal (such as walking 30 minutes every day, five days a week).

STEP 2: **Set a goal.** Perhaps you'd like to increase your count by 1,200 steps per day. Perhaps you'd like to reach 7,000 steps daily, or even 10,000.

STEP 3: **Decide how many steps you want to increase on a daily basis.** You may want to add 100 more steps per day every week. If you started at 4,000 steps as your daily average, for example, you would walk 4,100 steps each day the first week, 4,200 steps each day the second week, etc. Try not to make big changes all at once, like increasing from 5,000 to 10,000 daily steps in one week. Small, incremental changes are the most likely to become habitual.

STEP 4: **Choose ways you're going to increase your daily step count.** Adding a daily walk is a great idea. A walk of 20 minutes at a moderate pace is about 2,000 steps (2,000 steps = 1 mile). You can also break that up into two shorter walks. Walking a dog is a great way to get more steps in. Along with the many other benefits of owning a dog, research shows that dog owners walk an average of 2,760 more steps per day than people who don't own dogs. If you don't want your own dog, you can volunteer to walk dogs at a local animal shelter.

There are also many "little" ways to increase your step count—and they add up…
- **Walk while talking on your phone.**
- **Instead of driving,** walk to a destination, like a store.
- **If you drive,** park farther away from your destination and walk the rest of the way.
- **In a parking lot,** park the farthest distance from the entrance.
- **Avoid drive-throughs**—get out of your car and walk inside.
- **Empty wastebaskets every day.**

GET SOCIAL SUPPORT

Walking with a family member or friend is a wonderful way to help motivate yourself to achieve your daily step goal. Similarly, devices such as Fitbit allow you to make friends or join a like-minded group on the Fitbit platform and report your daily steps. People who do so take about 700 more steps a day than people who don't. Similar apps include SocialStepsApp.com. There are also online walking communities on Facebook and other social media, such as the Pacer Pedometer and Walker Tracker pages on Facebook.

If you enjoy walking alone, try listening to your favorite music, podcast, or audiobook, but be sure to remain aware of your surroundings.

Best Time to Exercise Varies by Gender

Study of 30 adults led by researchers at Skidmore College, Saratoga Springs, New York, published in *Frontiers in Physiology*.

For women, exercising in the morning is better for reducing fat, especially abdominal fat, and improving blood pressure…exercising in the evening is best for increasing strength. For men, time of day mattered less for improving strength…but evening exercise improved heart and metabolic health.

Best Walking Break for Prolonged Sitting

Study titled "Breaking Up Prolonged Sitting to Improve Cardiometabolic Risk: Dose-Response Analysis of a Randomized Cross-Over Trial," led by researchers at the Center of Behavioral Cardiovascular Health, Columbia University Medical Center, New York City, published in *Medicine & Science in Sports & Exercise.*

When the saying "sitting is the new smoking" was coined by James Levine, M.D., Ph.D., specialist in obesity, it seemed like a stretch. Now it's not so far-fetched, especially as manual labor is replaced by technology and more bodies face computers for hours. Health risks from prolonged sitting include an increased risk of high blood pressure, type 2 diabetes, and obesity. It makes sense for people to get up and move at regular intervals, but few studies have tried to answer the questions of how much moving and how often to get up to counteract the health hazards of sitting too long.

Researchers from Columbia University's Vagelos College of Physicians and Surgeons have reported on a study that looked at the effects of four short periods of walking, called exercise "snacks." This is the first study to compare several exercise options that could easily be done by people who are at risk from prolonged sitting.

The study is published in *Medicine & Science in Sports & Exercise*, the journal of the American College of Sports Medicine. The study is called a randomized cross-over trial because each person entered in the study randomly completed four exercise options during five separate days of sitting for eight hours under study conditions.

Eleven middle- and older-age adults completed the study. In addition to the exercise options, each subject completed one day of uninterrupted sitting to be compared to the exercise options. Results of this day were used as the baseline or control. On all the days of the study, blood sugar and blood pressure were monitored, and the participants were asked about any changes in energy or mood. Subjects were all given the same meals. While sitting, the people were in comfortable ergonomic chairs and were allowed to read, talk on the phone, or use a laptop computer. Exercise breaks were light-intensity walking on a treadmill.

The key results of four exercise options as compared to the control day showed that one minute of walking both every 30 minutes and every hour of sitting significantly reduced blood pressure. Five minutes of walking every hour of sitting also showed a significant reduction in blood pressure...and five minutes for every 30 minutes of sitting significantly reduced blood pressure and blood sugar.

So the obvious winner for the research team to lower blood pressure and blood sugar is walking for five minutes every 30 minutes. All the walking options significantly improved mood and fatigue, except walking one minute every hour. The researchers note that the obvious benefits may encourage "sitters" to take their walking breaks.

Previous studies have shown that prolonged sitting is bad for your health even if you exercise regularly when you are not sitting. When you sit for eight hours without exercise breaks, your large muscles use very little sugar for energy, increasing your risk of high blood sugar, type 2 diabetes, and other health problems. Taking a five-minute walking break every 30 minutes may be a simple way to reduce these risks.

You're Never Too Old to Build Strength

Sharlyn Green, MBA, national trainer at Tivity Health; the owner and manager of Core Connection LLC, Peoria, Arizona; and the campus director of resident programs, Freedom Plaza Care Center Peoria. She earned her MBA in management and healthcare administration.

Focused strength training is one of the best ways to reverse the loss of muscle mass and to build muscle. Effective strength training can include a variety of options: body-weight exercises, such as squats and push-up variations; group exercise classes such as yoga or mat Pilates; weight training with barbells, hand weights, or strength-training machines at the gym; and resistance training with tools like elastic tubing. Functional body weight exercises—like squats, lunges, and pushups—are very effective for building total body strength because they are multi-joint movements that work larger groups of muscles.

Some of the symptoms of "old age" are not actually the result of aging. They are the result of inactivity. In every stage of life, and at all ages, exercise is proven to be beneficial, but some seniors may not feel comfortable with traditional strength training. Are there exercises for people who may feel intimidated by the idea of weightlifting?

These three strength-focused exercises are a great place to start your strength-training journey. Make sure to pay attention to how you feel and progress to a more difficult option once you can complete the more basic exercise with perfect form.

•**Chair Squat or Sit to Stand.** Standing up from a seated position is something most of us do multiple times each day. We can build lower body strength and core strength, protecting our joints and maintaining mobility, if we pay attention to form and alignment.

How to perform a chair-based squat. Sit in a chair and scoot forward, making sure your knees are directly over your feet and your feet are about hip-distance apart. Press down on the four corners of the chair to stabilize, and engage your core by drawing your belly button in. Sit up, lengthening your spine, and hinge forward slightly at the hips, allowing your upper body to begin to shift forward while keeping your chest up and your gaze forward. You can support your back by placing your hands on your thighs, progressing to rising from the chair without support.

Adding hand-weights creates more challenge. Make sure to maintain proper form and neutral postural alignment while pressing up to a standing position and while you descend back into the chair. This movement can also start from a standing position, right in front of the chair, moving into a mini squat and progressing until you come to a completely seated position. Squats can be combined with upper body movements, such as biceps curls and

Joints Are Meant to Move

Some seniors believe that strength training will make their joints hurt more. The truth is that our joints are designed to move! Painful, achy joints may make you think twice about movement and exercise, but severely limiting movement can cause your muscles to weaken, which affects posture and core strength. Lack of movement can even make joint pain worse in the long run. Some of the common causes of chronic joint pain—osteoarthritis, poor posture, past injuries, inactivity, and poor movement form and mechanics—can be addressed by strengthening the muscles that support your joints along with a gentle flexibility and stretching practice. The right exercises can go a long way to helping to support your body and improve joint function.

Your joints are more resilient with regular exercise. Over time, with a regular strength-training routine, you may find that your joint range of motion improves and your strength increases, making it easier, and more fun, to do the things you enjoy. *Some tips for a joint-friendly workout…*

•**Be kind to your joints,** and take time to heal any current injuries.

•**Warm up before strength training.** Dynamic, gentle moving stretches and low-intensity, low-impact movement is best for those with joint pain.

•**Don't push through sharp or acute pain.**

•**Slow and steady progression is important when dealing with joint pain.**

•**It can be helpful to begin with movements that strengthen your core muscles.** Strengthening core muscles will help improve your posture and give you a foundation of strength to move forward.

•**Try working with an exercise professional** to make sure you move with proper form and alignment.

•**Give your body the time it needs to recover after workouts,** especially more intense or challenging workouts, so you can return to strength training with energy, fully recovered and ready to go.

front raises or lateral raises, which target shoulder muscles, for more upper body challenge.

•**Farmer's Walk.** Walking is something we do every day. A Farmer's Walk adds resistance, training your lower body, upper body, and stabilizing core muscles.

Find a place where you have room to walk. Choose weights that are manageable, not too heavy, to begin this exercise. Starting at a neutral stance, with eyes forward and a tall spine, hold the weights next to your hips. Brace your core before you begin to walk at a slow and steady pace. Keep your chest lifted as though there is a string lifting the sternum up gently toward the ceiling, and find a tall, neutral spine. Be careful to stop completely before turning carefully to return to your starting point. Start with 30 seconds to five minutes, depending on your ability level. You can progress with heavier weights, or increase your time performing the Farmer's Walk, as you feel stronger.

•**Tree Pose.** Not only does this yoga pose help build balance and confidence, but it also builds lower body and core strength.

Standing by your chair or countertop, find a focal point straight ahead. Gently engage your abdominals and adjust your posture until you feel tall and aligned. Shift your weight toward your right foot as you lift your left heel, noticing the balance challenge. Keep the knee on your standing leg slightly bent, not allowing it to lock. Open the hip by opening your left knee toward the left side, engaging your gluteal muscles in the back of your hip.

You can kickstand the left heel above your right ankle or place the sole of the left foot on your right calf for more balance challenge. Try adjusting your hold on the chair or countertop until you feel challenged, but in control and safe. Eventually, you can try lifting one or both arms up like the branches of a tree.

START LOW AND SLOW

One key to a safe and effective strength-training routine is to start with lower resistance,

Exceeding the Exercise Guidelines Increases Longevity

Meeting the minimal recommendation of 300 minutes of moderate physical activity weekly or 150 minutes of vigorous activity is associated with at least a 19 percent lower risk for early death.

Recent finding: Doubling or even quadrupling those numbers reduces risk by up to another 13 percent. Check with your doctor before starting an exercise program.

Edward Giovannucci, M.D., professor of nutrition and epidemiology at Harvard University, Boston, and coauthor of a study published in *Circulation*.

progressing slowly as you get stronger. Don't jump right in and overdo it with heavy weights or high repetitions. This can lead to soreness and injury. It's important to train with proper form and alignment so you don't reinforce poor posture and movement patterns that can create pain.

Make sure to work with a trainer or instructor who has the proper training to keep you moving in the right direction for years to come. When starting a new exercise program, especially if you're new to exercise, if you haven't exercised in a while, or if your health status has changed, consult your health-care provider for advice on how to get into the swing of things safely so you can reap the most benefits from your efforts.

Finding a regular exercise program that you enjoy will help keep you motivated and consistent. At SilverSneakers.com, you'll find a variety of exercise classes, including classes that focus on strength training. In fact, we have over 110 live virtual classes each week that can help keep you healthy strong and connected. You can check your eligibility at https://tools.silver sneakers.com/Eligibility/CheckEligibility

CHAPTER 10

Get the Best Medical Care

Yes...You Can Be Treated at Cleveland Clinic, Yale, or Johns Hopkins

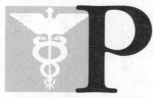Patients interested in seeking care from the Mayo Clinic, Johns Hopkins, Memorial Sloan Kettering Cancer Center, or another big-name medical institution often think they need some sort of connection or "in" to do so.

Reality: Anyone may request an appointment at one of these recognized facilities, regardless of geographic location or personal connections...and very often no physician referral is necessary, although it might make things easier.

We asked patient advocate Annette Ticoras, M.D., how to get the best medical treatment...

•**Pick your place.** Do you have friends or family members who have been successfully treated at a certain big-name medical center? Have you read about a promising treatment protocol being used at a specific iconic hospital? Start researching that institution. You also can ask your current doctor for a recommendation by saying, "I trust your diagnosis/ treatment recommendation, but before I start this process, can you recommend a hospital that specializes in cancer/autoimmune/organ transplant?"

•**Call your insurance carrier.** Most renowned hospitals accept insurance, including Medicare. Search the hospital's website for a list of its accepted insurance companies, then double-check with your insurance carrier. Also ask the insurer if a referral is necessary. If your hospital of choice isn't in-network, ask your insurance company, "If my current in-network physician writes a referral, does that change my coverage at all?"

•**Contact the hospital.** On the hospital's website, look for the "Make an Appointment"

Annette Ticoras, M.D., physician, board-certified patient advocate, and owner of Guided Patient Services, Inc., Westerville, Ohio. GPSColumbus.com button, typically prominently placed on the home page…or call the hospital directly. You will be connected with a care adviser or an intake coordinator who will walk you through the initial steps, including reviewing insurance coverage and outlining what medical records the facility will need.

•**Share your medical records.** You may be able to download your medical records yourself from your patient portal or simply call your health-care provider's office and request them. If your current doctor's office uses Epic's My-Chart electronic health record platform, there's a good chance that the new institution does as well, which means that the new provider can easily access your biopsy results, imaging scans, and more.

•**Plan your travel.** The hospital you choose will offer a packing checklist (including seasonal items, such as a winter coat if you're traveling from Georgia to, say, Minnesota in January) and a detailed list of medical documents to bring, including a list of all your medications and your Medicare or insurance card. The hospital's medical concierge team can help you coordinate travel details and hotel or lodging, often at discounted rates. In some cases, lodging even may be physically connected to the hospital itself.

If staying onsite for treatment isn't an option: If staying near the hospital is cost-prohibitive or you'd simply prefer to be treated at home, ask if the hospital can provide you with a treatment plan that your local medical team can carry out. The local physician has to agree to this new plan and have the means by which to provide that care safely or he/she may be able to find a system nearer to your home that offers the new preferred treatment plan.

•**Consider getting a virtual second opinion.** If having an expert from a top hospital review your arthritis, cardiac, or cancer case will help you feel rock-solid confident about your diagnosis and/or treatment plan but travel isn't in the cards, there is another option. Yale Medicine, Massachusetts General Hospital, Duke Health, Cleveland Clinic, University of Chicago Medicine, and more offer virtual second-opinion programs, also called "remote

second opinion programs." Insurance likely won't cover this, but you usually can use funds from your Health Savings Account or Flexible Spending Account. Rates range from around $700 (Stanford Medicine) to $2,400 (Dana Farber).

Procedures vary, but generally you create an account with the institution…are assigned a care coordinator…and send in the requested medical information. You will receive a written diagnosis or treatment plan several days to a week or so later. Some programs also include a telehealth or phone consultation.

Note: A handful of states do not permit second opinions over state lines. Check your program's website to be sure.

Emergency Health-Care Documents: How to Get Them in a Hurry

Ray Prather, JD, CPA, partner of the law firm Prather Ebner Wilson, Chicago. PEWLaw.com

What happens if you're in an accident or have a sudden illness that requires risky emergency surgery—but you haven't named anyone to make medical decisions for you in the event that you can't do it yourself?

If you don't already have a health-care proxy and other documents in place, the medical decision-making usually will fall to your spouse…your adult children…or your parents, in that order.

Problem: If that rubric leaves the decision-making to multiple people or to someone you're not comfortable with, you may need to create a health-care proxy document, a living will, and an estate will quickly.

GET THE RIGHT DOCUMENTS…FAST

•**Health-care proxy.** Also called a health-care power of attorney, this document names someone to make medical decisions for you. The process for getting the right paperwork varies by state. Often, you can simply print

Beware of ER Misdiagnoses

More than seven million misdiagnoses occur in US emergency rooms every year, killing or disabling 370,000 patients. Bring an advocate with you…ask to see the physician in charge…don't accept discharge if you're not feeling better. Be skeptical of diagnoses such as stress/anxiety, panic attack, and "viral syndrome" that share symptoms with serious often misdiagnosed conditions such as heart attack, stroke, and kidney infection.

Joel Cohen, M.D., medical director at the primary medical-care practice DoctorCare, Scottsdale, Arizona, commenting on a report from the US Department of Health and Human Services' Agency for Healthcare Research and Quality. DoctorCareAZ.com

a health-care proxy form from the Internet and sign it before a witness. But you will need guidance about which decisions it covers in your state and what's required to make it legally binding, so get an estate attorney on the phone or ask the hospital's patient advocate.

•**Living will.** In some states, the health-care proxy also extends to end-of-life decisions such as removing medical care or withholding life-sustaining treatments. In other states, you'll need a separate living will, also available on the Internet. Again, check with an estate attorney or the hospital's patient advocate.

•**Do-Not-Resuscitate order (DNR) or Physician Orders for Life-Sustaining Treatment (POLST).** If you don't want CPR, you'll need a document specific to that effect, separate from the living will. Withholding CPR must be ordered by a physician, so consult your doctor to complete one.

•**Will and durable power of attorney.** If you don't have a will and durable power of attorney in place, you might want to quickly draw them up to indicate your wishes regarding your property. But be sure to consult an attorney so you don't introduce complications for your heirs. Many estate-law firms will help you in an emergency…and several states—with many more soon to follow—have be-

gun accepting electronic wills, which further speeds the process.

PREVENTION

Of course, the best scenario is to have all these documents in place long before an emergency. The price for having these documents drawn up varies based on the market, but a reputable estate attorney will give an estimate of the fees before you hire him/her.

Beyond COVID…The Age of Self-Testing—Is It Right for You?

David Sherer, M.D., retired anesthesiologist, patient advocate, and author of Hospital Survival Guide: The Patient Handbook to Getting Better and Getting Out *and* What Your Doctor Won't Tell You. *DrDavidSherer.com*

Not long ago, at-home health tests were only for pregnancy and glucose monitoring. But advances in understanding of the human genome have opened the door to a wide-reaching array of DNA tests. And the shrinking number of medical providers has contributed to the explosion in the number of home tests available to detect chronic conditions that we used to rely on office visits to pick up. There are at-home tests for everything from cholesterol to testosterone now.

But beware: With many tests, you could be wading into murky waters. *Patient advocate and longtime Bottom Line Personal contributor David Sherer, M.D., says to proceed with caution…*

THE GOOD, THE BAD…THE INACCURATE

There are advantages and disadvantages to at-home tests.

On the positive side…

•**You don't have to go to a doctor.** These days, seeing a doctor could involve waiting months for an appointment. At-home tests are especially helpful for people living in areas where there are doctor shortages. Keep in mind, though—only a limited number of at-home tests can be done entirely from home…

the more common scenario is to purchase a test online and go to a lab for a blood draw.

•**You can test or prescreen if you're at risk for certain conditions**—perhaps heart disease runs in your family. Testing before any symptoms develop allows you to get ahead on the treatment curve.

•**You can monitor chronic conditions with fewer doctor and lab visits.** Certain home tests, such as measuring your blood pressure with a cuff and monitoring blood glucose, can help you make adjustments in diet and exercise or talk to your doctor about changes in a treatment plan.

On the negative side…

•**You can get false-positives or false-negatives,** especially from tests that haven't been approved by the FDA or if a test kit wasn't handled properly. Results also may be inaccurate because of timing.

Example: If you think you were exposed to HIV and test yourself for antibodies sooner than three to six months after exposure, you could get a false-negative. Also, it can be confusing to do a home test accurately—some people find it hard to do a finger prick for a blood sample and do not get enough blood.

•**Some tests give an incomplete picture of disease risk.**

Examples: Many tests for BRCA gene mutations—which indicate risk for breast cancer—check for only the three most common mutations even though there are thousands of possible ones. Some cholesterol tests measure only total cholesterol, which can be misleading.

•**You might misinterpret the results of any test—positive or negative.** It is always best to review your results with your medical provider, who can compare them to past results.

•**Your privacy could be at risk if the testing company enters your results into a database that could be compromised.** Always read through all disclosures on the testing company's website, and limit what it can do with your results.

•**You have to pay for them.** With the exception of the COVID-19 test, which is reimbursable, at-home tests are not covered by insurance, though you may be able to use FSA or HSA dollars.

TO GET THE RIGHT RESULTS

Careful research can help you avoid many of the disadvantages listed above…

•**Buy only FDA-approved tests.** Many at-home tests are "lab-developed tests" (LDTs), which are not FDA-approved. If a test has been approved by the FDA, it's likely to say so on the package and the company website. A Google search should let you know for sure.

•**Look for companies that work with, or are themselves, a well-known lab**—such as Quest Diagnostics or Labcorp. There should be a phone number that you can call with questions or to get online help with how to do the test. For some companies, like those mentioned here, test requests and results are reviewed by an independent physician who you might be able to speak with.

•**Beware of surprising consequences of your results.** Though the costs of at-home tests aren't typically reimbursed by insurance, you should call your plan administrator to find out if your results might impact your coverage in any way.

Example: If a genetic test shows that you have a BRCA gene mutation, will your insurance accept the result and cover more frequent mammograms?

•**Read the directions once…twice… three times.** Test accuracy depends on the manufacturer's ability to produce a quality test and your ability to do the test correctly. Even something as common as blood sugar testing can be inaccurate if you don't prick your finger as directed.

People with diabetes: The FDA recently cleared the POGO Automatic Blood Glucose Monitoring System, the first one-step monitor—you place your fingertip on the pad of the device, and a built-in lancet and the device do the rest.

•**Don't decipher the next steps on your own.** A doctor should interpret your results and review them with you.

Safer Self-Testing

The two US testing giants Quest Diagnostics and Labcorp have made a variety of direct-to-consumer screening and diagnostic tests available through their specialty divisions, QuestDirect (QuestDirect.Quest Diagnostics.com) and Labcorp On Demand (OnDemand.Labcorp.com). Both services let you shop for, order, and pay for tests online. You then make an appointment to have blood drawn at one of their facilities and set up a private online account through a patient portal for access to the results. Independent physicians review all tests and may be available to speak with you about results by phone.

—David Sherer, M.D.

Also: Because of liability factors, he/she may insist on repeating the test—this also will reassure you that the results are accurate.

Caution: Test results for life-altering diseases such as HIV or a genetic mutation for cancer can be emotionally devastating. It's crucial to have the proper interpretation and care from a medical professional.

•**Understand the test's limitations.**

Examples: Cologuard can pick up certain markers for cancer, but it's not a substitute for a colonoscopy, especially for people at high risk. Many cholesterol tests give only your total cholesterol count, but you need to know the breakdown of LDL, HDL, the ratio and triglycerides to determine whether your numbers are in the safe zone. Look for an FDA-approved "complete lipid panel test," such as the one from Solana Health.

Genetic tests, which were started to help people learn more about their heritage, have expanded into assessing risk for certain illnesses, perhaps based on family history. But this isn't something you should leave to home testing.

•**Be wary of tests with dubious science behind them.** Some types of tests are simply of unproven value.

Example: DNA testing to uncover the best diet for you based on your genes (a twist on the 1990s' fad of eating according to your blood type, a concept that was completely debunked). A study on this topic, published in *JAMA* in 2018, found no association between a person's genotype and whether he/she would have success on either a low-carb or low-fat diet.

Also be wary about at-home testing for diet sensitivities and allergies. Non-FDA tests may give you faulty results, and if you stop eating certain food groups based on incorrect information, you could end up with a nutrient deficiency.

Your Adult Vaccination Checklist

William Schaffner, M.D., medical director of the National Foundation for Infectious Diseases (NFID) and professor of preventive medicine and infectious diseases, Vanderbilt University Medical Center, Nashville. VUMC.org

We all are weary of the constant messaging to get COVID-19 vaccines—but that doesn't make the need for immunizations for other infectious diseases any less important. *Bring this checklist to your next health-care appointment to make sure you are up to date on all of your vaccinations…*

•**Flu.** Everyone six months and older should be vaccinated against influenza annually. Certain people are at high risk for flu complications, including older adults and those with chronic illnesses. Optimal time to get the vaccine is October through early November for maximum protection from December to February, when flu season peaks.

For people age 65+: Three types of flu vaccine are recommended for older adults—a high-dose shot…an adjuvant vaccine, which provokes a stronger immune reaction…and a recombinant vaccine, which is safe for people with egg allergies. All of these work better than the standard flu shots given to adults under age 65.

•**Pneumonia.** All adults ages 65 and older should get vaccinated for pneumonia. If you are younger than 65 but have an illness or risk factors, ask your doctor if you should get a pneumonia shot sooner.

•**Shingles.** This infection causes painful blisters and nerve pain. It is caused by the chickenpox virus, which lies dormant in the body after childhood infection until something triggers it. Two shots separated by two to six months are recommended for all adults over age 50.

•**Hepatitis B.** Adults up to age 60 should receive a hepatitis B vaccine to prevent liver disease caused by this virus, which is spread through contact with blood, semen, and bodily fluids, typically during sexual contact or use of contaminated needles. Hepatitis B virus (HBV) also can be spread through household contact with HBV-infected people. You're unlikely to get it after age 60, but if you have diabetes and monitor blood sugar via finger sticks or give yourself insulin injections, ask your doctor if you should get the vaccine.

•**Tetanus and diphtheria.** A booster of this vaccine is needed every 10 years.

•**COVID-19.** Updated vaccines by Pfizer/ BioNTech and Moderna are recommended by the CDC to replace the original vaccines. Both have been adapted to the primary COVID-19 strain and subsequent variants. Both vaccines are authorized for people as young as six months old. The CDC recommends that everyone age six or older should receive one vaccine. People younger than six or older than 65 or those with a compromised immune system may need additional doses.

For added protection: If your previous shots were all of one brand, try a different brand if you are over the age of 60. Check with CDC.gov for COVID vaccine updates.

To find vaccine locations: Visit Vaccines. gov.

•**Monkeypox.** This disease rarely causes death, but it can necessitate quarantine for several weeks. Monkeypox spreads through prolonged close contact such as hugging or touching or via shared clothing and towels. Vaccines are available only to high-risk people through state and local health departments.

•**Polio.** If you weren't vaccinated as a child, were incompletely vaccinated, or are traveling to a place where you could be exposed to poliovirus, the CDC recommends a series of up to three shots, several months apart.

Treating Skin of Color

Kassahun Bicha, M.D., FAAP, dermatologist with U.S. Dermatology Partners and the co-chair of the National and International Committee for Skin of Color Society.

Dermatology is a visual field. In many cases, a skilled physician can make a diagnosis based solely on what something looks like.

But there's a glaring gap in dermatology education: Many physicians are trained on what diseases look like on white patients only. In fact, a study published in the *Journal of the American Academy of Dermatology* found that only 4 to 18 percent of the images in dermatology textbooks show black or brown skin. Some books don't have a single example of acne, psoriasis, or dermatitis on dark skin.

A physician who has been trained to recognize eczema by how it looks on white skin may struggle to recognize this common disease when it looks different on black and brown skin, Kassahun Bicha, M.D., FAAP, told us.

COMMONLY MISSED CONDITIONS

Part of the diagnostic dilemma is that darker skin may not look red when it is inflamed or irritated. *This simple difference can affect the diagnosis of a variety of issues...*

•**Cellulitis** can look purplish or brown.

•**Eczema** can look brown, violet, or gray. Further, darker-skinned people with eczema are more likely to develop bumps on their arms, legs, and torso, as well as dark, bumpy circles under the eyes—something not often seen in white patients.

•**Psoriasis,** usually red or pink on white skin, is often salmon-colored with a silvery-white scale on brown skin. It can be dark brown or violet with a gray scale on black skin.

•**Melanoma.** People with darker skin often develop melanoma lesions on the soles of their feet, palms of the hand, fingernails, toenails, or inside the mouth. A dermatologist who is looking for lesions on sun-exposed skin can easily miss these, which may help explain why skin cancer is often diagnosed late and has a poor prognosis in people with black or brown skin.

Several skin conditions are more common in Black and Brown patients...

•**Post-inflammatory hyperpigmentation** consists of darkened patches of skin located at the site of previous inflammation or injury.

•**Pseudofolliculitis barbae** occurs when hairs either leave the hair follicle and curl back into the skin or penetrate the skin before leaving the hair follicle. The body reacts by causing inflammation and bumps.

•**Melasma** appears as brown-gray patches of skin on and around the cheeks, lips, chin, nose, and forehead

•**Acne keloidalis nuchae** is a long-term inflammatory condition that leads to inflamed plaques and papules on the head or neck.

•**Dermatosis papulosa nigra** causes benign skin growths on the neck and face that may be skin-colored or hyperpigmented.

•**Keloids.** People with darker skin are more prone to develop these raised scars.

•**Vitiligo** affects people of any skin color, but the white or lightened patches it causes are more obvious on darker skin, making the condition more distressing.

IMPROVE CARE

When it comes to skin health, Black and Brown patients need to be proactive, informed, and persistent to get the right diagnoses and treatments.

•**When researching skin conditions online,** look for photos of skin conditions on your own skin color. (See the sidebar for websites to try.)

•**Don't settle for the first diagnosis you get.** If you're unsure about a diagnosis or a treatment isn't working, get a second (or third) opinion.

•**There are a growing number of dermatology practices that specialize in**

Photographic Resources

You and your dermatologist can now find a wealth of photos showing how common skin conditions look on Black and Brown patients. *Here are a few to try...*

Black & Brown Skin

BlackAndBrownSkin.co.uk

Brown Skin Matters

Instagram.com/brownskin matters/?hl=en

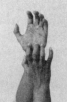

black and brown skin. Try the doctor finder feature on the Skin of Color Society website https://skinofcolorsociety.org.

•**If you can't find a local provider,** consider a doctor who offers video appointments that you can do over the phone or computer.

•**Once you find a dermatologist that you trust, undergo routine skin checks.**

•**Ask your hairdresser or barber to tell you if they notice any suspicious spots.** He or she may be the first person to spot evidence of skin cancer on your scalp, neck, or face.

•**Use a broad-spectrum, water-resistant sunscreen of at least SPF 30 every day.**

Best—and Worst—States for Retiree Health Care

Jeff Smedsrud, cofounder of HealthCare.com, a health insurance comparison tool that publishes the online Medicare resource MedicareGuide.com. He previously was senior vice president of the insurance company IHC Group.

Choosing where you will live in retirement isn't just about picking a state with low taxes and lots of sunshine. As the years go by, the odds go up that the health-care system will play a major role in your life—and the cost, quality, and availability of health care varies dramatically. While some people consider health care when selecting a destination, their analysis rarely goes further than confirming there's a well-regarded hospital nearby. While a state might have highly regarded hospitals, it also might impose relatively steep out-of-pocket costs on Medicare enrollees… or many doctors might not accept Medicare. MedicareGuide.com ranked the 50 states plus the District of Columbia* on 24 measures related to quality, cost, and accessibility of health care available to seniors. *Among its findings…*

OVERALL RANKINGS

First place: Minnesota

Last place: Oklahoma

Key takeaway: Whatever climate, region, and population density you have in mind for your retirement destination, you can find a suitable state that offers top-tier senior health care.

When it comes to delivering health care to seniors, the two states at the very top of the rankings also are at the very geographic top of the country—Minnesota and North Dakota. *These states receive high marks in a range of health-care–related measures…*

North Dakota has the lowest prescription-drug prices and the fewest doctors who don't accept Medicare. Minnesota has the second-highest ratio of home health aides per capita and the third-highest life expectancy. If those brisk Midwestern locales aren't what you have in mind, warm Hawaii and California make the top 10…as do wealthy Northeastern states Massachusetts and Connecticut…mountain meccas Colorado and Montana…and two more Midwestern options—Nebraska and Iowa.

The main connection among these states: Most made an effort to improve their health-care systems in the 1980s and 1990s, suggesting that state government initiatives can improve health-care quality, but doing so takes time.

Worst states for senior health care: Oklahoma, Georgia, D.C., Mississippi, Louisiana, West Virginia, North Carolina, Alabama, Tennessee, and South Carolina.

If you're wondering about popular retirement destinations that aren't in the top or bottom 10, Maine lands at 12…Arizona at 15…

New Mexico at 18…Vermont at 19…Florida at 23…Texas at 35…and Nevada at 37.

HEALTH-CARE COSTS

First place: Utah

Last place: D.C.

Key takeaway: High-cost-of-living states aren't always high-cost-of-health-care states for seniors.

States with the lowest overall senior health-care costs include Utah, California, South Carolina, Kansas, Minnesota, Iowa, Arizona, Arkansas, New Mexico, and North Dakota. It might come as a surprise to see California—known for its high costs—on that list, but senior health-care costs can be counterintuitive, with government subsidies and spending creating unexpected distortions.

Examples: North Carolina, California, and Hawaii have the lowest prescription-drug prices—even though Hawaii and California are expensive places. California also has the lowest average Medicare Advantage maximum out-of-pocket amounts, followed by Wisconsin and North Dakota. And pricey New York and New Jersey take two of the four top spots on the list with the lowest average Medicare Part D deductibles, joining Missouri and Wisconsin.

More low health-care cost leaders: New Mexico and South Carolina have the lowest average monthly Medicare Supplement plan premiums…South Carolina and Arizona, the lowest average Medicare Advantage plan premiums…Utah and Arizona, lowest overall out-of-pocket medical spending per capita.

Least affordable health-care overall: D.C., Delaware, West Virginia, Connecticut, Vermont, New York, Maryland, Alaska, Alabama, and Georgia.

OVERALL HEALTHFULNESS

First place: Connecticut

Last place: Mississippi

Key takeaway: Consider health outcomes when evaluating a state's health-care system, not just whether there's a highly regarded hospital nearby.

Assessments often focus on the overall quality of a state's hospitals. According to ratings

*Washington, D.C. is treated as a state for the purposes of these rankings. Rankings are from October 2021.

from the Centers for Medicare & Medicaid Services, Hawaii, Delaware, Alaska, and Idaho have the best public hospital systems, while Louisiana, Georgia, Texas, and Oklahoma have the worst.

The overall quality of a state's public hospital system doesn't necessarily reflect the quality of a hospital that you would choose. Even states that have poorly regarded public hospital systems contain a few hospitals with strong reputations.

Checking on Local Health Care

The quality of a state's health-care system doesn't tell the whole story. Sometimes what matters is what is available close to your home.

•**Confirm there's at least one well-regarded hospital.** Use the hospital ratings from *US News & World Report* (Health. USNews.com) and Medicare's Care Compare online tool (Medicare.gov/care-compare).

•**Confirm there are well-regarded doctors in specialties that you require.** Several websites compile patient ratings of doctors, including Healthgrades.com, Vitals. com, and RateMDs.com. Consider it promising if there are multiple well-reviewed local doctors in the specialty.

•**Confirm there are high-quality nursing homes—even if you don't need one now.** Medicare's Care Compare tool provides nursing home ratings.

•**Confirm your insurance or Medicare will work there.** Original Medicare is nationwide, but if you have a Medicare Advantage or Medigap plan, you might have to change plans when you relocate. Contact Medicare (800-633-4227) and/or the provider of your Medicare Advantage or Medigap. If you're covered through a former employer's plan, ask the benefits department whether the plan would provide coverage.

Charles B. Inlander, consumer advocate, and health-care consultant based in Fogelsville, Pennsylvania. He was the founding president of the People's Medical Society, a nonprofit consumer-advocacy organization, and author or coauthor of more than 20 consumer-health books.

Examples: Tulane Medical Center in New Orleans…Emory University Hospital in Atlanta…Houston Methodist Hospital in Houston…and St. Francis Hospital in Tulsa, Oklahoma, are a few.

Perhaps the more meaningful measure of health-care quality is the outcomes of that state's residents.

Example: People live longest in Hawaii, California, Minnesota, and New York…and die youngest in Mississippi, West Virginia, Alabama, and Oklahoma. When you focus on the percentage of adults who have type 2 diabetes, the lowest rates are in Colorado, South Dakota, and Montana…the highest in Alabama, West Virginia, and Mississippi. As for the heart disease death rate—Minnesota, Massachusetts, and Hawaii fare best…D.C., Oklahoma, and Mississippi worst.

When MedicareGuide grouped together seven factors that reflect on states' general healthfulness, the top 10 were Connecticut, Massachusetts, New Jersey, Hawaii, New York, Colorado, Alaska, California, New Hampshire, and Nebraska. The bottom 10 were Mississippi, Oklahoma, West Virginia, Alabama, Tennessee, Louisiana, Arkansas, Kentucky, South Carolina, and Georgia.

ACCESS TO HEALTH CARE

First place: Maine

Last place: Nevada

Key takeaway: Seniors should consider whether there's an adequate supply of the health-care providers they might need later in retirement…and whether those providers accept Medicare.

Recent retirees may need a skilled nursing facility or home health aides down the road. Vermont, Maine, and Idaho have the highest rate of skilled nursing facilities per capita…while New York, Virginia, and North Carolina have the lowest. New York, Minnesota, and D.C. are at the top of the list when it comes to home health aides per capita…while Florida, Georgia, and Alabama land at the bottom.

Another measure: The share of doctors who accept Medicare. Top on this list are North Dakota, South Dakota, and West Virginia…California, New York, and Texas bring up the rear.

When the scores for nine senior-health-care-access-related factors were added up, Maine, Vermont, Minnesota, North Dakota, West Virginia, Connecticut, Nebraska, and Iowa fared best.

Note: Most of these states are relatively rural. Big cities may have prestigious hospitals, but you don't have to sacrifice health care to retire to a rural low-population state.

Worst for health-care access: Nevada, Georgia, South Carolina, Utah, North Carolina, Virginia, Oklahoma, Texas.

States with the Best Hospitals

NiceRx.

Pennsylvania tops the list of states with the best hospitals, according to a report from NiceRx. Researchers looked at each state's patient safety data, number of hospitals on the *U.S. News* honor roll, number of hospitals in Healthgrades' America's top 50, number of hospitals per million people, and number of staffed hospital beds per million people. The data were used to create a state health-care score on a scale of one to 10. Pennsylvania earned a score of 8.04, with four hospitals in America's Top 50 and one hospital on the *U.S. News* honor roll. Pennsylvania has 2671.5 staffed beds and 13.8 hospitals per 1 million residents. Other top states included Illinois, Ohio, Michigan, and Massachusetts.

Getting the Help You Need When You Have a Disability

Darrell Jones, interim executive director at National Council on Independent Living, Washington, D.C. NCIL.org

Just thinking about it can be devastating. What if you—or a loved one—sustain a catastrophic injury or experience an ill-ness that makes you unable to return to the workforce? Besides having to adjust to your new capabilities, there's a mountain of other considerations—*How will I accomplish daily tasks? Will I have to move? Do I need a different mode of transportation? How will I pay my medical bills? Will my family member have to quit his/her job to take care of me?*

But there is help, says Darrell Jones of the National Council on Independent Living (NCIL). There are a host of programs available to people with disabilities, but finding your way through them can be confusing, especially for someone still coming to terms with new limitations. *Here are some ways to get started on that journey...*

•**Reach out to people who understand what you're going through.** One of the most helpful resources is the Center for Independent Living (CIL). This is not a place to live but a resource center that provides information, referrals, advocacy, life-skills training, and peer support. CILs are available in hundreds of cities and towns across the U.S. They empower individuals with disabilities to exercise their freedom of choice. You will find other people with disabilities who have learned how to manage day-to-day life.

The CIL staff will know the systems you have to deal with and can help you navigate them.

Examples: They can help you find resources to make modifications to your home... avoid placement in a nursing facility or help you relocate to a community if you now live in a nursing home...access the financial benefits you are entitled to...even find a church group that builds wheelchair ramps or a community organization that offers accessible recreational opportunities. The CIL knows the ins and outs of your area as well as your state and the federal government.

To find the CIL nearest to you: Use the directory at ILRU.org, or contact the NCIL at 844.778.7961 or ncil@ncil.org.

•**Check out other resources.** Adjusting your life to your new disability can be full of uncertainty. It's natural that you'll begin to question your identity. Your family and friends may begin to see you differently, which can hurt. If you can no longer do the same work, it will take some time to come to terms with your changed abilities. *Consider...*

•A mental health counselor may help you deal with the emotions that could affect your decision-making and quality of life. Check with the local CIL to see if it has a list of recommended mental health professionals.

•Organizations that represent people with specific disabilities, such as United Spinal Association (UnitedSpinal.org)...the National Federation of the Blind (NFB.org)...National Association of the Deaf (nad.org)...and American Stroke Association (Stroke.org), may be helpful. For other disabilities, do a web search for support groups in your area or call the United Way (United Way.org).

If there's no CIL or similar organization in your area, seek information from churches, the public library, or the firehouse. Even in remote areas, resources may exist, but you'll need someone to help you find them.

AVAILABLE RESOURCES

•**Employment.** Many people who become disabled assume that their working days are over. And for some, that may be true...but for others, it's a matter of redefining what work might look like. Maybe you won't be able to do your old job or perhaps even work in the same field, but there could be work that you can do and find fulfilling.

•Vocational Rehabilitation (VR) programs. Every state has a VR program that can connect you with assistive technologies, retraining, job placement, and other forms of support to get you working again. Find contact information for your state's Rehabilitation Services Administration at RSA.ed.gov/about/states.

•The Social Security Administration (SSA. gov) offers two programs for people with disabilities who would like to return to work—the Plan to Achieve Self-Support (PASS)...and Ticket to Work, which help recipients save up for the tools and equipment they need to re-enter the workforce.

•Financial benefits. Disability can be financially draining. Besides possibly losing your own income, your spouse may have to stop working to care for you. Medical bills can be astronomi-

cal. Durable medical equipment is expensive, as are home and vehicle modifications.

The Social Security and Supplemental Security Income disability programs are the largest of several federal programs that provide assistance to people with disabilities who meet certain medical criteria.

•Social Security Disability Insurance (SSDI) pays benefits to you and certain members of your family if you worked long enough before your disability and paid Social Security taxes. Eligibility is based on your work history and whether you have a disability that meets Social Security's definition. Generally, you are entitled to benefits if you cannot work for one year or more because of a disability.

•Supplemental Security Income (SSI) is geared specifically toward people with limited financial means. It has maximum-income thresholds for eligibility.

Depending on your circumstances, you may be eligible for SSDI and SSI at the same time.

•If you're denied coverage, the CIL can guide you on how to appeal or put you in touch with people who can help. You also can perform a web search for "Disability Advocates" in your area.

•Temporary financial assistance. Depending on your case, it can take a year or more to be approved and receive Social Security benefits. To fill the gap, many people apply for Temporary Assistance for Needy Families (TANF), which is federally funded but administered through the individual states. To apply, visit your state's welfare agency. Once your Social Security kicks in, you'll be dropped from TANF.

•**Medical insurance.** If you're already insured, you'll want to find out what benefits you're owed by your insurance company. If you're having trouble securing the benefits that you believe are your due, contact your local CIL or your state's insurance department. There's a searchable listing of these departments on the website of the National Association of Insurance Commissioners (NAIC.org).

•Medicaid might be the best option for securing health-care coverage. If you've been approved for SSI, you may get Medicaid coverage automatically, depending on which state you live in. In some states, you're automatically enrolled...in others, you're automatically qualified but still must apply...and in a handful of states, you're neither automatically enrolled nor automatically eligible but most likely will qualify. If you need Medicaid but don't get SSI, you can apply at HealthCare.gov/medicaid-chip.

•Medicare Part A is available to people under 65 if they have certain qualifying disabilities, and those individuals may then be eligible for Part B. For more information, visit Medicare.gov.

•**Housing.** One of the primary goals of the NCIL is expanding options for accessible, affordable housing that enables disabled people to stay out of institutions and live in the homes of their choice. You can reach out to your local CIL for guidance—it can connect you with federal, state, county, and local housing-assistance programs.

•The U.S. Department of Housing and Urban Development (HUD) offers subsidized rental assistance for disabled people under Section 811 of the National Affordable Housing Act. Non-Elderly Disabled (NED) Housing Choice Vouchers (HCVs) help people secure housing in the private market. To find out what options are available, check the HUD website for a directory to help you contact your local housing authority.

•**Food.** The federal Supplemental Nutritional Assistance Program (SNAP) is the key resource for obtaining help with food. SNAP has special eligibility rules for disabled people. Generally, if you receive Social Security disability benefits, you're eligible for SNAP, but you still must apply via your state agency, which you can contact at your local SNAP office.

•**Transportation.** Depending on the state and where you live, you may be eligible for non-emergency medical transportation services. Both Social Security and Medicaid provide for free transportation to and from doctors' appointments. Local communities often have paratransit services with free or reduced fares for disabled people. To find out what transportation options are available in your community, check in with your county transportation department or Human Services office.

Get a Second Opinion

David Sherer, M.D., retired anesthesiologist, patient advocate, and author of *Hospital Survival Guide: The Patient Handbook to Getting Better and Getting Out* and *What Your Doctor Won't Tell You.* DrDavidSherer.com

Perhaps you have been diagnosed with something as serious as cancer or something less serious such as a torn rotator cuff. You might trust your doctor—and his/her diagnosis—completely. But what if you don't? Perhaps you want a second opinion—to explore other treatment options or just to confirm your original doctor's diagnosis and treatment plan.

You might feel awkward about asking your doctor if you should get a second opinion... but the truth is, doctors are asked about second opinions a lot more often than you might think. And under many circumstances, you might not even need to tell him/her in advance.

WHY GET A SECOND OPINION

Sometimes insurance companies make it easy for you and mandate a second opinion before a procedure is covered, but even when it's your choice, getting one can help you better understand your condition and treatment options. This is especially important if the proposed treatment comes with serious side effects and/or potential long-term consequences...or there are new treatment options available.

Example: If you seek a second opinion from a specialist at a major medical center known for treating your problem, you may have access to newer therapies or clinical trials...or you may find alternatives to surgery.

There are even more compelling reasons to get a second opinion...

•**Your condition is life-threatening or life-changing.** The more serious the medical problem, the more valuable a second opinion. This is particularly true if you have cancer or an autoimmune disease—severe illnesses that require a lot of nuance and complicated therapies.

Many forms of cancer are treatable if you get the right diagnosis and prompt treatment.

Research published in *Annals of Surgical Oncology* that focused on patients with breast cancer found that a second review by a multidisciplinary tumor board at a National Cancer Institute–designated center changed the diagnosis in 43 percent of cases and that translated to more accurate treatment.

Second opinions also can be valuable for noncancerous conditions. A study at University Medical Center in Utrecht, the Netherlands, published in *PLOS One* found that over half of patients with internal-medicine issues, such as abdominal pain, fatigue, or weight loss, who asked for a second opinion received a more complete diagnosis and 13 percent got a new diagnosis. For many of them, a new medication was started and symptoms improved.

•**You're unsure about the first doctor.** You should have faith in your primary doctor's opinion. But if you don't, seek a second opinion.

•**Your doctor suggests a radical procedure.** A second opinion can help you evaluate invasive treatments, such as surgery, and those with potentially serious side effects, such as going on a biologic drug that can alter the immune system.

•**Your condition has not improved after three to six months.** If you expected your condition to improve but it hasn't, you should question whether the diagnosis or treatment plan is flawed.

•**There are alternatives to the proposed treatment.** It is easy to understand why you need treatment if you have a torn rotator cuff or significant degeneration in a knee joint and your doctor shows you the problem on imaging tests. But in some cases, there may be nonsurgical alternatives that can yield the same or better results. Surgeons tend to be biased in favor of surgical solutions. Consider practitioners who take a conservative approach such as physical pain specialists and physiatrists.

DON'T BURN YOUR BRIDGES

There's no rule that says you must disclose to your original doctor that you're getting another opinion…and trampling on any doctor's ego should not be your primary consideration.

Also, keep in mind, doctors often consult with other doctors to form their opinions.

You may be able to access your medical records on your own from your health-care system's patient portal. Print them and bring them to the new doctor. For images of radiology tests, you often can get a copy from the facility where the tests were done. Keep in mind—even if you provide all your records, the second doctor may need to do follow-up tests.

If there's no way to get your records other than to inform your existing doctor, you might say, "I respect your opinion but want another opinion because my health is at stake" or if the diagnosis is more serious, "…my life is in jeopardy." If your doctor has a problem with that, you might question his motives.

If your first diagnosis was from your primary provider and you're looking for a specialist's opinion, consider asking your primary for a referral. Your care could involve a collaboration, and you'll want everyone on the same page.

FINDING A SECOND OPINION

Whether you need surgery or nonsurgical treatment, take the following steps…

•**Check to see if your insurance limits you to providers in its plan or if you can cast a wider net.**

Example: You might be able to look out of state at major medical centers that have cutting-edge techniques.

•**Use all the tools available to you,** from word of mouth to online research, to look for doctors who have extensive experience with your health issue.

•**Check to see how many times any doctor has performed the procedure** and whether he has written or lectured about it. If you can't find the information you want online, contact the doctor's office manager to ask questions about the doctor's practices.

Note: Doctors within the same institution but not within the same practice office should be unbiased in their opinions, but if there is only one specialty practice in your area or affiliated with your local hospital, you might want

---

Where to Be Treated

If the doctor you choose is affiliated with more than one hospital, you might have to select where you will be treated. Do the same research that you used to find your second opinion. Ask how often the procedure you'll be having is performed at that facility and what outcomes have been documented. Ask about the availability of advanced equipment and treatment techniques.

These questions usually can be answered by the hospital's patient navigator.

Also see what medical experts, reviewers, and media reports have to say about the facility. If time allows, ask about taking a hospital tour.

—David Sherer, M.D.

---

to find a doctor in another health network who is also covered by your insurance.

WHEN OPINIONS DON'T AGREE

Having similar opinions can strengthen your trust in your original doctor. But when opinions differ, answers to key questions can help determine which direction to go. *Ask the second doctor...*

• **What led you to this conclusion?**

• **Why is this treatment better than my original doctor's treatment?**

• **What outcome can I hope for based on research and the doctor's experience?**

• **Is the latest therapy available?**

For a non-life-threatening issue, you might feel more comfortable choosing a less aggressive approach, such as physical therapy rather than surgery. But for a cancer diagnosis, get the fullest explanation possible for the new opinion so that you can compare it with the one given by your initial doctor.

Of course, it's possible to look for a third opinion—sometimes fourth or fifth opinions with rare and unusual or "orphan" diseases—but you'll have to weigh the pros and cons of the delay in treatment that this will cause.

Protect Yourself from Anesthesia Errors

David Sherer, M.D., retired clinical anesthesiologist and inventor based in Chevy Chase, Maryland. He is lead author of *Hospital Survival Guide: The Patient Handbook to Getting Better and Getting Out* and *What Your Doctor Won't Tell You*. DrDavidSherer.com

If you've ever had a biopsy, colonoscopy, joint replacement, or heart procedure, you've experienced the miracle of anesthesia firsthand. Medication that prevents patients from feeling pain (or remembering it afterward) has come a long way since the days of taking a shot of whiskey or breathing in a chloroform-soaked cotton pad. Thanks to advancements in the medications and delivery methods, patient deaths attributable to anesthesia have plummeted from one in 10,000 cases in 1980 to less than one in 250,000 today.

Still, when it comes to helping a patient navigate a procedure without pain, there is the possibility of unpleasant—even dangerous—side effects. It's important to arm yourself with information before you hit the operating table.

AVOIDING ANESTHESIA ERRORS

Just because anesthesia is safer today than ever before doesn't mean that side effects or mistakes don't happen. *Here are some ways to protect yourself...*

• **Be honest in your pre-anesthesia interview.** Just prior to receiving general or regional anesthesia, you'll meet with your anesthesiologist and/or be asked to fill out a pre-anesthesia questionnaire. This information can help your health-care team predict how you will respond to certain drugs. Some questions will duplicate those you've already answered for your doctor, but this time your answers are being reviewed by different providers for a specific purpose. And answering these questions even may help you remember a detail that you forgot to share with your doctor, such as an over-the-counter product you have been using or a bad reaction to anesthesia during your wisdom tooth extraction or C-section decades ago.

•**Be honest when answering questions about your drinking and smoking habits** (both increase risk for complications and delay recovery)…whether you take medicine for erectile dysfunction (which can cause blood pressure to drop dangerously low when combined with anesthesia)…if you've recently had a cold or the flu…and anything else he/she might ask.

Some patients are more likely to develop complications due to pre-existing conditions, so make sure your anesthesiology team knows if you've been diagnosed with diabetes…heart disease, high blood pressure or stroke…allergies…kidney disease…a lung condition, such as asthma, COPD or have a history of smoking…obesity…or seizures or other nervous system complication.

•**Tell the anesthesia team if you have loose or chipped teeth or recently underwent cosmetic dental work.** Dental injuries are one of the more common complications of general anesthesia. Loose teeth can be dislodged during intubation. If you recently had a crown or implants placed, let the anesthesiologist know, so extra care can be taken to avoid damaging your new work…or you may be asked to wear a plastic mouth guard during the procedure.

•**Tell the anesthesia team if you use more than one pillow at night or a CPAP machine.** People who need to prop themselves up to sleep well (perhaps due to reflux, obesity, or sleep apnea) generally don't tolerate lying down for prolonged periods, as is required during surgery. It changes the way weight is distributed on your diaphragm and/or can cause your tongue or neck tissue to obstruct the airway. Letting your team know you need extra pillows at home puts them on high alert for challenges.

If you use a CPAP machine: Let your doctor know before the day of your procedure. You may be asked to bring it to aid your breathing in the recovery room.

•**Tell the anesthesia team if you easily become nauseated, carsick, or seasick.** Anesthesia stimulates an area of the brain called the *chemoreceptor trigger zone,* which is linked with nausea. People who tend to experience nausea in day-to-day life may be more likely to experience it after surgery. You can request that anti-nausea medications, such as *ondansetron* (Zofran), *granisetron* (Kytril), and *dolasetron* (Anzemet), be administered during surgery to prevent post-op nausea. Or order the FDA-approved ReliefBand wristband device, and ask for it to be put on your wrist after surgery.

•**Ask family members if they've ever had a negative experience with anesthesia.** Several anesthesia-related problems tend to run in families. If you've never gone under anesthesia before, it's crucial for you to warn your anesthesiologist if any family members, especially your parents, have experienced problems.

ANESTHESIAS AND RISKS

•**General anesthesia is for surgeries of the head, chest, spine, and abdomen.** It involves a combination of preoperative sedatives, narcotic painkillers, muscle relaxants, and sleep agents to render you unaware and immobile. Most of these are given via IV right before the operation.

Possible side effects: Sore throat…nausea and vomiting…and lingering grogginess.

Rare serious risks: Brain damage due to lack of oxygen, nerve or dental injury, aspiration pneumonia, or death.

•**Regional anesthesia** is used to numb the entire lower part of the body or numb a specific region (such as a shoulder, foot, or toe). It's often used alongside sedating drugs, which make you so relaxed that you barely realize you're in surgery.

•**Spinal anesthesia,** one type of regional anesthesia, is injected through the back into the spinal fluid. Spinal anesthesia with sedation often is used for hip and knee surgeries, hernia repairs, and transurethral resection of the prostate (TURP).

Possible side effects: Headache, feeling short of breath and a rapid, but temporary, drop in blood pressure. Serious but rare risks include pain, bleeding or infection at the injection site, nerve injury, or a debilitating headache.

One benefit: A small catheter can be placed to allow the medicine to be delivered continuously over hours or even days.

Note: If the doctor wants the patient awake during surgery, he/she may use spinal anesthesia (also known as a spinal block) with some sedation to ease the patient's anxiety. Called *awake spinal surgery*, it results in shorter operating time, quicker recovery, and fewer side effects.

•**Epidural anesthesia** is similar to spinal anesthesia. Anesthetic is injected through the back into an area near the spinal cord. Epidurals take effect more slowly than spinals and are

less likely to produce a sudden, rapid drop in blood pressure. A catheter also can be placed to administer the medicine continuously.

•**Nerve blocks**—a third type of regional anesthesia—are good for hand, arm, leg, and foot procedures, as well as cosmetic procedures such as face-lifts. Local anesthesia is injected into a specific nerve to numb the region or limb. Patients can remain awake and speak with their surgeon. Rare risks include nerve injury or seizures if the medicine is accidentally injected into the bloodstream.

•**Local anesthesia** is typically used in procedures involving isolated areas, such as during LASIK or cataract surgery, breast biopsies, or mole removal. The risk of side effects is extremely low.

•**Monitored anesthesia care (MAC)** is a combination of local anesthesia plus sedation. MAC often is used during outpatient diagnostic procedures or therapeutic procedures such as colonoscopies, breast biopsies, and minor orthopedic procedures including carpal tunnel surgery. Various levels of anesthesia, ranging from light to heavy, may be used to control pain, along with sedating and antianxiety drugs.

Advantage: You remain semiconscious ("twilight sleep") and can respond to verbal commands.

Potential side effects: Post-procedure nausea and drowsiness. While MAC has been proven to be overwhelmingly safe, there are rare and isolated instances in which dosing errors have harmed patients.

Post-Op Cognitive Problems

One-quarter of patients over age 65 may experience problems with thinking, learning, judgment, and perception in the weeks and months following surgery. Called *postoperative cognitive decline* (POCD), it's thought to be caused by the release of inflammatory toxins that can occur when anesthesia is administered.

Recent finding: A 2020 study by the University of South Australia found that nearly 40 percent of patients continue to experience POCD one to five years after coronary bypass, one of the most common heart procedures. POCD impacts older adults more often because an aging brain doesn't bounce back from anesthesia easily.

Reduce your risk of POCD by regularly practicing brain-healthy habits such as following the Mediterranean diet...getting regular exercise...maintaining a healthy weight...managing stress...and getting sufficient sleep.

Also ask your doctor about possible risks of your specific surgery...how deep your level of anesthesia will be (POCD is more likely to occur following longer, more complicated procedures using general anesthesia than quick outpatient ones)...and what medications will be used during and after the surgery. Opioids, for instance, may increase risk for POCD.

—David Sherer, M.D.

Meet Post-Hospitalization Needs

Charles B. Inlander, consumer advocate and healthcare consultant based in Fogelsville, Pennsylvania. He was the founding president of the nonprofit People's Medical Society.

Hospital stays are getting shorter and shorter. Thirty years ago, the average stay was seven days. Today, it's down to 4.5 days and falling.

A shorter stay is beneficial in many ways: It reduces your risk of acquiring a hospital-caused infection. It means you can go home quicker and enjoy the comfort of your own home and bed. And it reduces your cost.

But shorter hospital stays and same-day surgery have some downsides. In most cases, you need time at home to recover after hospitalization or an outpatient procedure. That may require the help of a family member or friend. You may need significant follow-up procedures. Depending on your capabilities, you may have to manage a slew of new medications on a short- or even long-term basis.

Most people are not prepared for post-hospital care. We tend to overestimate our capabilities and don't have a plan. As a result, your recovery might be slowed, or you might even need to be re-hospitalized. *Here are some things you should do to make sure your post-hospitalization needs are met, and you have a successful recovery…*

•**Plan ahead.** If you know you are going to be hospitalized, discuss with your doctor what you should expect once you are discharged. Will you need help taking care of your medical needs, such as changing bandages, monitoring vital signs, or taking medications at specific times? Will you need any special equipment, such as a walker, lift chair, or hospital bed? Will you need transportation for follow-up physician appointments or post-hospitalization procedures such as chemotherapy, cardiac rehab, radiation, or physical therapy?

•**Be realistic.** Be honest with yourself about your capabilities. Remember, you are not expected to be 100 percent when you come home from the hospital. Assess your home needs. For example, will you be able to use stairs to reach your bedroom or bath? Can your spouse meet your care needs while recovering? Do you have help to do food shopping or meet other daily needs? Do you have a reliable group of family members and friends who can provide transportation to your appointments?

•**Before discharge.** When you are admitted to the hospital, a social worker should be assigned to your case. Based on your needs, your social worker should develop and help oversee your discharge plan. The plan should be written and include any prescriptions your doctor wants you to take and other specific actions, such as wound monitoring, physical therapy, or follow-up appointments. Your social worker should go over this plan with you and determine the help you may need in implementing the plan at home. The social worker should also be ordering the medical equipment you may need and arranging for visiting nurses (if necessary) to come to your home to deliver care.

•**Have an advocate.** Don't be afraid to have a friend or family member with you through this entire process. Many of us are afraid to ask questions or feel intimidated talking with doctors and nurses. Having someone you trust with you can make a world of difference and allow you to focus solely on having a complete recovery.

An Endodontist Can Save Your Teeth…and Your Money

Natasha Flake, DDS, Ph.D., MSD, vice president of the American Association of Endodontists. Dr. Flake is an associate dean and professor in the department of endodontics at University of Washington School of Dentistry, Seattle. Dental.Washington.edu

You're eating ice cream with your grandchild when a sudden, intense jolt of pain shoots through your molar and lingers for the rest of the afternoon. Or while attempting to rip open the plastic packaging on a new refrigerator filter several months ago, you unknowingly cracked your front tooth and now it's starting to ache. Or perhaps you were diagnosed with a cavity just before the COVID-19 pandemic hit and never had it treated because you were scared to be maskless in a medical setting…now you can barely chew food without searing pain.

For each of these scenarios, most people would dial their general dentist…and chances are that he/she could squeeze you in and craft a treatment plan. But there is an alternative when it comes to painful dental emergencies—an endodontist…and he/she may be better equipped to fix the problem.

WHAT IS AN ENDODONTIST?

Endodontists are dentists who have undergone two or more additional years of advanced training beyond dental school, during which they become experts in tooth pain, infection, and disease. All endodontists are dentists, but less than 3 percent of dentists are endodontists. An endodontist's practice focuses on treating the inside of teeth—the pulp, which includes blood vessels, nerves, and connective tissues. ("Endo" is Greek for "inside" and "odon" is Greek for "tooth.")

These highly specialized dentists do everything they can to save damaged or infected teeth and prevent them from being pulled. Damage may happen when bacteria sneak into the pulp through a long-neglected cavity or a crack created by dental trauma such as a fall, a car accident, or even just biting down on something the wrong way. When bacteria infiltrate a tooth, they can cause inflammation, infection, lingering sensitivity to hot or cold temperatures, pain (especially when eating sticky or crunchy foods and particularly on the release portion of the bite), and even tooth loss. You may also find a pimple-like bump on the gum, which is evidence of the buildup of bacteria in and around a tooth.

This is where endodontists come in. *They are experts at saving teeth using two procedures in particular…*

•**Root canal.** This in-office procedure is designed to save natural teeth. A root canal starts with a hole being cut in the top of the affected tooth so that the endodontist can access the pulp. Through that hole, the inside of the tooth is cleaned and disinfected. The tooth is then sealed, and a new filling or a crown is placed. This procedure takes only one or two visits.

Endodontists perform up to 25 root canals a week. Most general dentists perform two or fewer a week.

In many cases, diseased teeth that would have been pulled can be saved with endodontic treatment. That's important, because missing teeth allow remaining teeth to shift,

affecting your ability to chew and significantly changing the aesthetics of your smile. A pulled tooth can be replaced with a replica of some sort—an implant, denture, or removable partial denture—but the artificial tooth will never function as well as the original one.

Unfortunately, root canals have a bad reputation, making them among the most feared medical procedures. A recent study by the American Association of Endodontists (AAE) found that 53 percent of US adults would rather have a snake in their lap for 15 minutes than get a root canal…62 percent would rather run a marathon…and 54 percent would rather sing the national anthem at a sporting event.

When given the choice between having a root canal or having a painful, infected tooth pulled, patients usually opt for the extraction.

Reason: They think having a tooth pulled will hurt less and cost less.

Reality: The opposite is true. An endodontist's skill in administering anesthetics and using cutting-edge dental technology means that the procedure can be virtually painless. Most patients remain awake during root canals, which are done under local anesthesia. Particularly anxious patients may opt for nitrous oxide, also known as laughing gas, or an oral antianxiety medication to help them through the procedure. The negative, painful connotations that root canals have earned usually are due to the pain associated with the tooth before the treatment, not during it.

Tooth extraction, on the other hand, frequently hurts more than the infection itself and is more traumatic to the mouth and gums. Root canal patients are six times more likely to describe the procedure as painless compared with patients who have a tooth pulled, according to the AAE.

Replacement of a natural tooth also requires multiple dental visits that can quickly add up cost-wise, as prosthetics such as implants and bridges must be placed and then maintained over the years. When an endodontist saves a natural tooth, he/she also is saving the patient the future expenses and time associated with pulled teeth.

Sometimes a tooth is too damaged or diseased to be saved and must be pulled, but whenever saving it is possible, an endodontist will try.

•**Apicoectomy.** Calcium deposits in the pulp are a natural part of aging and can develop in response to trauma. When calcium deposits in the tooth make it difficult for traditional root canal instruments to be used effectively, an endodontist can perform a root-end resection, also called apicoectomy. This surgery also may be needed to help teeth that are causing trouble even after a root canal procedure…or to treat teeth with damaged roots.

Like root canals, apicoectomies are done in the endodontist's office under local anesthesia. Rather than approaching the pulp from the top of the tooth, the endodontist opens the gum tissue and enters the tooth through the base of the root to clear out any infected or inflamed tissue. A filling is then placed, and a few stitches are used to close up the gums.

NEW MEMBER OF THE TEAM

The sooner you treat a cracked, chipped, or infected tooth, the better your chances are of saving it. Under the best circumstances, your dentist and endodontist will work together to ensure the optimal dental outcome—general dentists refer about half of their root canal patients to an endodontist in an average year.

Your dentist can give you a referral to an endodontist, or you can find one using AAE's "Find My Endodontist" search tool at FindMy Endodontist.com or by asking friends for recommendations. Most insurance companies cover root canal therapy and other endodontic treatment, but call your insurer first to double-check.

Health-Care Worker Exodus

USA Today/Ipsos

A USA Today/Ipsos poll reported that 23 percent of American health-care workers say they are likely to leave the field soon. Respondents reported feeling "burned out,"

"anxious," and "angry." The poll surveyed 1,170 doctors, nurses, paramedics, therapists, home health aides, dentists, and other medical professionals.

Preserving Dignity at the End of Life

Lauren T. Starr, Ph.D., MBE, RN, postdoctoral fellow in palliative and end-of-life care, New Courtland Center for Transitions and Health, University of Pennsylvania School of Nursing, Philadelphia.

Hospice is a type of health care that moves away from curative treatments and instead focuses on relieving pain and symptoms, reducing suffering, and improving quality of life for people who are within six months of the end of their lives.

Hospice means shifting from the goal of a longer life through treatments to creating the best quality of life for the days one has left. It enables patients and families to prioritize symptom management over the pursuit of aggressive, often uncomfortable treatments that may or may not extend life.

In 90 percent of cases, this care is provided right in a patient's home. Nurses, nursing assistants, social workers, doctors, art and music therapists, chaplains, and other support staff travel to the patient and provide a range of resources to meet patient and family needs, from hospitals beds and lifts to medications, toileting supplies, and bandages.

SERVICES FOR FAMILY

Hospice doesn't just provide support for the patient: It also focuses on helping family caregivers by providing emotional and spiritual support in addition to hands-on help with caregiving tasks.

For limited hours a week, nursing assistants or volunteers may help with chores, food preparation, and laundry. Volunteers can sit with a patient while a family member runs errands, and many hospices also offer respite care, where they will care for the patient in a local hospital or other facility to give the family caregiver a break for a few days.

After the patient passes away, hospice will continue to check on and support surviving family members through trained bereavement care.

CORRECTING MISCONCEPTIONS

It can be difficult for people to accept stepping away from curative treatments, and that can create misconceptions around what hospice is. *Here's a look at some common concerns...*

MISCONCEPTION: **Hospice is giving up.** Stopping curative care can strike some people as giving up on the patient. But it is simply honoring the patient's wishes to prioritize quality of life and comfort. A person who has a poor prognosis may prefer to have 20 joy-filled days than 2,000 that are filled with discomfort or suffering.

MISCONCEPTION: **The doctor will tell you when it's time for hospice.** It can be difficult for physicians to recommend that their patients consider hospice services, as some doctors feel that they must try everything possible to prolong life at any cost. As a result, many people don't enter into hospice care until weeks or even days before their death. That means they're often deprived of care that could have eased pain and addressed their social, spiritual, and psychological concerns.

Some people wait for their doctor to initiate discussions about hospice, but patients and families can ask questions about hospice at any time (and should!).

MISCONCEPTION: **Hospice hastens death.** A person can go into hospice when a physician or nurse practitioner determines that they are likely to die in the next six months.

While it may feel like stopping curative treatments will make a loved one pass away sooner, that's often not the case. In fact, a study found that people with lung cancer lived about a month longer if they were in hospice care compared with those who continued with curative treatments. When patients have their emotional and physical needs met, they may have the strength and will to live longer.

MISCONCEPTION: **Hospice is expensive.** Hospice services are usually covered by Medicare, Medicaid, and most private insurers. Most patients have no copays. Drugs to manage pain and symptoms, clinician and social work visits, and various equipment to enable care at home are provided as part of the hospice benefit.

EMOTIONAL SUPPORT

If you're the patient in hospice, you may be frightened as you face the prospect of dying or you may feel regret about things you have or have not done in your life. Hospice providers, social workers, and chaplains are there to provide emotional support and can also facilitate family discussions and mediate when conflicts arise. They can help you talk to loved ones about how you feel, let go of things you can't change, and find peace and forgiveness.

TALK ABOUT IT
BEFORE YOU NEED IT

Because hospice can be a difficult concept, it's important to learn and talk about it before you need it.

Having conversations helps people make choices that align with their goals. Some people want aggressive treatment until they die, while others want an end-of-life experience that does not have pain. A person with a terminal illness may have a primary goal of spending as much time as possible with family. If aggressive medical treatment interferes with that, they may opt to forgo that treatment and instead focus on taking measures to improve quality of life and time with loved ones.

As you have these conversations, it's also a good time to make sure you have advance directives, medically binding documents that outline your wishes, such as who can make medical decisions on your behalf and under what circumstances you would want life-extending care and resuscitation. These documents may include living wills and durable and medical powers of attorney.

CHAPTER 11

Infectious Disease

Fend Off the Flu

For the past few years, influenza has taken a backseat to COVID. It's not just that people weren't paying attention, either: There were fewer cases of flu even though testing and reporting were up. The most likely explanation is that COVID prevention measures, like masking, handwashing, and social distancing, kept us safe from more than one virus.

But now that people have largely returned to prepandemic habits, the flu could become a problem once again. Even though the "pandemic winter" of 2021–2022 was a "light" flu season, there were still up to 170,000 hospitalizations and 14,000 deaths, according to estimates from the U.S. Centers for Disease Control and Prevention. *Here are some simple steps to stay well this winter...*

STAY HOME IF YOU'RE SICK

One of the silver linings of the COVID-19 pandemic is the normalization of people staying home when they're sick. It's no longer a badge of honor to drag your coughing, sneezing, and GI-disturbed self to work, now that people are more aware of just how risky it can be to share air with the sick.

In fact, you don't even have to cough and sneeze to spread germs. Researchers from the University of Maryland reported that people can spread the flu simply by breathing. Donald Milton, M.D., MPH, examined the exhaled breath from 142 people with influenza when they were breathing, speaking, coughing, and sneezing on the first three days they experienced flu symptoms. His team found that flu patients routinely shed infectious virus into aerosol particles small enough to present a risk for airborne transmission. Neither coughing nor sneezing appeared to contribute significantly to influenza virus shedding.

Cameron Wolfe, MBBS, associate professor of medicine, division of infectious disease, Duke University Medical Center.

VACCINATE

Since it's not practical to stay home all winter to try to avoid contracting the flu, the next best thing is to protect yourself as much as possible. Although it's only about 10 to 50 percent effective, the flu vaccine is still highly recommended as part of your prevention strategy. The vaccine's effectiveness depends on how well each year's formulation aligns with the prevalent strain of the year. (To have vaccines ready each year, scientists predict which strain will be active before flu season hits, and they don't always get it right.) For the 2023–2024 season, the flu vaccine will be based on the strain that predominated the year before.

The flu shot contains a dead virus and can't give you the flu. You may, however, feel a little run-down after getting the shot. As your body produces protective antibodies, you may have muscle aches or a fever for a day or two. It takes two weeks for the shot to provide full protection.

Antiviral Medications

If you do get sick, drink plenty of fluids, rest, and use over-the-counter medications to ease your symptoms. Also, call your doctor and ask about getting an antiviral medication. *Several medications were effective against last year's dominant flu strains…*

- **zanamivir** (Relenza)
- **baloxavir marboxil** (Xofluza)
- **oseltamivir** (Tamiflu)
- **peramivir** (Rapivab).

These drugs must be taken within 48 hours of the onset of symptoms, and they shave off about 24 to 32 hours of symptoms.

People who are over age 65, obese, or living in a long-term care facility have a higher risk of complications from the flu, including bacterial infections, viral pneumonia, and cardiac and other organ system abnormalities that require medical attention.

BUT I DON'T GET THE FLU

You've probably met someone who skips his or her yearly flu shot and still doesn't get sick. Researchers from the University of Michigan and Duke University who wanted to understand this phenomenon infected 17 people with the flu virus and made an interesting discovery. The people who stayed well weren't immune to the flu—in fact, they had a significant immune response to it—they just experienced it differently and with no symptoms. The researchers found that those people had differences in their biological metabolism and gene expression, explained study author Alfred Hero, M.D., in *PLoS Genetics*. And those differences, he noted, "had to do with antioxidants."

QUERCETIN

That specific study did not explore the effects of eating an antioxidant-rich diet, but several others have, and one particular compound stands out: quercetin, a flavonoid found in tea, chocolate, and red wine. In 2021, researchers reported in the journal *Biomolecules* that quercetin indirectly inhibits the influenza A virus, regulates the inflammatory response, and lessens the severity of illness.

While flavonoids have been found to have a variety of potential health effects, a study published in *Science* suggests that they may work best to limit the damage caused by flu in the presence of a specific intestinal microbe: *Clostridium orbiscindens.*

"It's not only having a diet rich in flavonoids; our results show you also need the right microbes in the intestine to use those flavonoids to control the immune response," the study's senior author, Thaddeus Stappenbeck, M.D., Ph.D., explained. While this is early animal study information, the authors noted that it certainly can't hurt to boost your intake of flavonoids. The researchers are now investigating ways to boost the gut health of people who don't have enough *C. orbiscindens*.

WHAT THIS MEANS FOR YOU

It's important to follow the CDC recommendations to wash your hands frequently, avoid touching your face, and keep surfaces

Eat This to Fight the Flu

Add these quercetin-rich foods to your fall diet to help stave off the flu...

FOOD	AMOUNT
Apples	4.7 mg/100 g
Asparagus	7.61 mg/100 g
Black Elderberry	42 mg/100 g
Blueberries	5.05 mg/100 g
Capers	233 mg/100 g
Cherries	2.64 mg/100 g
Cocoa Powder	20 mg/100 g
Onions	22 mg/100 g
Oregano	42 mg/100 g
Tea	1.99 mg/100 g

clean and disinfected, but those steps may not be enough to avoid getting the flu. For added protection, get an annual flu shot and eat plenty of antioxidant-rich foods. If you get sick, help protect others by staying home until your fever has subsided without medication for 24 hours.

RSV in Adults Can Be Serious

William Schaffner, M.D., professor of preventive medicine and infectious diseases at Vanderbilt University in Nashville. Vanderbilt.edu

Until recently, *respiratory syncytial virus* (RSV) was considered a pediatric illness. Now we know adults can get reinfected with this seasonal bug throughout their lives, developing cold and flulike symptoms. Seniors, people with compromised immune systems, and those with heart and lung problems can develop serious complications, resulting in nearly 10,000 deaths annually. The Food and Drug Administration approved the first RSV vaccine for individuals 60 years and older in early May 2023.

Pneumonia Is Still a Threat

William Schaffner, M.D., professor of preventive medicine in the Department of Health Policy and professor of medicine in the Division of Infectious Diseases at Vanderbilt University School of Medicine, Nashville. Vanderbilt.edu

With all the attention on COVID and influenza, it's easy to forget that pneumonia is a serious health threat. An infection that attacks the air sacs in the lungs, it is the most common flu complication. "Walking pneumonia," now called community-acquired pneumonia, is acquired outside a hospital and can be caused by multiple bacteria and viruses. Hospital-acquired pneumonia usually refers to pneumonia with resistant bacteria that develops in people on respirators who have been on antibiotics. Pneumonia often can be managed at home, but without prompt care, it can become serious quickly.

Symptoms: What distinguishes pneumonia from a bad cold or flu is that the cough produces sputum and you have chest pain and difficulty breathing. You might experience fatigue, nausea and/or vomiting, diarrhea and, in people over age 65, mental confusion and a lower-than-normal temperature.

Diagnosis: Your doctor will take a health history and do a physical exam. You might need a chest X-ray, a blood test, and/or sputum test to identify whether it is from a virus or bacteria.

Treatment: In addition to pain relievers and drinking fluids, you may need antibiotics if the cause is bacteria...or an antiviral if the cause is a virus.

Prevention: If you're 65 or older...or between 19 and 64 with underlying conditions... or are immunocompromised...you should get the pneumococcal vaccine, which targets different strains of the bacteria Pneumococcus. There are two types of Pneumococcal vaccine—Pneumococcal conjugate vaccines (PCV13, PCV15 and PCV20)...and Pneumococcal polysaccharide vaccine (PPSV23). Your doctor will know which is best for you. The vaccines are effective, but still take precautions to avoid infection even after vaccination.

PNEUMONIA AND COVID

Pneumonia can develop in lungs under siege from COVID. The most important way to avoid both is to be vaccinated and boosted against COVID. If you are diagnosed with COVID and are over 65 or have underlying conditions, treatment with Paxlovid can help prevent pneumonia. Paxlovid does increase the risk for rebound COVID, but it's a better scenario than being on a ventilator.

Viruses and Alzheimer's Disease

Tufts University.

The varicella zoster virus (VZV), which causes chickenpox and shingles, can activate the herpes simplex virus (HSV) and play a role in the development of Alzheimer's disease, new research suggests. HSV-1 normally lies dormant in the brain's neurons, but when it's activated, it leads to the accumulation of tau and amyloid beta proteins and the loss of neuronal function. Repeated cycles of activation can lead to more brain inflammation, plaques, and cognitive damage. COVID infection can also awaken dormant VZV and HSV, which may explain why some people experience long-term neurological effects after infection. The shingles vaccine considerably reduces the risk of dementia, possibly because it stops the cycle of viral reactivation.

HIV Cure May Be in Sight

Medscape Medical News.

A 66-year-old man appears to have complete clearance of the human immunodeficiency virus (HIV) after being treated for leukemia with a stem cell transplantation from an HIV-resistant donor, researchers reported at the 24th International AIDS Conference. The man discontinued antiretroviral therapy more than 20 months ago and has no detectable HIV-1 DNA. He is the fourth person to have complete clearance of the virus and the oldest person to do so. While the researchers are using the term remission, they say this suggests that an HIV cure is possible or even likely. Stem cell transplant procedures are complicated, however, and not suitable for all people with HIV.

Long COVID: How to Get Your Life Back

Jacob Teitelbaum, M.D., an expert in the fields of chronic fatigue syndrome, fibromyalgia, sleep, and pain. He is the author of numerous books, including *From Fatigued to Fantastic* (4th Edition). Vitality101.com

One study on the long-term risks of COVID-19, published in *Nature Communications* in October 2022, says it all: Of the tens of thousands of people studied, 40 percent of those who were sick with COVID had not fully recovered from their infection many months later. And 5 percent never recovered at all. In other words, 45 percent of those with the novel coronavirus ended up with long COVID.

The researchers identified more than 20 symptoms linked to long COVID, like breathlessness, heart palpitations, and confusion or difficulty concentrating. They also found a high incidence of disturbances in smell, taste, sight, and hearing; muscle aches; and other symptoms related to mental health, the heart, and the respiratory system.

This isn't the first or only study to find a high incidence of long COVID. In a study by researchers in England, 75 percent of patients who received care for the coronavirus were still suffering ongoing symptoms three months later. In another study in Ireland, more than half of 128 people reported persistent fatigue 10 weeks after their initial COVID symptoms.

THE CAUSE OF LONG COVID

As a lifelong expert in myalgic encephalomyelitis/chronic fatigue syndrome (ME/CFS) who has treated thousands of patients with the problem, I believe that long COVID is a form of postviral ME/CFS. (Many viruses cause this condition, including Epstein-Barr and human herpesvirus 6.) The common symptoms of post-viral ME/CFS include persistent, disabling fatigue, chills and sweats, body aches, brain fog and concentration issues, digestive issues, trouble sleeping, dizziness, and shortness of breath.

Why such a broad range of symptoms? Basically, post-viral ME/CFS affects the hypothalamus, a part of the brain that controls the dispersion of hormones throughout your body. ME/CFS also interferes with sleep and cripples the function of mitochondria, tiny structures within the cells that generate cellular energy. Those fundamental disruptions are why ME/CFS (and long COVID) affect multiple systems in the body—the brain, the heart, the lungs, the musculoskeletal system, the gastrointestinal system, the senses, and more.

About 10 percent of people will continue to have long COVID ME/CFS about a year after their infection. Fortunately, this is treatable with a patient-tested, science-backed protocol that has helped many people improve dramatically and even recover full health.

STEP #1: Shut down excessive inflammation

Chronic inflammation—caused by an overactive immune system that's still reacting to the virus—is a key feature of long COVID. A scientific summary published by the National Institutes of Health says that chronic inflammation is the likely "mechanism for the symptoms of long COVID." In a study published in *Current Medical Research and Opinion*, people with "post-COVID syndrome" (another name for long COVID) had high levels of four biomarkers of chronic inflammation.

Several key supplements taken daily for six to 12 weeks can rebalance the immune system and help tame chronic inflammation.

•**Take curcumin and glutathione daily.** Curcumin, the active ingredient in the spice turmeric, is a potent anti-inflammatory agent. Glutathione is a powerful antioxidant that neuters the free radical molecules that cause inflammation. I recommend 750 milligram (mg) daily of a form of curcumin with a high rate of absorption. For glutathione, I recommend 300 mg twice daily.

This combination is particularly effective for lung healing. However, it's important to note that lung damage from COVID tends to improve and often resolves after two years. I recommend monitoring your oxygen levels with a pulse oximeter so you can see improvement over time and feel reassured. These two supplements help speed the process.

•**If you're in pain, add Boswellia.** If you have significant pain, I recommend combining curcumin and the herb Boswellia. The curcumin balances the cyclooxygenase inflammation system, which affects the musculoskeletal system. The Boswellia balances the lipoxygenase pathway of inflammation, which plays an important role in the lungs and the gut. Take 750 mg of Boswellia two to three times daily in addition to the curcumin recommendation above.

•**Take omega-3 (fish oil).** The omega-3 fatty acids found in fatty, cold-water fish like salmon, sardines, tuna, and mackerel help balance the immune system. I recommend approximately 600 mg daily of a product that combines the essential fatty acids DHA and EPA.

STEP #2: Boost energy

I recently conducted a study on the herb red ginseng, a plant renowned for its ability to protect and restore physical and mental stamina. In the study, 188 people with ME/CFS or post-viral fatigue took a special form of red ginseng grown hydroponically with a style of cultivation to help the plant generate a maximum level of *ginsenosides*, the compound that gives red ginseng its restorative powers. The product used in the study was Red Ginseng HRG80, which comes in the form of chewable tablets. Three out of every five people who took the herb had improved symptoms, including significant increases in energy, mental clarity, and quality of sleep, and decreases in pain. Take one chew in the morning, with a second dose at lunch.

STEP #3: Consider the SHINE protocol

This protocol involves sleep restoration, hormonal support, infection treatment, nutritional supplementation, and exercise (as able). In a study published in the *Journal of Chronic Fatigue Syndrome*, the SHINE protocol improved fatigue, sleep, mental clarity, pain, and well-being in 90 percent of people with post-viral ME/CFS. *Key elements of the protocol include...*

•**Sleep restoration.** Getting seven to eight hours of sleep is important for healing. But 40 percent of people with long COVID have sleep disturbances, according to researchers at the Cleveland Clinic, who reported their findings at the 2022 annual meeting of the Associated Professional Sleep Societies. I have found the best sleep medications for people with post-viral ME/CFS include *zolpidem* (Ambien), *trazodone* (Desyrel), and *gabapentin* (Neurontin). Talk to your doctor about the medication and dosage that is right for you.

•**Hormonal support.** In a study published in *Endocrine*, people with long COVID had imbalances in thyroid and adrenal hormones. These changes seem to be involved in the persistent symptoms of long COVID, the researchers said. Based on a mix of symptoms and blood tests, but even with normal testing, I treat patients with post-viral ME/CFS with bioidentical hormone therapy for thyroid, adrenal, ovarian, and/or testicular hormones. (Bioidentical hormones are chemical twins for the hormones generated by the human body.) Talk to your doctor about whether hormonal treatment is right for you.

•**Infection treatment.** Most people with post-viral ME/CFS have weakened immune systems, resulting in multiple chronic infections. The most common infection is with the fungus *Candida albicans*. I have found that many ME/CFS patients benefit from six weeks of treatment with the antifungal *fluconazole* (Diflucan). Talk to your doctor about testing and treating for candida infection. Epstein-Barr (mono) viral reactivation is also common.

•**Nutritional supplementation.** To optimize nutrition, my post-viral ME/CFS patients take a daily multivitamin mineral supplement. Look for a powdered supplement (for easy absorption) that delivers 500 to 1,000 mg of vitamin C, about 50 mg of most B vitamins, 200 mg of magnesium, and 55 micrograms (mcg) of selenium.

•**Exercise.** For many people with post-viral ME/CFS, exercise beyond a certain point makes the patient feel more fatigued. In a study published in the *Journal of Translational Medicine,* the problem of "post-exertional malaise" in long COVID and CFS/ME were exactly the same. But exercise is also important for healing. To exercise with long COVID, begin with light exercise, such as walking (or if regular walking is too difficult, water walking in a heated pool). Walk only as much as you comfortably can (or start with five minutes). Then increase the time you walk by one minute every one to two days, as is comfortable. When you get to the point that exercise leaves you feeling worse, cut back to a comfortable level and continue that amount of walking each day.

You can find out more about the SHINE Protocol in my book *From Fatigued to Fantastic.* Or you or your doctor can email me at fatiguedoc@gmail.com and ask for free treatment tools, which include the SHINE Protocol overview, intake and treatment protocol checklists, quick screens, and more.

Long COVID Comes in Three Versions

Kings College London.

There are three distinct types of long COVID, researchers from Kings College London reported after analyzing data on 1,459 people who had ongoing symptoms for longer than 84 days...

•**Neurological.** Long-term fatigue, brain fog, and headache are the most common subtype among people infected with the alpha and delta variants.

•**Respiratory.** Long-term chest pain and severe shortness of breath are most common in people who were infected in the wild-type period when the population was unvaccinated.

•**Diverse.** A third group of people experience a range of symptoms including heart palpitations, muscle aches and pain, and changes in skin and hair.

The three subtypes were seen in all variants, but additional symptom clusters were subtly different between variants. These differences may not be due to variants themselves, but other factors, such as time of year, social behaviors, and treatments.

Don't Count on Antibody Tests

William Schaffner, M.D., professor of preventive medicine and infectious diseases at Vanderbilt University Medical Center, Nashville. Vanderbilt.edu

Antibody tests are not a reliable gauge of COVID immunity. Some people rely on these tests to decide if they should get a COVID booster, but no medical organization recommends this. There is no agreed-upon antibody level that has been shown to be protective against COVID and no standardization between tests on the market.

Intermittent Fasting Boosts Immunity

Valter Longo, Ph.D., professor of gerontology and biological sciences, Edna M. Jones Chair in Gerontology, Leonard Davis School of Gerontology, director of the Longevity Institute, University of Southern California, Los Angeles, and author of *The Longevity Diet*. ValterLongo.com

Skipping food for 12 hours followed by a mostly plant-based diet high in legumes and whole grains, with a little fish and dairy over the next 12 hours can significantly improve risk factors linked to heart disease and diabetes.

Also beneficial: Combine this intermittent fast with mini-fasts that involve consuming 800 to 1,100 calories per day for five days every three to six months. Fasting in this way may help reset the immune system, clearing out older infection-fighting white blood cells and replacing them with newer, stronger cells.

Addiction Drug May Ease Long COVID Symptoms

Reuters.

Low doses of naltrexone, a generic drug typically used to treat alcohol and opioid addiction, may help ease the pain, fatigue, and brain fog that can linger for months after a coronavirus infection. The drug has been used with some success to treat a similar complex, post-infectious syndrome marked by cognitive deficits and overwhelming fatigue called myalgic encephalomyelitis/chronic fatigue syndrome (ME/CFS). One study found that 74 percent of 218 patients had improvements in sleep, and reduced pain and neurological disturbances.

There are at least four clinical trials to test naltrexone in hundreds of patients with long COVID, and it is on the short list of treatments to be tested in the U.S. National Institutes of Health's $1 billion RECOVER Initiative, which aims to uncover underlying causes and find treatments for long COVID. Low-dose naltrexone, which has anti-inflammatory properties, may reverse some of the underlying pathology driving symptoms, Reuters reports.

At 50 milligrams (mg), 10 times the low dose, naltrexone is approved to treat opioid and alcohol addiction. Low-dose naltrexone must be purchased through a compounding pharmacy.

Stop the Pain of Recurrent UTIs

Suzette E. Sutherland, M.D., M.S., F.P.M.R.S., associate professor of urology at University of Washington School of Medicine, Seattle, and director of female urology at UW Medicine Pelvic Health Center (UW Medicine.org). She is a past president of the Society of Women in Urology and a member of the Education Committee for the American Urogynecologic Society.

You recognize the symptoms immediately—a relentless need to urinate, followed by a painful burning sensation when you do…unpleasant odor or cloudy color to your urine…and cramping or pressure in the lower abdomen. For millions of people —women and men—urinary tract infections (UTIs) are more than just a nuisance. They happen several times a year and may, although not commonly, travel into the kidneys, causing a more serious infection that comes with fever, nausea/vomiting, and even confusion. *We asked urology specialist Suzette E. Sutherland, M.D., what you can do to prevent these infections…*

•**Most women will experience at least one UTI in their lifetime**…between 20 percent and 40 percent of those who do will have a recurrence…and up to 50 percent of those women will have multiple recurrences. Men almost exclusively in their 50s and older also get UTIs.

•**UTIs happen when bacteria enter the urinary tract through the urethra,** the tube that carries urine out of the body. In most cases, antibiotics clear up the infection. But for some people, the UTI returns. Three or more UTIs within a year—or two within six months —are considered recurrent UTIs (rUTIs). Patients suffering from rUTIs often live in fear of the next infection.

Fortunately, there are strategies that may help prevent the next one…

RECURRENT UTIS IN WOMEN

Why UTIs happen: In women, the vagina and anus are colonized with billions of bacteria. This is normal and healthy and has nothing to do with hygiene. (Men are colonized with just as many bacteria.) The good bacteria usually outnumber the bad, preventing infections. But sometimes infection-causing bacteria make their way from the vagina or anus up toward the urethra. This can happen during sex or when wiping back to front.

Another little-known yet common cause of UTIs in menopausal women has to do with hormone levels. Estrogen helps the good bacteria, such as *Lactobacillus*, maintain the right balance in the vagina. As estrogen depletes during perimenopause and menopause, troublemaking bacteria get a leg up. Since a woman's urethra is only three inches long (versus seven to eight inches in men), once those bac-

---

Tailored Treatment for rUTIs

In the past, doctors often prescribed the same antibiotics to treat most UTIs. But overuse or incorrect use of these drugs has fueled antibiotic resistance, meaning that bacteria have learned to evade the drugs and continue thriving.

A new way of treating rUTIs involves performing a urine culture that identifies the specific organism causing the infection, such as *Escherichia coli* or *Staphylococcus saprophyticus*. The health-care provider then can select an antibiotic best suited for the particular bacteria and avoid mistreating. Urine culture results take a few days to process properly for accurate results.

While waiting for your results: You can find symptom relief with the pain-relieving drug *phenazopyridine hydrochloride* (Pyridium). Available over-the-counter as Azo or with a prescription, this oral medicine can quiet bladder symptoms, but it shouldn't be taken for more than a few days. And don't be alarmed—it turns your urine an intense orange.

—Suzette E. Sutherland, M.D., M.S., F.P.M.R.S.

---

teria move up from the vagina or anus, it's easy for them to reach the bladder.

A three-pronged approach that factors in the vagina, the anus, and the urethra-bladder complex can help women keep these bacteria in balance and under control, preventing rUTIs.

•**Vagina.** Local estrogen can make a big difference in minimizing rUTIs in menopausal women. It is available in three forms—vaginal cream (Estrace, Premarin)…vaginal suppository (Vagifem, Yuvafem)…and vaginal ring (Estring). These are not systemic estrogens, meaning they stay in the vaginal area and don't travel into the bloodstream and throughout the body. This helps avoid any of the risk for increased blood clots, heart attack, stroke, or breast cancer associated with larger-dose, systemic estrogens. Low-dose vaginal estrogen even can be used by women with a history of breast cancer. A urogynecologist or female urologist can explain how to use vaginal estrogen correctly.

Encouraging: In a 2021 study by researchers at University of South Florida, Tampa, nearly 70 percent of 167 postmenopausal women with rUTIs reported that vaginal estrogen cream improved or resolved their symptoms.

•**Anus.** *The following strategies can help minimize the number of bad-for-you bacteria in and around the anus…*

•Avoid constipation. As stool builds up in the rectum, more bacteria proliferate. Keep things moving by slowly increasing daily fiber intake, aiming for 25 grams a day from plant-based, fiber-rich foods such as beans, produce, nuts, and popcorn. You also can try a fiber supplement such as Metamucil or Citrucel or take 400 milligrams (mg) of magnesium citrate a day to stimulate the bowels.

Caution: Avoid laxatives—they can cause diarrhea, introducing even more problematic bacteria into the perineal area, and can cause long-term bowel dysfunction due to laxative dependence.

•Consume bowel-friendly probiotics. Probiotics are good-for-you bacteria found in fermented beverages and foods such as kefir, yogurt, sauerkraut, and kimchi.

Try: Lifeway Kefir and Activia yogurt.

If you opt for probiotic supplements: Look for ones that are specifically marketed for bowel and digestive health.

•**Bladder and urethra.** *The following techniques keep your bladder and urethra healthy…*

•Stay hydrated. Dehydration is the number-one cause of UTIs. That's because the less you drink, the less often you need to use the bathroom, and urinating helps flush bacteria from the urinary tract. Aim for at least two liters of fluid a day, with about half of this being water.

Goal: Drink enough that your urine is a light-yellow color and any bacteria that do make their way to the urethra are diluted and carried away.

•Try proanthocyanidin supplements. You've heard that cranberry juice helps prevent UTIs. That's only partly correct. Cranberry juice—more so than the skin, seeds, and stems—contains a soluble bioavailable compound called *proantho-cyanidin* (PAC) that attaches to UTI-causing bacteria, preventing them from latching on to the cells that line your urinary tract. These immobilized bacteria are flushed out during urination.

Some products contain high amounts of PAC…some have very little. Look for products that contain 36 mg of PAC in a single serving… are derived from pure cranberry juice and not the whole cranberry…and are labeled "soluble" or "bioavailable," which are most easily used by the body and most effective at fighting bacteria.

Products to try: Ellura capsules ($49.50 for 30 capsules, Amazon.com) or Utiva Cranberry PACs ($39.99 for 30 capsules, UtivaHealth.ca). Take one a day for prevention (not treatment) of rUTIs.

Drinking regular cranberry juice may help, but it's difficult to determine the PAC content. Make sure it's unsweetened pure cranberry juice. You can temper the bitterness by mixing it with some club soda, but not too much, or it will dilute the PAC concentration.

•Urinate after sex. This can help flush out any bacteria that have migrated up the urethra. Women who tend to develop UTIs after sex can take one to two capsules of PAC-containing supplements before sex and again the following day for additional protection.

RECURRENT UTIS IN MEN

Men also have billions of bacteria residing all over their body, including below the belt. But the most common reason older men develop rUTIs involves an enlarged prostate gland, also called benign prostatic hyperplasia (BPH), which makes it difficult to empty the bladder. That means urine sits in the bladder for prolonged periods, allowing bacteria to multiply. BPH is the most common prostate problem affecting men over age 50.

Men with BPH can help reduce the frequency of rUTIs by fully emptying their bladder as regularly as possible. *This can be facilitated by treating BPH, which can be accomplished by…*

•**Taking prescription medication to shrink the prostate gland.** *Finasteride* (Proscar), a 5-alpha reductase inhibitor, is commonly used for this reason.

•**Taking medication to relax the muscles at the bladder opening** (bladder neck) and part of the urethra that runs through the prostate. These alpha blockers make it easier for urine to flow and for the bladder to empty completely. *Tamsulosin* (Flomax) is a popular one.

•**Having the prostate removed in a procedure called a transurethral resection of the prostate.** Risks include retrograde ejaculation (semen flows into the bladder during sex), urinary incontinence, and erectile dysfunction.

Men with rUTIs also should stay hydrated, use PAC supplements, avoid constipation, and consume probiotics.

The Right Toothpaste for You

Meredith Worthington, Ph.D., executive editor of ConsumerLab.com, LLC, an independent group based in White Plains, New York, that tests and reports on the quality of health and nutrition products. ConsumerLab.com

There are plenty of toothpastes on store shelves, each boasting dental-care benefits and listing unpronounceable ingredients. *But which claims should you believe? Facts worth knowing about toothpaste…*

•**Fluoride is the most important toothpaste ingredient.** Instead of the word "fluoride," you may see the terms "sodium monofluorophosphate"…"sodium fluoride"…or "stannous fluoride" on fluoridated-toothpaste labels—these are the three forms of fluoride that the U.S. Food and Drug Administration recognizes as clinically effective for cavity prevention.

Note: Some people seek out fluoride-free toothpastes because they are concerned that fluoride causes cancer, but dozens of studies indicate those concerns are misplaced.

•**The "ADA Accepted" seal ensures claims on packaging are legit.** The American Dental Association (ADA) won't issue this seal to a product unless the manufacturer can provide lab tests and/or clinical trials to back its claims. This seal also ensures that the tooth-

Brush Your Teeth Before or After Breakfast?

Before breakfast—mouth bacteria are at peak levels when you wake up, which is the reason for bad breath. Eating breakfast, especially if it contains sugar, causes bacteria to multiply. Brushing before breakfast clears the bacteria away and boosts tooth-protective saliva…and the fluoride in toothpaste protects against acids in breakfast foods. *Brushing after breakfast*—fluoride will not be displaced by chewing food. Wait 30 minutes after eating before brushing to avoid damaging tooth enamel, especially if you consume acidic beverages such as coffee or orange juice.

Apoena de Aguiar Ribeiro, DDS, MS, Ph.D., pediatric dentist and microbiologist…Rocio Beatriz Quinonez, DMD, MPH, MS, professor of pediatric dentistry, both at University of North Carolina, Chapel Hill. Dentistry.UNC.edu…Carlos González-Cabezas, DDS, MSD, Ph.D., dentist, professor, dean for academic affairs, University of Michigan School of Dentistry, Dent.UMich.edu

paste doesn't contain flavorings that could contribute to tooth decay.

Helpful: Check products in the ADA Seal Chairside Guide (https://bit.ly/3txYUjH) for ADA-accepted products.

•**"Natural" toothpastes aren't necessarily safe.**

Example: The natural toothpaste Redmond Earthpaste includes calcium bentonite clay, which can contain heavy metals such as lead. And many natural toothpastes don't contain the most important ingredient—fluoride.

Best natural product: The natural toothpaste Tom's of Maine Whole Care contains fluoride—as the company notes, fluoride is natural and found in ocean water, soil, rocks, and living creatures including humans. (Some other Tom's of Maine toothpastes don't contain fluoride.) There is no official definition of the word "natural" on toothpaste labels.

•**"Sensitive teeth" toothpastes should contain stannous fluoride or potassium nitrate.** These ingredients can reduce sensitivity to touch and the movement of breath over the teeth, but stannous fluoride has the added benefit of fighting gingivitis.

Warning: For some people, stannous fluoride may cause difficult-to-reverse tooth staining. Stannous fluoride toothpaste stabilized with zinc phosphate, which should appear in the list of inactive ingredients on the toothpaste label, may be less likely to cause staining.

Products to try for sensitive teeth: Colgate Total SF and Crest Pro-Health, which contain stannous fluoride…or Sensodyne Deep Clean Sensitive Toothpaste, Colgate Sensitive Prevent and Repair or Hello Sensitivity Relief, which contain potassium nitrate. Colgate Total also contains zinc phosphate.

•**Whitening toothpastes can cause discomfort.** They can contain irritating abrasive agents and/or chemical whiteners.

For surface stains: We recommend Tom's of Maine Simply White Clean Mint Toothpaste, which contains mildly abrasive hydrated silica but does not contain the potentially irritating tartar-control agent pyrophosphate.

For nonsurface stains: Whitening toothpastes have only modest benefit, so on deeper stains, we recommend using whitening strips, which have better effects. We recommend Crest 3D Whitestrips, the only product that has been accepted by the ADA.

Discontinue use if either of these causes significant discomfort.

Reusable Contact Lenses Boost Risk of Eye Infection

Ophthalmology.

People who wear reusable contact lenses are nearly four times as likely as those who wear daily disposables to develop *Acanthamoeba keratitis* (AK), a rare sight-threatening eye infection. The most severely affected patients (a quarter of the total) end up with less than 25 percent of vision or become blind following the disease and face prolonged treatment. Overall, 25 percent of people affected require corneal transplants to treat the disease or restore vision. Showering with lenses in increased the odds of AK by 3.3 times, while wearing lenses overnight increased the odds by 3.9 times. Among daily disposable wearers, reusing lenses increased their infection risk. Having had a recent contact lens check with a health professional reduced the risk.

Refreeze Meat Safely

U.S. Department of Agriculture (USDA). USDA.gov

Centers for Disease Control and Prevention (CDC), Atlanta. CDC.gov

Thawed, raw, or cooked meat is safe to refreeze—however, refrozen meat may lose some moisture when thawed and the texture and taste may be affected.

Safety warning: Do not refreeze meat that has been unrefrigerated for more than two hours (one hour if the temperature is above 90°F).

Best: Thaw meat in the refrigerator—thawing it on a countertop can cause mold, bacteria, and other harmful microbes to grow.

Another option: Thaw meat outside of the fridge by sealing the meat in a plastic bag and putting the bag into cold tap water, making sure to change the water every 30 minutes until the meat is thawed…or microwave it just before cooking to defrost it. Also, meat that has been in the freezer for a long time may develop ice crystals—also called freezer burn—but the meat is still safe to eat.

Information: CDC.gov/foodsafety/keep-food-safe.html

Wash Your Kitchen, Not the Chicken

North Carolina State University.

Washing chicken is thought to spread bacteria in the kitchen, but a new study finds that even unwashed chicken can contaminate other foods. Researchers invited 300 home cooks to prepare chicken thighs and a salad in a test kitchen. Half of the participants were sent information advising them against washing chicken. The chicken thighs were inoculated with a harmless strain of bacteria that the researchers would be able to detect.

Researchers swabbed the kitchen and salad before the chicken was cooked, after the meal was finished, and after the kitchen was cleaned to identify any potential contamination. They discovered that people who *did* wash the chicken and people who *didn't* wash the chicken had similar levels of contamination from the raw chicken in their prepared salads.

"Regardless of whether people washed their chicken, the kitchen sinks became contaminated by the raw chicken, while there was relatively little contamination of nearby counters," said Ellen Shumaker, PhD. "This study demonstrates the need to focus on preventing contamination of sinks and emphasizing the importance of hand-washing and cleaning and sanitizing surfaces."

Plant Flavonoids May Fight Mosquito-Borne Illnesses

Study led by researchers at University of Tsukuba, Japan, published in *BMC Biology*.

Flavonoids disrupt larval development of *Aedes aegypti* mosquitoes—the kind that carries Zika, yellow fever, and dengue—which have been developing resistance to traditional insecticides.

Virus Can Cause Face Paralysis

J. Wes Ulm, M.D., Ph.D., Harvard Medical School. Dr. Ulm is a nationally and globally renowned physician-scientist with a longstanding history as a respected expert and pioneer in gene therapy, virology, molecular biology, and drug discovery and repurposing.

Ramsay Hunt syndrome (RHS), a complication that comes from prior infection with the *varicella-zoster* virus (VZV), which also causes chicken pox and shingles, can cause face paralysis. Once you are infected with VZV, the virus can lie dormant for decades in structures of the human nervous system such as the cranial nerves (which mostly emanate from the brainstem at the bottom portion of the brain) and clusters of nerve cells just outside of the spinal cord.

The virus can then be reactivated under conditions of stress or reduced immune function. This is known, in general, as shingles, especially when it results in a painful, blistery rash in a stripe-like pattern on the torso. RHS is a subset of shingles that snarls a specific nerve in the face, known as the facial nerve or cranial nerve VII.

SYMPTOMS OF RHS

The first symptom is usually pain in the ear and one side of the face. That is followed by blistery-appearing lesions and, of particular concern, paralysis of the facial nerve of varying severity and duration. This paralysis makes itself known in the form of an asymmetry on one side of the face (with the cheek and mouth dipping below the other side), along with difficulty in smiling and partial loss of taste. Some people also experience ringing in the ear, hearing loss, dizziness, and dry eyes.

PROGNOSIS

RHS eventually resolves on its own, with full or at least partial restoration of function. Full resolution occurs in 70 percent of RHS cases. In Bell's palsy, a much more common form of facial nerve paralysis, full resolution of the symptoms occurs in 90 percent of cases.

Herpes Refers to How a Virus Stores Information

RHS is a subset of herpes zoster. The herpes in the term is simply a reference to the virus's classification as a member of the broader human herpesvirus family of viruses that store their genetic information in double-stranded DNA, unlike viruses such as COVID-19 that use RNA.

Treatment is designed to mitigate symptoms and, where possible, to reduce the load of the virus that causes the disorder. The latter is achieved with common antiviral drugs used for the herpes family of viruses, including *acyclovir* or *valacyclovir* or, in some cases, *famciclovir*, for at least a week. A doctor may also prescribe corticosteroids. Artificial tears and eye drops can be helpful in some cases, while patients with more severe or persistent symptoms may require more intensive follow-up by a physician and care team.

Painkillers are a basic part of management. If over-the-counter analgesics like acetaminophen, aspirin, or ibuprofen are insufficient, a physician might prescribe stronger painkillers and, in some cases, a drug like *gabapentin*, which is used for neuropathic pain involving the affected nerves (especially in the event of postherpetic neuralgia, a painful complication of shingles or RHS).

PREVENTION

While prevention is difficult to guarantee, patients obtaining the shingles vaccine are at reduced risk of RHS as well. Steer clear of anyone with an active chicken pox infection (since the virus is spread through a respiratory route or by saliva or mucus), and be careful around anyone with an existing case of shingles or RHS, since the vesicles also contain active virus particles.

New Tick-Borne Disease Concern

Study by researchers at Emory University, Atlanta, Georgia, published in *Emerging Infectious Diseases*.

Heartland virus, a disease spread by lone star ticks, has been found in one of every 2,000 ticks sampled in Georgia. The disease was first found in Missouri in 2009, and since then about 50 confirmed cases in 11 states have been reported. Of particular concern is that the disease found in Georgia ticks has a different genome from what has been found elsewhere—possibly indicating that the virus is evolving as it spreads. Symptoms include fever, fatigue, and muscle and joint pain. Patients may require hospitalization, and the virus is potentially fatal.

Problem: The disease is still not well understood, so it is possible that many more people have been infected but had only mild symptoms.

First U.S. Vaccine for Tick-Borne Encephalitis (TBE)

Sam Telford, ScD, professor of infectious disease, global health, biology, and epidemiology at Tufts University in North Grafton, Massachusetts. Tufts.edu

TBE, a virus carried by ticks found in Asia and Europe, attacks the brain and spine and can cause disability or death. The vaccine TICOVAC should be considered for people ages one and older who will be traveling to affected areas abroad. Given in three injections, it has been shown to be safe with no serious side effects. TBE does not occur in the U.S., and the vaccine does not protect against Powassan encephalitis, which does occur in the U.S.

Monkeypox Is Not Dangerous or as Transmissible as COVID

William Schaffner, M.D., professor of preventive medicine at Vanderbilt University School of Medicine in Nashville.

Typically confined to Africa, the virus has spread to Europe and North America. At press time, there have been slightly over 30,000 confirmed cases in the U.S. Transmission occurs through broken skin or respiratory droplets via prolonged physical contact (not through sex). Symptoms include fever, muscle aches, and a rash, sometimes on the genitals and/or anus. The antiviral *tecovirimat* and the monoclonal *brincidofovir* are approved treatments. The Jynneos vaccine will be deployed in a targeted way.

Best Mosquito Repellents

Research by Health.com.

Best overall—Off! Deep Woods Mosquito Repellent Spray. *For hiking*—Ben's 100 Max DEET Tick & Insect Repellent Spray. Wipes—Repel 30 percent DEET Wipes. *For sensitive skin*—Sawyer Family Controlled Release Repellent Lotion. *Best long-lasting*—Sawyer Picaridin 20 percent Continuous Spray. *Best-smelling*—Natrapel 20 percent Picaridin Eco Insect Repellent Spray. *Best oil-of-lemon-eucalyptus*

(OLE)/natural option—Repel Lemon Plant-Based Eucalyptus Insect Repellent. *For babies and kids*—Babyganics Natural Insect Repellent. *For pets*—Vet's Best Mosquito Repellent for Dogs and Cats. All are available from Amazon, Walmart, REI, and other online and retail stores.

How Risky Is Using a Public Toilet?

Charles Gerba, M.D., professor of microbiology and immunology, the University of Arizona, Tucson. Arizona.edu

Research links public toilets with infections such as norovirus, salmonella, and hepatitis A. The pathogens that cause these illnesses deposit on surfaces in restrooms primarily when toilets are flushed and microbes are dispersed in an aerosolized plume—so risk depends on how well the toilet is ventilated and how well and how often it is cleaned.

Risk-reducing strategies: Although sitting on a contaminated toilet seat is not likely to make you sick, using a disinfecting wipe on the seat before sitting might reduce likelihood of infection. Toilet seat covers don't offer much protection and likely are contaminated by spray from toilet flushes.

Most important thing you can do: Thoroughly wash your hands after using any bathroom.

Also: Do not put a bag or purse on the floor of the stall—that often is the dirtiest area of the bathroom.

CHAPTER 12

Medical News Alerts

Protect Your Health on a Changing Planet

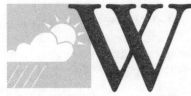

When you think of climate change, you probably think of problems with ecological health, like drought, rising sea levels, and wildfires. But climate change can also take a toll on personal health, both physical and mental. We spoke with Micah B. Hahn, Ph.D., MPH, to learn more.

"The climate crisis is a human health emergency," Jonathan Patz, director of the University of Wisconsin–Madison Global Health Institute (GHI), and colleagues wrote in an editorial in the *Journal of the American Medical Association*. The editorial points out that "numerous climate-sensitive health risks are scientifically established," including the risk of death from heat waves, respiratory illness from smog and ozone (which increase when there is more nitrogen dioxide from car exhaust in the air), higher levels of pollen that cause more allergies, physical and mental effects from wildfires, and exposure to infectious diseases like West Nile Virus.

The health impacts of climate change are so pervasive that an article in the March 2021 issue of *Academic Medicine* called for medical education to include curricula on "climate change and its effect on health." But you don't have to wait for your doctor to get up to speed when it comes to climate change and health. You can start protecting yourself today by taking simple precautions and actions.

WARM SPELLS AND HEAT WAVES

The higher temperatures we are seeing and will continue to see increase the risk of cardiovascular and respiratory illness—and death. Researchers from the University of Wisconsin–Madison estimate that warmer average tempera-

Micah B. Hahn, Ph.D., associate professor of environmental health in the Institute for Circumpolar Health Studies at the University of Alaska Anchorage, and a former epidemiologist at the Centers for Disease and Control and Prevention, in the Climate and Health Program.

tures caused by climate change could result in 11,562 additional annual deaths among Americans 65 years and older, who are more sensitive to heat stress and more likely to develop heat illness.

There are two types of heat risks: 1) a single day with higher-than-normal temperatures, such as the 108° Fahrenheit recorded in Seattle in June 2021; 2) multiple, consecutive days of warm weather, like the "heat dome" that set-

Climate Change and Mental Health

Climate change can change your outlook—and not for the better. A study of Alaska's Swan Lake fire, which burned for nearly four months in the summer of 2019, found that it affected mental health in many ways. As the fire burned, people were anxious for their lives and property. Some people felt claustrophobic, because smoky skies kept them indoors for months. Over the four months, people felt increasingly stressed. The following summer, many experienced stress as other natural disasters like earthquakes struck the area. There was also grief, a sense of loss and helplessness, and mourning for the shattered beauty of the natural environment, as 170,000 acres of trees were reduced to blackened toothpicks. *When residents of the area were asked about the best ways to lessen wildfire-related mental health problems, they frequently mentioned…*

1. Early communication about the disaster

2. More information about the disaster

3. A community-based preparedness program

4. Community support for evacuation planning

5. Better emergency shelters

6. Talking with others about the connection between the disaster and prolonged stress

7. Support groups consisting of people who've been through the disaster

8. Grief counseling.

tled over the West in September 2022 for about a week, setting heat records throughout California, Arizona, and other states in the region.

If you're faced with high heat, there are several steps you can take to lower your risk…

•**Pay attention to heat alerts.** The National Weather Service issues heat alerts, which can tell you in advance when a hot day or heat wave is coming—so you can limit exposure. You can find more information at Weather.gov.

•**Limit exposure.** When it's excessively hot outside, try to stay inside. If you must go out, avoid strenuous activity, such as exercising. Wear a wide-brimmed hat (to keep the sun off your face) and loose, lightweight, light-colored clothing.

•**Buy cooling devices in advance.** Don't wait until a heat wave to buy a fan or air conditioner. It's likely they'll be sold out. Plan ahead for excessive heat.

•**Drink lots of water.** Staying hydrated is one of the best ways to reduce the effects of excessive heat. During a hot day or heat wave, try to drink at least 50 ounces of water per day.

•**Go where it's cool.** If you can't cool down your home or apartment, go to places in your community that are cool, such as an indoor mall, movie theatre, public library, or cooling center.

•**Be extra careful if you're in a high-risk group.** People who are extra-sensitive to heat include those ages 60 and older, pregnant women, people with chronic kidney disease, and people with cardiovascular or respiratory disease, such as asthma or COPD.

•**Check on your neighbor.** If you have a neighbor who lives alone and is elderly or has a hard time moving around, check up on them during a heat wave to see if they need help.

WILDFIRES

Exposure to smoke is the most direct health impact of a wildfire. Exposure isn't limited to people near the wildfire. Smoke from wildfires can spread downwind, putting communities far from the fire at risk.

Breathing wildfire smoke can increase your risk of heart attacks, arrhythmia (irregular heartbeat), long-term heart disease, respiratory

---

**Do Your Part to Slow
Climate Change**

Just as there are many simple ways to reduce the personal health risk of climate
change, there are many ways to personally
reduce the greenhouse gases that cause
climate change.

• **Walk and bike more, and drive less.**

• **Decrease flying.** Airplanes are a huge
source of emissions.

• **Use all the food you buy.** Food waste
(uneaten food) accounts for about 8 percent
of global greenhouse gases.

---

distress (shortness of breath), asthma attacks,
and even cancer.

In one study, researchers at the University
of California, San Diego, looked at visits to the
emergency room during wildfires in Southern
California and found more than double the normal rate of asthma diagnoses, and more than
triple the normal rate of shortness of breath.

Here's how to lower your risk...

• **Evaluate air quality.** When wildfires are
burning, visit AirNow.gov and enter your ZIP
code to learn the air quality where you live.
If the quality is below good or moderate, stay
indoors.

• **Use an air filter.** When wildfires are burning, use an air purifier indoors, preferably with
a HEPA filter, which removes the fine particulate matter in smoke from the air. Brands
favored by a site that specializes in evaluating
consumer products for performance and cost
include Coway, Winix, Blueair, and Levoit.

• **Use other ways to reduce particulates
indoors.** Close the windows. Get new filters
for your central air conditioner. Damp-mop the
floor. Wash sheets and clothes more often than
normal.

• **Increase your intake of olive oil and
fish oil.** It can't hurt and, according to scientific research, it may help. In studies conducted
at the University of North Carolina at Chapel
Hill, both olive oil and fish oil protected blood

vessels from the damage typically caused by
inhaled fine particulate matter.

• **Wear a mask when you go outside.**
Wearing an N-95 or P-100 mask can block fine
particulates from smoke.

VECTOR-BORNE DISEASES

As the globe warms, ticks, fleas, and mosquitoes that were confined to a particular area
expand their range, putting more people at risk
of diseases carried by these insects. For example, West Nile virus was once confined to
Africa, but it's now the most common form of
mosquito-caused disease in the United States.

Take these steps to lower your risk...

• **Wear mosquito repellant, long sleeves,
and pants.** Try a product with 20 percent
picaridin, a safe, EPA-approved synthetic compound that is as effective as DEET but without
the toxic side effects. Put it on your skin and
your clothes.

• **Eliminate standing water around your
house.** It's a breeding ground for mosquitoes.

• **After walking through tick country,
dry (don't wash) your clothes.** Research
shows that putting clothes directly into the dri-
er on high temperature for 50 minutes can kill
ticks by desiccating them. (Putting them in the
washer doesn't.) Taking a shower and doing a
tick check is also important in order to remove
ticks that are crawling or feeding.

Urban Trees Fight Climate Change Better Than Forest Trees

Study led by researchers at Boston University, published in *Global Change Biology*.

Trees in "edge" zones between forests and
developed areas grow nearly twice as fast
as trees 100 feet or more inside woods—and
bigger trees remove more carbon dioxide from
the atmosphere, mitigating the effects of climate change.

Lessons Learned from the Pandemic

Barry A. Franklin, Ph.D., director of Preventive Cardiology/Cardiac Rehabilitation at Beaumont Health in Royal Oak, Michigan. He is past president of the AACVPR and the ACSM. DrBarryFranklin.com

The pandemic appears to be finally winding down, and we can now take a moment to reflect on what we have learned and apply those principles should a new variant or entirely new pandemic strike in the future.

While the pandemic has been devastating in the United States, not all citizens have been affected equally. Cultural and societal factors have placed some populations at increased risk of contracting and dying from COVID-19.

•**Race.** After adjusting for age, Hispanics, Blacks, Native Americans, and individuals of lower socioeconomic status account for a disproportionately high percentage of COVID hospitalizations and deaths.

This may be partially attributed to social factors that affect health, including personal lifestyle choices, income and wealth disparities, inequalities in health-care access and use, occupational vulnerability, public transportation transmission, and living in multi-family housing.

Additionally, these demographic groups have a higher prevalence of underlying hypertension, diabetes, obesity, cardiovascular disease, and pulmonary conditions—all of which can worsen COVID-19 illness.

•**Living in rural areas.** Rural Americans are more likely to die from COVID-19 infections than their urban counterparts. This heightened mortality may be attributed to higher age, lower socioeconomic status, limited access to health care, and greater incidence of underlying chronic disease. Further, people living in rural areas have lower rates of vaccination against COVID-19. Even when access to the vaccine is not limited, rural Americans tend to express less enthusiasm for the vaccine's safety and value.

According to numerous reports, the scientific evidence is overwhelming: COVID vaccines are generally safe and highly effective in preventing COVID-related hospitalization and death.

•**Medical misinformation.** The spread of medical misinformation is extensive. For example, numerous studies have definitively proven that wearing a mask does not expose the wearer to dangerous levels of carbon dioxide, but that remains a concern among some people.

In July 2021, U.S. Surgeon General Vivek Murthy, M.D., commented that nearly every recent death due to COVID could have been prevented. Dr. Murthy emphasized that: "Health misinformation...can cause confusion, sow mistrust, harm people's health, and undermine public health efforts. It's one of several reasons why people are not getting vaccinated."

•**Poor baseline health.** Even before the pandemic, Americans had a high prevalence of unhealthy lifestyles, risk factors, and chronic disease, as well as the shortest life expectancy among all high-income countries.

According to one landmark study, adhering to a healthier lifestyle could prolong the life expectancy by up to 14 years for women and 12 years for men.

The 4Ws

To reduce the risk of viral transmission—whether it is COVID-19 or a future threat, follow the 4Ws...

•**Wear a mask if you are in an area with high transmission.**

•**Wash your hands.**

•**Watch your distance (≥6 feet).**

•**Walk briskly (ideally 2.5 to 3 miles per hour or faster)** to maintain a baseline of fitness.

Think of these protective interventions as slices of Swiss cheese: Every slice has holes, but each layer covers some of the holes of the one underneath it.

The Role of Diet

The Mediterranean diet, which has been shown to decrease inflammatory markers, may also help decrease COVID-19 incidence, severity, and mortality.

Foods that increase levels of nitric oxide, such as beets, leafy greens, and lean meats (e.g., bison) have also been shown to improve vascular health.

For overweight and obese individuals, losing just 5 percent of body weight confers health benefits.

NEED FOR GREATER SELF-RESPONSIBILITY

Both the pandemic and our poor health as a nation can be improved with a time-honored American value: self-responsibility. Failure to take responsibility for our own health unequivocally increases the life-threatening risks of COVID, and it leads to many of the underlying chronic illnesses that worsen the impact of the virus, such as obesity, type 2 diabetes, and coronary artery disease. Small, positive changes to what we eat, how often we exercise, and avoiding cigarette smoking can add years and quality to our lives.

•**Exercise.** Regular physical activity prevents and treats chronic disease, boosts immune function, decreases inflammation, and maintains or reduces body weight and fat stores. Plus, getting just 150 minutes of moderate-intensity exercise per week (or 75 minutes of vigorous activity) is associated with a reduced likelihood for hospitalization, intensive care unit admission, and death among patients with COVID-19. Higher levels of aerobic fitness also appear to confer more favorable COVID-19 outcomes.

•**Smoking.** Because COVID-19 targets the lungs, quitting smoking is imperative.

The sooner we embrace the 4Ws, get vaccinated, and get boosted, the sooner COVID-19 will be over.

The Surprising Science of Happiness

Brendan Kelly, Ph.D., professor of psychiatry at Trinity College, Dublin, and consultant psychiatrist at Tallaght University Hospital. He is author of *The Science of Happiness: The Six Principles of a Happy Life and the Seven Strategies for Achieving It.*

What does it mean to be truly "happy"? Few concepts seem as simple—even young children can tell you if they're happy—but the deeper you dig, the more enigmatic true happiness becomes. And it seems that even when people have a good sense of what makes them happy, they often fail to prioritize those things. Research has found that placing a high value on happiness actually can make people less happy. Finland, for example, is the happiest country in the world…yet it also has a high suicide rate.

We asked happiness researcher Brendan Kelly, Ph.D., to give us a better understanding of what happiness is and how you can achieve it…

•**Life is least happy in the middle.** One might be the loneliest number, but 47 is the saddest age. When a Dartmouth College economist examined data from 132 countries, he discovered a remarkably consistent pattern—happiness has a U-shaped trendline as people age, with the lowest point arriving at age 47 virtually everywhere in the world.

Why are the late 40s the least happy years? Most likely because that is when people tend to be under the most pressure—supporting families, paying mortgages, and struggling to advance their careers. Naturally some people's life events will alter their personal happiness trends, and of course, younger and older people face pressures, too, but when you look at societies as a whole, the data are clear—the late 40s are when happiness is hardest to achieve.

What to do: Don't mistake midlife malaise for a downward happiness spiral that will drive you deeper into despair…and don't assume that you must change careers or spouses to rediscover joy. Life likely will start to be happier soon simply because that's what usually happens as 47 disappears into the rearview mirror.

●**There are two different types of happiness.** *Hedonic happiness* is pleasure in the moment, such as splurging on a weekend trip to Las Vegas. *Eudaimonic happiness* is more akin to contentment, such as the sense of fulfillment derived from saving money and making progress toward a financial goal. Which of these matters? Which is true happiness?

The answer is…both. People who balance hedonic and eudaimonic happiness are better off than those who derive pleasure exclusively from one or the other, according to University of Rochester psychologists. That balance becomes an issue for some people as they age—there's a tendency to drift excessively toward eudaimonic happiness later in life.

What to do: If your life is largely without hedonic happiness, borrow some exultation from others. Spend time with your children, for whom joy in the moment is natural and contagious…or adopt a dog or cat—pets can radiate spontaneous joy.

Another option: Prioritize forming new friendships—to the brain, this is a form of hedonic pleasure.

●**Placing a high value on happiness makes happiness less likely.** Here's some troubling news if you're reading this because you very much want to be happier—if you put a high priority on happiness, you hurt your chances of obtaining it. A series of recent studies have made this paradoxical finding—in fact, prioritizing happiness even seems to be a risk factor for depression. One theory is that striving for any one specific emotion—in this case, happiness—is a less effective path to long-term happiness than is accepting one's emotions. Another possibility is that people who put a very high priority on happiness set their expectations so high that even good times disappoint.

What to do: Be aware of what makes you happy, and let this guide your day-to-day decisions…but don't see sadness as failure. It isn't reasonable to expect to be joyous all the time.

●**We dread disappointment more than we desire happiness.** Investors have heard about the risk-aversion trap—many investors cost themselves returns because their fear of losses exceeds their desire for profits.

A similar problem pops up with happiness: Many people fail to take advantage of opportunities to do things that are likely to make them happy because they're too worried about the possibility that these things could go wrong. In particular, they're often concerned that they'll look foolish in other people's eyes if, for example, they try a new hobby but flub the attempt.

What to do: If you're tempted to decline a potential source of happiness for fear of looking foolish, you should know that it's much harder to appear foolish than you think.

Reason: Almost no one is paying attention to you—they're all caught up in their own lives.

●**Money is the secret to happiness…up to a point.** The old adage "money can't buy happiness" is wrong—a pair of Princeton researchers found a strong link between people's income and their self-reported evaluation of their happiness. But more money doesn't always equal more happiness—these researchers discovered that additional income beyond $75,000 stops providing additional happiness. Further research from Purdue University has set the limit at anywhere from $60,000 to $95,000, depending on how happiness is measured. In fact, annual income above $95,000 seems to be linked to slightly reduced happiness, though these figures can vary based on local cost of living and other factors.

There is some logic to this. It's likely to undermine your happiness if you don't have enough money to meet your basic needs and feel secure about your future…but once you achieve financial security, additional income might not provide enough upside to offset the additional workplace pressures and responsibilities required to earn it.

What to do: If you earn significantly more than $75,000 to $95,000 per year, reflect on your work/life balance. Would you be happier if you worked less even if that meant you earned less?

Artificial Intelligence and Your Health

AI Can Diagnose Heart Disease

An artificial intelligence tool can identify and distinguish between two life-threatening heart conditions that are often easy to miss: hypertrophic cardiomyopathy (thickening and stiffening of the heart) and cardiac amyloidosis (deposits of an abnormal protein in the heart). The tool can detect and differentiate the diseases before they can affect health outcomes and allow for earlier treatment.

Cedars-Sinai Medical Center.

AI Program May One Day Be Able to Detect Early-Stage Alzheimer's Disease (AD)

An artificial intelligence program may one day be able to detect early-stage Alzheimer's disease (AD). The AI program GPT-3, created by OpenAI, is currently known for its ability to produce a human-like response to any task that involves language, from writing poems and essays to responding to simple questions. Researchers at Drexel University have found that it can also be trained to detect speech patterns that are associated with dementia, improving the early diagnosis of AD. Investigators are now working to develop a web application that could be used at home or in a doctor's office as a prescreening tool.

Drexel University.

•**Religion and politics affect happiness.** There is a strong link between people's core beliefs and how happy they are. Studies have repeatedly found that religious people tend to be happier than nonreligious people—a 2017 review of the research on the subject conducted at Sultan Qaboos University found that this was true across religions and around the globe. A 2019 Pew Research Center survey found that 36 percent of actively religious Americans described themselves as "very happy" compared with 25 percent of inactively religious and nonreligious Americans.

What to do: No one should change his/her deeply held convictions based on these findings, but you can understand that certain convictions could make you less happy. Someone deeply committed to political causes might be well served to cultivate nonpolitical interests as well.

•**People living in societies with shared values tend to be especially happy**—if they're part of the "in crowd." Not only is Finland the happiest country in the world, the other Nordic nations invariably land near the top in happiness surveys as well. These countries have a great deal of "social cohesion"—their citizens tend to feel unified, which contributes to happiness. But there's a dark side to social cohesion—people who feel excluded from the mainstream in very unified societies often are tremendously unhappy, which likely explains Finland's steep suicide rates.

What to do: If you're part of the in crowd in a close-knit community, reach out to people who seem outside the mainstream. Not only could your gesture help those outsiders feel included, it could make you happier, too. The person who does a favor typically gains more happiness from it than the recipient.

Developing a Pill Bottle for Parkinson's

CBC Radio. CBC.ca

Jimmy Choi usually uses social media to highlight his incredible feats of athleticism. Recently, however, he shared a different kind of video: one showing how difficult it is for him to take a pill out of a bottle. Choi has Parkinson's disease.

Then something interesting happened: A man who saw the video, Brian Alldridge, responded by designing a bottle that can dispense

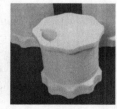

Credit: David Exler

a single pill with the turn of a knob. Alldridge learned how to use a 3D modeling program called Fusion 360 to develop the design, but he didn't have a 3D printer to try it out, so he posted his design online and offered to share his files with anyone who wanted to improve upon it, print it, and test it out. He says he woke up "to a million views and thousands of people offering to print it."

One of those people was engineer David Exler, who started creating bottle prototypes (see photo) and sharing them with Choi for testing. Exler also offered to print and ship pill bottles to 50 people in exchange for $5 donations to the Michael J. Fox Foundation for Parkinson's Research.

Alldridge, in the meantime, is hoping to meet with manufacturers about mass-producing the bottles cheaply. "It has less plastic in it than your average McDonald's toy, and should be priced as such," he explained. All of the proceeds will go to nonprofit organizations.

"There's a lot of negativity out there," Choi said in an interview with CBC Radio. "But people need to see the positive side that social media can be used for good things and for things that are helping and making an impact, not just on one person, two people, but we're talking thousands of people that this will have an impact on."

When It Comes to Joint Replacement, Age Is Nothing but a Number

Raymond Hwang, M.D., MEng, MBA, assistant clinical professor of orthopedic surgery at Tufts University School of Medicine, Boston, and medical director at Hinge Health, a digital musculoskeletal clinic for back, neck, joint, and other musculoskeletal pain. HingeHealth.com

Have you stopped playing golf because your knee hurts too much…or find yourself sitting out because of hip pain when the grandkids come by to play? Many people live with joint pain because they think their age means they can't have any type of joint-replacement surgery. And that's under-standable—historically, the average age for these procedures has been in the mid-to-upper 60s.

But even as we age, we still want to walk, run, bike, and otherwise stay active for as long as possible. Nonsurgical interventions, including physical therapy (PT), should be the first line of treatment for the majority of chronic joint pain conditions and may be the best solution for joint pain.

But if additional treatment is needed, advancements in technology that limit the time under anesthesia…reduce infection risk…and get patients on their feet mere hours after surgery make it possible even for people in their late 70s, 80s, and 90s to thrive after knee- or hip-replacement surgery. In fact, in May 2022, a 102-year-old man in India underwent a successful partial hip replacement following a fracture that resulted from a fall. The surgery took 20 minutes, and he was back on his feet within just 24 hours.

WHY REPLACEMENT SURGERY?

Joints deteriorate for several reasons…

• **Arthritis is the most common reason for a knee or hip replacement**—specifically osteoarthritis, painful wearing out of joint cartilage that occurs with age. According to a 2019 study by researchers at Peking University, Capital Medical University in Beijing, and Harvard Medical School, the number of global cases of osteoarthritis increased by 113 percent between 1990 and 2019, from about 248 million cases worldwide to 529 million cases, respectively.

• **Obesity,** an epidemic in the U.S., is commonly associated with osteoarthritis. Excess weight puts more stress on joints, which tends to accelerate the wear-and-tear process that eventually leads to inflammation of that joint. And obesity itself is pro-inflammatory, so it can worsen the inflammation related to osteoarthritis. Lastly, joint pain often causes people to be less active, which can increase risk for obesity.

• **Injury.** Older adults often need hip replacement following a fall that results in a hip fracture. One out of every four U.S. adults age 65+ will suffer a fall, with more than 300,000 of them being hospitalized for hip fractures, per the Centers for Disease Control and Prevention.

HEALTH TRUMPS AGE

For many older adults, knee and hip replacements can be safely performed regardless of their age. In fact, it's less about a person's *chronologic* age (the number of years he/she has been alive) and more about his *physiologic* age (how well his body functions thanks to lifestyle choices, genetics, and existing diseases—also called comorbidities). A patient can be 55 years old and very fragile, with heart disease, diabetes, and the beginnings of osteoporosis…or 85 years old and quite robust thanks to a lifetime of physical activity, healthy eating, and fortunate genes. The 55-year-old patient would be a less ideal candidate for a joint replacement given his comorbidities, despite his relative youth, while the 85-year-old may have a lower risk for complications given her good health.

Regardless of chronological age, patients with no major comorbidities and who are physically active should have the stamina and health required to recover from a knee or hip replacement if surgery is required. They even may be able to go home the day of surgery (rather than going to a rehabilitation facility for weeks) and usually can recover with the help of in-home virtual or outpatient PT specifically designed for people recovering from surgery.

Advancements that made this possible…

•**Alternatives to full knee or hip replacements.** Traditional knee replacement, called *total knee arthroplasty* (TKA), involves replacing three different components, or compartments, of the knee with metal and plastic parts. If a patient has arthritis in only one of these compartments, he may be a candidate for a partial knee replacement, which means that only the diseased area is replaced. This makes for an easier recovery…helps maintain the knee's range of motion…and tends to result in less blood loss.

Similarly, some patients may be candidates for a partial hip replacement, called a *hemiarthroplasty,* during which the ball part of the hip joint is replaced but not the socket in which the ball sits. This is a shorter, less invasive operation than a total hip arthroplasty (THA), in which both the ball and socket are replaced.

•**Robotic joint replacement.** No, a robot isn't calling the shots during this surgery, but this cutting-edge technology does involve robotic equipment guiding your doctor. With the help of 3-D imaging, your doctor can "see" your anatomy and program a to-the-millimeter procedure path, meaning that your joint replacement can be positioned with more precision. Incisions are smaller, and recovery often is faster.

•**Regional anesthesia instead of general anesthesia.** General anesthesia, during which patients "go to sleep" and need medical equipment to breathe for them, has historically been used during knee and hip replacements, but it is risky for older adults. Heart arrhythmias—quickened, slowed, or irregular heart rates—can occur during and after surgery using general anesthesia, and that risk increases with the patient's chronological age. Patients also can develop pneumonia or a collapse of the air spaces in the lungs due to general anesthesia. Additionally, there is a risk for post-operative dementia and post-operative delirium. Among patients age 65 years and older, up to 65 percent develop post-op delirium and 10 percent experience long-term cognitive decline after noncardiac surgery, according to a 2019 study in the *British Journal of Anaesthesiology*. Most often, these cognitive effects wear off, but they can be permanent…and they hit patients with preexisting cognitive decline harder.

To avoid these complications, more doctors are using regional anesthesia, such as spinals or nerve blocks, instead of general anesthesia. The patient is mildly sedated and breathing independently, so there aren't the same negative effects on the brain. Regional anesthesia also has been associated with less postoperative pain, shorter hospital stays, and lower risk for blood clots and infections.

BOOST YOUR ODDS

Because of these improvements, there are no strict upper age limits for joint replacement. But you can improve your odds of success even further by asking your doctor what you can do before surgery to speed your recovery. *Examples…*

• **Pre-op PT** (also called pre-hab) can build strength and endurance, leaving you optimized to handle the stress of surgery and even give you a head start on postoperative rehabilitation. Today's virtual PT options allow people to do exercises in the comfort of their home.

• **Meet with a registered dietitian** and formulate a well-rounded nutrition plan for the days and weeks prior to surgery.

• **Minimize narcotics.** Ask your doctor to minimize the use of narcotic pain medications—they can cause confusion, nausea, slowed breathing, and constipation regardless of age. While it's often necessary to take these medications for some period after major surgery, the doses and duration should be as low and short as possible.

Also: A long-lasting local anesthetic allows patients to return home sooner and more comfortably.

Caution: Patients ages 65 years and older who use benzodiazepines such as Xanax (*alprazolam*) and Klonopin (*clonazepam*)… first-generation antihistamines such as Benadryl (*diphenhydramine*)…and antipsychotics such as Seroquel (*quetiapine)* and Abilify (*aripiprazole*) are at increased risk for cognitive changes after anesthesia and should ask their doctors about possibly discontinuing use until after the procedure. (Never stop any medications without first consulting your doctor.)

WHO SHOULDN'T HAVE REPLACEMENT SURGERY?

Certain individuals are at a higher risk for complications, including people with poorly controlled diabetes, smokers, and individuals with obesity.

Patients who cannot or choose not to have joint-replacement surgery can explore alternatives, including steroid injections and PT. Moving soon after surgery is critical to reduce the risk for blood clots, infections, and pneumonia, so individuals with limited mobility from issues in addition to the arthritic knee or hip, such as balance problems or obesity, may prefer to explore these alternatives.

Because many comorbidities get worse with age, older patients should ask their physicians about possible concerns…consider their own personal risk tolerance…and make the decision together. The point of these surgeries is to relieve pain and get patients back to doing the things they love—gardening, traveling, playing tennis and golf, running after their grandkids—as well as functioning independently on a day-to-day basis.

Electrical Implants Regenerate Knee Cartilage

Study led by researchers at University of Connecticut, Storrs, published in *Science Translational Medicine.*

In rabbits with damaged joint cartilage, an implant that generated electrical current from the animals' movements stimulated the growth of new cartilage cells.

Toeing the Line: Advances in Bunion Surgery

Georgeanne Botek, DPM, podiatric surgeon within the orthopedic surgery department of the Cleveland Clinic. ClevelandClinic.org

Until recently, surgery to remove a bunion—that unsightly, bony bump on the joint at the base of the big toe—was painful, invasive, and required a very lengthy recovery. But recent advances in bunion surgery have changed all that. *We asked Georgeanne Botek, DPM, podiatric surgeon at the Cleveland Clinic, about the new options for bunion removal…*

FIRST—IS SURGERY NECESSARY?

Not every bunion—or *hallux valgus*, as it's called medically—should be corrected, and surgery should not be done for cosmetic reasons alone. If a bunion doesn't cause you pain or interfere with your daily life, then work with a skilled podiatrist to prevent it from getting worse by wearing proper shoes and foot inserts, doing certain exercises, and making other lifestyle changes.

If a bunion causes your foot to consistently or chronically ache and throb even when you're at rest, surgery likely is warranted.

Other reasons to have surgery: When the deformity starts to affect the position of your second toe…or you are experiencing changes to the way you walk, your gait and/or your balance.

TODAY'S BUNION SURGERY

A bunion forms when the joint at the base of the big toe moves out of place and causes changes in the adjacent smaller toes such as creating a hammertoe. The aim of bunion surgery—bunionectomy—is to realign the joint (and possibly the tendons and ligaments) and put the bones back in place. The traditional or open surgery involves making an incision on the top or inside medial border of your great toe, shaving down the bone and cutting the metatarsal bone. Recovery usually takes at least six to eight weeks.

There are more than 150 surgical techniques for bunion surgery—Chevron, McBride, Lapidus, Juvara, open wedge, etc. Surgeons often are trained in multiple systems because not every approach is right for every patient. The best bunion-removal surgery technique for you depends on several factors, including how much deformity your bunion has caused and your overall health.

New approaches for bunion removal require smaller incisions and less time in surgery, depending on the severity of the bunion. Recovery also is easier—with a smaller scar and a compressive screw, the patient typically can walk on the foot in a boot anywhere from one to three weeks after surgery and possibly start wearing shoes in six to eight weeks. Being immobile for a shorter period means less chance of stiffness as you recover.

Bonus: Today's longer-acting local anesthetics and regional nerve blocks can manage pain for up to 48 to 72 hours after surgery…and judicious use of recommended over-the-counter medications means that many patients no longer need narcotics after the block wears off.

The newest approach to correcting a bunion is *lapiplasty*, in which the surgeon uses 3D imaging to reposition the joint and toe bones back in place before securing the joint with a titanium plate. Cuts to the joint help correct the misalignment. This surgery may require a larger or multiple incisions. The outpatient procedure itself may take up to two-and-a-half hours, depending on the surgeon. After a few days in a bandage, you'll switch to a surgical walking boot. You may be able to bear weight on the foot within one week…be back at work within two to three weeks…and be able to wear shoes in six to eight weeks. Lapiplasty is as effective as the open procedure for mild-to-moderate-size bunions…provides cosmetically pleasing results…and has a recurrence rate of less than 30 percent.

RECOVERY AND RISKS

Whatever procedure you have, you won't be able to go on your treadmill or walk your dog immediately after, but your surgeon may encourage low-impact exercise videos, riding a stationary bike, and doing resistance and flexibility work that won't affect the surgical site.

One thing that hasn't changed: Bone healing still takes time. Full recovery is a year-long process as your foot bones remodel and your body adjusts to the foot being back in its normal position. Follow-up instructions will include not going barefoot or wearing high heels and adding appropriate arch support to shoes if you have flat feet.

Risks: Swelling, stiffness, infection, numbness, and slower-than-expected healing. Bunion surgery is safe for patients of most any age, but it can be more complex when there is bone thinning from osteoporosis or osteopenia.

For the best outcome: Optimize your health before the surgery—the recovery period will only aggravate any existing health issues because you will be less mobile than usual.

Examples: If you have diabetes, get your blood sugar under control…lose weight if you need to…make sure your levels of vitamin D are in the normal range…if you have any other foot problems, such as swelling, address them with your doctor before you have any bunion procedure.

FIND THE RIGHT DOCTOR

Like most medical procedures, the key to successful bunion surgery is the surgeon's expertise. There is a steep learning curve, and any surgeon you choose should have done at least 50 procedures on real patients.

Before deciding on a surgeon and a specific bunionectomy technique, talk to multiple doctors. Word of mouth also can be helpful—ask other people who have had a bunion operation for their opinions about the surgery and the surgeon.

At each consultation, ask the health-care provider for a realistic assessment of what to expect, including what your foot will look like and, if any bone will be removed, whether your big toe will be shorter than before and by how much.

Virus Discovery Leads to Multiple Sclerosis Breakthrough

Marwa Kaisey, M.D., assistant professor of neurology, Cedars-Sinai, Los Angeles. She specializes in multiple sclerosis and neuroimmunology.

In January 2022, a scientific study garnered the kind of attention normally reserved for celebrity gossip. Researchers reported that multiple sclerosis (MS), an autoimmune inflammatory disease that causes the body to damage neurons in the brain and spinal cord, is most likely caused by a virus. While this startling news took many people by surprise, MS researchers were not among them.

"We've known about this link for decades," Marwa Kaisey, M.D., told us. What was different was the sheer size of the study (10 million people) and the credibility of the journal it was published in (*Science*). We asked Dr. Kaisey what these findings mean for people with MS.

THE VIRUS LINK

The virus in question is called Epstein-Barr virus (EBV), and almost everyone has been exposed to it. It is most well-known for causing mononucleosis, but it can also cause mild cold-like symptoms or no symptoms at all. And it appears that it can cause MS in some people, too.

The team that published the study in *Science* looked at blood samples from 10 million healthy people on active duty in the U.S. military and found that exposure to EBV—but no other viruses—increased the risk of MS 32-fold. Furthermore, they found an increase in a biomarker of MS-related nerve damage only after EBV infection.

While this convincingly points to EBV as a contributor to MS, it doesn't mean that it is a singular cause. About 95 percent of people have been exposed to EBV, but only 0.21 percent of Americans have MS. But among the people who do have MS, 100 percent have EBV. It appears that it is impossible to have MS without having had EBV.

This poses exciting questions about prevention. If a vaccine could prevent EBV, could we put an end to all future cases of MS? That's one of the avenues researchers are already looking at.

ATA188 FOR PROGRESSIVE MS

Researchers are also exploring a treatment called ATA188. They hypothesize that, in people with MS, the immune system can't adequately get rid of the virus. Instead, the EBV lingers inside "nests" of B cells. The immune system wants to attack these stowaways, but it can't differentiate between the virus and healthy cells. As a result, T cells attack healthy cells in the brain and spinal cord instead.

Enter ATA188. In this experimental treatment, T cells are taken from healthy people who have recovered from EBV and engineered so they can cross the blood-brain barrier and destroy the nests of B cells that are harboring the lingering virus.

In a small, yearlong study of people with progressive MS, the treatment looked promising. Out of 24 people, 13 were stable, seven improved, and four got worse.

A year is a short time to look at the effects of the drug, so the people staying stable was to be expected. But seven was an unexpectedly high number of people who got better. Re-

A Common Misdiagnosis

Research suggests that many people are incorrectly diagnosed with MS. Dr. Kaisey looked at 241 people who had been diagnosed with MS and referred for specialty care at either Cedars-Sinai or UCLA. Among them, about 18 percent didn't have MS at all. After further investigation, those patients were diagnosed with migraine (16 percent), radiologically isolated syndrome (9 percent), spondylopathy (7 percent), and neuropathy (7 percent). Those patients were inappropriately given MS medications for about 110 patient-years. (A patient-year is the sum of the number of patients multiplied by the number of years. If 10 patients are given a medication for 5 years [10 x 5], it would represent 50 patient-years.) About 60 percent of those patients were inappropriately given a disease-modifying treatment and 48 percent were exposed to a drug with a known risk of a rare brain infection called progressive focal leukoencephalopathy.

A possible solution is on the horizon: a new type of MRI that can differentiate between MS and other conditions. (Currently available MRIs cannot.) Being able to quickly diagnose MS with an MRI could lead to faster treatment and less damage to the nerves.

A team of researchers based out of Cedars-Sinai and the Cleveland Clinic are currently working on two fronts: They're testing the validity of new MRI technology and developing artificial intelligence technology to help community radiologists use the MRI for rapid diagnosis.

searchers followed the patients who improved and found that the results lasted for at least four years. The team is now enrolling 80 more patients into a phase 2 trial called EMBOLD.

ATA188 is particularly exciting for people with progressive MS, which has few treatment options available. Treatments for *relapsing* MS, however, are rapidly evolving.

RELAPSING MS

The treatment landscape for relapsing MS has changed dramatically in the last 30 years. Even in the last five years, a lot of new medications have come to market. Getting diagnosed in 2023 is very different than getting diagnosed in 2012.

But that doesn't mean physicians are keeping up. Doctors who went to medical school a decade ago may not have learned about the latest innovations. In fact, they may still be under the assumption that MS is a difficult disease to treat. That's simply not true anymore.

Today's drugs, also called disease-modifying therapies (DMTs), are more powerful than ever. They reduce the number of relapses, delay the progression of disability, and limit new disease activity. Many don't even have to be taken daily. There are now treatments that you can take every month, every six months, or even yearly. For one called *alemtuzumab* (Lemtrada), you can take a short course in the first year, a short course in the second year, and then be done indefinitely. While nothing can take away the diagnosis of MS, physicians increasingly have the ability to stop it in its tracks.

IMMUNE MODULATORS AND MORE

DMTs fall into two camps: immune modulators and immunosuppressives. Immune modulators work to rebalance the immune system. (MS is essentially an imbalance that causes the immune system to attack otherwise healthy brain and spinal cord tissue.) Immune suppressants take away a small portion of the immune system. Because different medications take out different portions of the immune system, they have different risks, benefits, and strengths.

During the pandemic, patients and physicians were more likely to avoid drugs that could diminish the immune system and leaned toward immune modulators. But now that we have vaccines and treatments for COVID-19, immune suppressants can safely re-enter the treatment arsenal.

New Treatments for MS

There are more than a dozen new FDA-approved disease-modifying therapies (DMTs) to treat multiple sclerosis (MS). These DMTs work by modulating and/or suppressing the overactive immune system response in relapsing onset MS, the most common form, characterized by alternating periods of inflammatory activity and remission. Some DMTs also help people with progressive MS and are most effective if taken early in the course of the disease.

Downside: DMTs can cause side effects, including progressive multifocal leukoencephalopathy (PML), a rare but potentially fatal brain infection.

On the horizon: New drugs to manage both forms of MS, including promising stem cell therapies and neurorepair/protective interventions.

Caution: Stem cell therapies—cures promised at freestanding stem-cell centers separate from clinical trials—are scams.

Scott Newsome, DO, MSCS, FAAN, FANA, associate professor of neurology, codirector, Multiple Sclerosis Experimental Therapeutics Program, Johns Hopkins Hospital, Baltimore, and president of Consortium of Multiple Sclerosis Centers. MSCare.org

STARTING FROM THE TOP

With more powerful medications, there are more risks. But more risk can lead to more reward. In the past, physicians started with the safest and often least powerful drugs and worked their way up the ladder if needed.

But now the thinking has shifted to the opposite: If a powerful drug can stop the disease in its tracks and lessen or prevent damage to the brain and spinal cord, it could be worth some added risk.

To tease out which of these approaches is best, two clinical trials are comparing them right now: Treat MS (Traditional Versus Early Aggressive Therapy for Multiple Sclerosis) and Deliver MS (Determining the Effectiveness of Early Intensive Versus Escalation Approaches for Relapsing Remitting Multiple Sclerosis).

FUTURE EFFORTS

No treatments can reverse the damage of MS once it's done, but they could be on the way. Scientists have learned that some people have a limited ability to heal themselves by building back myelin sheaths that protect nerve cells. (MS destroys the myelin sheaths.)

Researchers are investigating how myelin is formed to try to better understand how they can amplify that process and create drugs that will undo the damage.

Stem cell therapy is also being investigated as a one-time treatment. In a small study of 24 people, close to 70 percent remained free of symptoms five years after undergoing treatment. Stem cell therapy is not covered by insurance, as it's considered to be experimental, but your doctor may know of clinical trials in which you may be able to participate.

Fat Plus Fructose Is Bad for Your Liver

Molecular Nutrition and Food Research.

Adding beverages sweetened with liquid fructose to a high-fat diet increases the risk of nonalcoholic fatty liver disease (NAFLD), researchers reported in the journal *Molecular Nutrition and Food Research*. Fructose, unlike other sugars, is processed in the liver. When we eat fruit, a common source of fructose, the fiber slows absorption and gives the liver time to do its job. But the fructose used in food manufacturing is artificially concentrated, and liquid fructose is rapidly absorbed and overwhelming to the liver. It changes how the liver forms fats through sugar (a process called de novo lipogenesis). NAFLD is often asymptomatic, but it can lead to serious illnesses such as steatohepatitis and cirrhosis.

Fixing Our Drinking Water

U.S. Drinking-Water Infrastructure Is at Risk

Every two minutes, a crack develops somewhere in the 2.2 million aging pipes carrying drinking water across the country. And the 145,000 U.S. water-treatment facilities that send water from reservoirs and rivers are decaying.

American Society of Civil Engineers (ASCE), Reston, Virginia. ASCE.org

Dogs Help Conserve Water

Age, corrosion, and freezing ground can cause public water pipes to leak—and that can be difficult to detect when the pipes are buried underground.

Solution: Dogs in the U.K. that are trained to sniff out the chlorine in treated water are helping water companies detect leaks in underground pipes so they can be fixed faster.

Mary Schwager, television and print investigative journalist, WatchDogMary.com, reported in *Dogster*.

Time-Restricted Eating Influences Gene Expression

Salk Institute.

Gene expression is the process through which genes are activated and respond to their environment by creating proteins. To see how the timing of eating affects this process, researchers fed two groups of mice the same diet. One group was given free access to food, and the other group was restricted to eating within a nine-hour window. After seven weeks, the investigators found that 70 percent of mouse genes responded to time-restricted eating, including 40 percent of genes that are important for hormonal regulation. Hormonal imbalance is implicated in many diseases, from diabetes to stress disorders. This study suggests that time-restricted eating may help manage these diseases.

Reducing the Risk of Low-Birthweight Babies

Study titled "Weighting of Risk Factors for Low Birth Weight: A Linked Routine Data Cohort Study in Wales, U.K.," led by researchers at Swansea University, Wales, published in *BMJ Open*.

When a baby's born, a significant indicator for health is birth weight. Low birthweight (LBW) has been linked to a higher rate of illness and death in babies as well as developmental disabilities and poor academic achievement. According to the World Health Organization, a LBW baby weighs less than 2,500 grams (5.5 pounds) at birth. Low birthweight is common, occurring in about 8 percent of babies in the United States and the U.K., and about 20 million births globally.

WHAT ARE THE MODIFIABLE RISK FACTORS FOR LBW

LBW has several risk factors that could be managed to reduce risk, called modifiable risk factors. The WHO has called for a global effort to reduce LBW 30 percent by 2025. To understand what the most important modifiable risk factors are for LBW, researchers from the National Centre for Population Health & Wellbeing at Swansea University in Wales, U.K., have analyzed the risk factors leading to LBW for more than 25 years in close to 700,000 babies born in Wales. The research team used existing data collected by the Welsh National Community Child Health Database.

The study found that the highest risk factor for LBW was having more than one baby (twins, triplets, or more). Multiple births only occurred in about 3 percent of the births, but these babies had over 20 times the risk of LBW as single birth babies. Having a pregnancy within one year of a previous pregnancy was another significant risk. This interval of pregnancy more than doubled the risk of LBW. Treatable mental health conditions of the mother, including anxiety or depression, was another major risk for LBW. *Other key maternal and modifiable risk factors occurring during pregnancy that increased LBW risk included...*

•**Diabetes** (doubled the risk)

•**Anemia** (26 percent increase)

•**Use of an antidepressant** (doubled the risk)

•**Domestic abuse** (nearly doubled the risk)

•**Smoking** (80 percent increase)

•**Hospital admission for alcohol abuse** (60 percent increase)

•**Substance abuse** (35 percent increase)

HOW TO IMPROVE RISK FACTORS

The research team concludes that their findings can help shape guidelines to reduce the risk of LBW. These guidelines could include avoiding multiple egg implantations at fertility clinics (to avoid multiple births), discouraging short pregnancy intervals (less than one year), and addressing the mental and physical health needs of mothers. One of the limitations of the study was unavailable data that may also influence LBW, such as diet, exercise, and stress.

The average birth weight in the U.S. is eight pounds, but LBW has become more frequent. The primary cause of LBW is premature birth, which is before 37 weeks. Other risk factors can include intrauterine growth restriction (IUGR) and maternal age under 15. IUGR means that a baby does not grow enough in the womb due to problems with the placenta or the mother's health. Although not includ-ed in the U.K. study, African-American babies have twice the risk of LBW as white babies.

Life Really Might "Flash Before Your Eyes"

For the first time, electroencephalography (EEG) captured the brain activity of an 87-year-old seizure victim as he died of a heart attack, revealing brain waves typical of "rapid memory retrieval" in the moment just before death.

Study led by researchers at University of British Columbia, Vancouver, published in Frontiers in Aging Neuroscience.

Your Body Parts Don't All Age at the Same Rate

Study of biological age of seven organs and body systems of 480 adults led by researchers at National University of Singapore, published in *Cell Reports*.

The age of some organs is tied more to a person's chronological age than is the age of other organs. This could help predict onset of disease.

Example: The age of the cardiovascular system is most closely linked to an individual's age in years, while the gut microbiome age is least linked.

CHAPTER 13

Medication Smarts

Are You Taking Too Many Meds?

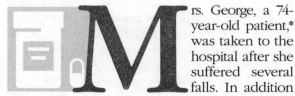

Mrs. George, a 74-year-old patient,* was taken to the hospital after she suffered several falls. In addition to her recently diagnosed dementia, she had hypertension, depression, daily headaches, acid reflux, and irritable bowel syndrome (IBS). After reviewing Mrs. George's medications, pharmacist Barbara Farrell identified that her dizziness and cognitive decline could be side effects of drugs she was taking (some of her antihypertensive medications, one prescribed for IBS, one for depression, one for headaches, and a sleep aid). Mrs. George was taking 14 medications each day.

That is not surprising. According to a 2020 report by the Lown Institute, a health-systems think tank that tracks prescription trends, 42 percent of older Americans routinely take five or more prescription drugs a day and close to 20 percent take 10 or more.

This practice of prescribing multiple medications is called *polypharmacy*. Doctors often feel pressured to prescribe (especially common when patients demand an antibiotic even though they likely have a virus that an antibiotic won't treat). Making matters worse, many health-care providers simply renew prescriptions without checking to see if they still are necessary...or the patient is afraid to stop taking a drug...or the original prescriber is no longer practicing, and the new provider continues filling it. Also, since most people have more than one doctor, unless those physicians

*Composite patient.

Barbara Farrell, PharmD, BScPhm, FCSHP, pharmacist who practices clinically in the Bruyère Geriatric Day Hospital in Ottawa, Canada, and assistant professor in the department of family medicine at University of Ottawa. Dr. Farrell is a member of the Ontario Pharmacy Evidence Network, cofounder of the Canadian Deprescribing Network and codeveloper of the website Deprescribing.org.

are in communication with one another, they may not know how many medications a patient is taking.

Polypharmacy also results when medications are taken to treat new symptoms that are side effects of other drugs the patient is taking—a prescribing cascade.

Example: A patient is prescribed a calcium channel blocker for high blood pressure. That drug causes ankle swelling, so a diuretic is prescribed. The diuretic causes dehydration or orthostatic hypotension, a type of low blood pressure that can cause blurred vision, nausea, heart palpitations, dizziness, fainting, and falls when you stand up...and it can cause low potassium levels, necessitating potassium supplements, which can cause nausea, which then needs to be treated with yet another drug.

Solution: Deprescribing—the supervised process of reducing or stopping medications that may no longer be helping or even might be hurting a patient.

OVERPRESCRIBED MEDICATIONS

Every day, 750 older adults in the U.S. are hospitalized due to adverse drug events (ADEs). In 2018, five million older adults sought out medical attention for adverse medication side effects, and the chances of developing a serious ADE increase by up to 10 percent with each additional prescription.

Older adults are particularly vulnerable due to age-related changes in the body's ability to metabolize drugs. The kidneys and liver take longer to clear drugs from the system, so blood levels of these medications can remain higher for longer periods.

Example: A dose of *digoxin* or *metoprolol* that effectively managed atrial fibrillation at age 60 likely will be too high for the same person at age 85 and could cause unwanted and potentially dangerous side effects.

The following drugs tend to be overprescribed and overused by older Americans...

• **Antidepressants.** Over the past 30 years, antidepressant use has been on the rise in older adults. People stay on them for years, even though they may no longer be needed. These drugs can cause significant side effects

that should be considered when weighing benefit and risk. Tricyclic antidepressants, such as *nortriptyline* (Aventyl) and *amitryptiline* (Elavil), have high anticholinergic activity, meaning that they affect the brain in a way that can worsen memory and increase fall risk while also causing constipation, urinary retention, decreased sweating, dry mouth, blurred vision, and increased heart rate. Other anticholinergic drugs include medications that treat gastrointestinal and sleep disorders, chronic obstructive pulmonary disease, and some bladder disorders...as well as the over-the-counter allergy or sleep medicine *diphenhydramine* (Benadryl, Nytol) and other common antihistamines.

Caution: When a person takes multiple anticholinergics, side effects skyrocket, increasing the risk for polypharmacy because those additional symptoms may be treated with different medications.

• **Benzodiazepine and "Z-drugs" (BZRAs).** Often used to manage anxiety and insomnia, BZRAs include benzodiazepines such as *lorazepam* (Ativan), *alprazolam* (Xanax), and *diazepam* (Valium) and Z-drugs such as *zolpidem* (Ambien), *zaleplon* (Sonata), and *eszopiclone* (Lunesta). BZRAs are meant to be used for only around four weeks, but people can develop a dependence that makes it hard to stop taking them. These drugs work by slowing activity in the brain—side effects include memory issues, daytime fatigue, and falls, all of which increase with age. The cognitive side effects can be severe enough that they can contribute to a diagnosis of dementia.

• **Proton Pump Inhibitors (PPIs).** This class of drugs, which includes OTC *lansoprazole* (Prevacid) and *esomeprazole* (Nexium), is used to reduce stomach acid, and treat heartburn and stomach ulcers. Except in rare cases, they should be used for no more than eight to 10 weeks, but some people end up taking them for eight to 10 years. In fact, up to 65 percent of long-term PPI users have no documented long-term indication for the medication. Chronic PPI use can contribute to headaches, nausea, and diarrhea...and may increase risk for deficiencies of the essential nutrients vitamin B$_{12}$ and magnesium.

•**Type 2 diabetes drugs.** Insulin, *glyburide* (DiaBeta), and other anti-hyperglycemic medications lower blood sugar in people with diabetes. But too-low blood sugar levels can cause falls, confusion, and seizures in older adults. Ask your doctor about the appropriate blood sugar targets for your age. Complicating matters, older type 2 diabetes patients often have other health conditions such as hypertension and heart disease, raising the risk for polypharmacy.

HOW DEPRESCRIBING CAN HELP

The goal of deprescribing is to reduce the harm caused by certain medications while maintaining or improving a patient's quality of life. If you—or a loved one—are taking any of the medications above, ask your doctor if deprescribing might be a smart option. In some cases, deprescribing is uncomplicated and involves slowly reducing the dose.

Example: With acid-reducing medications, such as PPIs, a patient who is eligible for deprescribing may start by taking them once daily instead of twice a day…halving the dose…or taking the PPI every other day for a few weeks before stopping altogether. Ideally, any residual heartburn or reflux will be managed by dietary and lifestyle changes.

BZRAs are harder to stop. The tapering process can cause anxiety and sleep issues. It can take days, weeks, or months for cognition to improve. Good sleep hygiene often is sufficient to manage insomnia, and cognitive behavioral therapy can be as effective as medication.

HOW TO PROCEED

Don't ever stop taking a medicine without first checking with your health-care provider. He/she may recommend tapering to an effective minimum dose or down to nothing at all…switching to a medication with fewer side effects…or stopping abruptly.

Ask your doctor, "Are there any medications I'm taking that I no longer need?" Whenever you are prescribed a new drug, ask, "Will it interact with my other medications?" and "Do the benefits outweigh the risks?" Push for a specific answer—"It's for your heart" is too vague, but "It will reduce your heart attack risk by 20 percent" is informative. You also can ask your pharmacist.

Reminder: Mention any vitamins, supplements, or OTC medicines you take.

As for Mrs. George—her medical team created a deprescribing regimen. Over 15 weeks, her IBS medication and antidepressant doses were reduced and stopped…her nighttime sleep aid was stopped…headache medication and acid-reducing medication were reduced and eventually stopped. She started keeping an IBS diary and using a laxative or antidiarrheal only when needed. Her cognitive functioning improved substantially within just a few weeks of these changes. Her bowels improved with minimal need for her "as-needed" medications. Her headaches resolved…balance improved (no more falls). Based on these changes, she was referred for a reassessment of her memory and cognition, and the dementia diagnosis was reversed.

The Healing Power of Psychedelics

Matthew Johnson, Ph.D., professor of psychiatry, and the Susan Hill Ward Professor of Psychedelics and Consciousness at the Johns Hopkins University School of Medicine. He is the author of over 50 scientific papers on psychedelics, and published psychedelic safety guidelines in 2008, helping to resurrect psychedelic research in people. HopkinsPsychedelic.org

---

In the last decade, there's been a surge of scientific interest in the healing power of psychedelics—mind-altering drugs like psilocybin, LSD, mescaline, ayahuasca, ketamine, and MDMA (3,4-methylenedioxymethamphetamine). Currently, there are more than 300 government-approved clinical trials testing the use of these drugs in many disorders and diseases—disorders for which they can provide relief even when no other treatment has worked.

Some of the strongest scientific evidence supports the use of psilocybin for depression, anxiety, alcoholism, and tobacco addiction, the use of ketamine for depression, and the use of MDMA for post-traumatic stress disorder (PTSD).

But researchers are also looking at psychedelics for a wide variety of other conditions, including obsessive-compulsive disorder, burnout, suicidality, eating disorders, opioid addiction, ADHD, mild cognitive impairment, and Alzheimer's disease, Parkinson's disease, diabetes, liver disease, migraine, and cluster headaches, phantom limb pain, and even the symptoms of COVID-19.

But don't expect your doctor to be prescribing a psychedelic anytime soon. None of these drugs are approved for use by the United States Food and Drug Administration (FDA), except for *esketamine* (Spravato), a ketamine-derived nasal spray for treatment-resistant depression. And under federal law, the use of psychedelics is illegal, except in government-approved clinical trials. (Several cities in the United States have decriminalized psilocybin, such as Washington, D.C., Denver, Seattle, and Oakland. The state of Oregon has legalized it for both personal and therapeutic use. These local laws do not nullify federal law.) However, in the context of the hundreds of government-approved clinical trials being conducted around the United States, these drugs present a future option you should know about.

HOW PSYCHEDELICS WORK

So-called "classic" psychedelics like psilocybin, LSD, mescaline, and ayahuasca work by binding to the 2A receptor for serotonin, a brain chemical (neurotransmitter) that regulates fundamental brain activities like mood, emotions, sleep, and sex drive. This receptor is only the first "domino" in a lengthy series of falling dominoes that produce a wide range of psychological and biological effects. (One of those dominoes is the neurotransmitter glutamate, which is the first receptor for "non-classic" psychedelics like ketamine.)

The result is that many parts of the brain are activated that are not normally activated, and some parts of the brain—like the prefrontal cortex, which regulates cognitive control—are far less active. Additionally, when you take

a psychedelic, the way the brain communicates with itself is radically changed. There is a massive increase in what scientists call "global connectivity"—parts of the brain that don't normally communicate with each other now do so.

Think of it this way: Normally, "local networks" in the brain mostly communicate with their next-door neighbors. When you take a psychedelic, those same networks communicate less with the neighbors and more with the people across town.

MYSTICAL EXPERIENCE

This increase in connectivity may be the reason why a psychedelic often has a profound effect on your sense of reality, including your sense of self. In studies at the Center for Psychedelic Research and Consciousness at Johns Hopkins University School of Medicine, this subjective experience is called a "mystical experience." Such experience is characterized by a positive mood, a sense of wholeness and connection within oneself and with the outside world, a sense of direct knowledge of the nature of reality, a sense of everything being sacred or holy, transcendence of time and space, and a sense of ineffability, or the fact that reality is beyond definition and language.

Research shows that those who have a mystical experience while taking a psychedelic are more likely to experience positive therapeutic effects. Their depression and anxiety are often relieved—even depression and anxiety after a terminal diagnosis, such as cancer. Their desire for an addictive substance, such as alcohol, cigarettes, or opioids, subsides.

Bottom line: A mystical experience while taking a psychedelic can grant a new perspective on life and self that allows a person to have a fundamental psychological resolution of their condition or disorder.

In many cases, the result is more like a cure than a reduction in symptoms. You might take a psychedelic one, two, or three times, rather than taking a drug every day for the rest of your life, as an antidepressant. That's one of the key advantages of these remarkable drugs.

Many scientific studies and papers present the power and potential of psychedelics to heal.

DEPRESSION

A study in the *Journal of Pharmacology*, published in February 2022, tested psilocybin on 27 people with major depressive disorder. Each person received two doses of psilocybin with supportive psychotherapy. After a year, three out of four patients had more than a 50 percent reduction in depression, and 58 percent had complete remission. The experience of "personal meaning, spiritual experience, and mystical experience" during the psychedelic session predicted the subsequent level of well-being.

In a meta-analysis of nine studies on ketamine and depression, researchers found that adding ketamine more than doubled the response, compared with placebo, with a 63 percent improvement in symptoms and a 64 percent improvement in remission. In the March 9, 2022, issue of *Expert Opinion on Drug Safety*, the researchers wrote that the treatment is "effective, safe, and acceptable."

LIFE-THREATENING CANCER

In a study in the December 2016 issue of the *Journal of Pharmacology*, 51 cancer patients with a life-threatening diagnosis and symptoms of depression and anxiety took either a therapeutic dose of psilocybin or a very low dose. Those who took the higher dose had large decreases in depression and anxiety, an increase in the quality of life, life meaning, and optimism, and a decrease in anxiety about death.

SUBSTANCE ABUSE

Researchers from Johns Hopkins University School of Medicine studied more than 400 people with an average of 4.5 years of substance use disorder (SUD). The abused substances included opioids, cannabis, and stimulants. After taking a psychedelic, 73 percent of participants no longer had SUD. The results were published in the January 2020 issue of *Frontiers in Psychiatry*.

POST-TRAUMATIC STRESS DISORDER

There are more than a dozen studies on the use of MDMA for PTSD. In a major study authored by 38 researchers in the United States, Canada, and Israel, 90 people with severe PTSD were given either MDMA or a placebo. Those taking MDMA had a 42 percent greater reduction in symptoms. In the June 2021 issue of *Nature Medicine*, researchers describe it as a "potential breakthrough treatment."

Important: As a street drug, MDMA is called "Ecstasy"—but research shows illegally purchased Ecstasy may not contain MDMA, and may contain other illegal drugs.

HEALTH BEHAVIORAL CHANGE

In a scientific paper published in the January 2022 issue of the *Journal of Psychopharmacology,* an international team of researchers theorized that the next frontier for research into psychedelic therapy might be health behavioral change—using the therapy to improve diet, exercise, and stress reduction practices, all of which can contribute to physical and psychological well-being.

SAFETY AND LEGALITY

Many people use psychedelics on their own—with a study estimating more than 30 million Americans have used a psychedelic during their lifetime. *But there are many risks from taking a psychedelic outside the context of an FDA-approved clinical trial…*

●**Legality.** Except for ketamine for depression—if you take a psychedelic outside the context of a clinical trial, you're breaking the law.

●**Improper compound.** If you're taking a psychedelic, you want confidence in the purity and dose of the compound you're taking. Having that kind of confidence is nearly impossible outside the setting of a clinical trial.

●**Health safety.** The safest way to protect your health when you take a psychedelic is to receive a real medical screening before the event, in which you're checked for physical risk factors such as elevated liver enzymes and psychological risk factors such as a family history of schizophrenia.

How to Find a Clinical Trial

If you're interested in legally taking a psychedelic for a disorder or disease, you can apply to participate in an FDA-approved clinical trial. You can find the database for clinical trials at Clinicaltrials.gov.

•**Under "Status,"** check "Recruiting and not yet recruiting studies."

•**Under "Condition or disease,"** enter your health problem, such as "depression" or "migraine."

•**Under "Other terms,"** enter the word "psychedelic."

•**Under "Country,"** enter "United States" or the country where you live.

•**Once "Country" is entered,** the database gives you the option to enter your state and city, and the distance from the trial you're willing to travel, like 50, 100, 200, or 300 miles.

•**Alternatively, you can enter the word "psychedelic" in the "Other terms" field—**and review the more than 370 studies currently listed on the website.

•**Cardiovascular.** People have died taking psilocybin. If you have severe heart disease, you shouldn't be taking the drug, which can modestly raise blood pressure.

•**Lack of support.** Psychedelics can cause a "bad trip," in which you are overcome by delusion and paranoia. Such an outcome is far more likely if you take a psychedelic by yourself rather than in a controlled and supportive setting. Also, a setting outside of a clinical trial may not provide any support during or after taking the psychedelic—when a person may have trouble integrating experiences that come up, like those related to trauma.

•**Abuse.** Taking a psychedelic puts you in one of the most vulnerable situations you've ever been in, and some people have been the victims of sexual or psychological abuse.

If you're determined to take a psychedelic outside the safe and legal bounds of a federally approved clinical trial, there are "psychedelic retreats" in countries like Mexico, Costa Rica, and Jamaica. The "Multidisciplinary Association for Psychedelic Studies" lists more than 300 therapists and a mission that includes helping "people to benefit from the careful uses of psychedelics." (*Please note:* It is technically illegal to travel overseas to engage in an activity that is illegal in the United States.)

The Power of the Placebo Effect

Yoni K. Ashar, Ph.D., doctor of psychology, neuroscientist, and a National Institutes of Health–funded researcher at Weill Medical College, Cornell University, New York City.

During World War II, Henry Beecher, M.D., a Harvard-trained anesthesiologist, ran out of morphine to use for anesthesia. He turned to a placebo and began injecting patients with saline instead. That simple salt water worked well enough for him to perform surgery on many of his patients. The reason? They believed it would.

The placebo effect is a phenomenon in which patients can take a nonmedical substance, whether it's a saline injection or a sugar pill, and experience a positive response. In 1955, Dr. Beecher estimated that 35 percent of any treatment success was due to the placebo effect. Today, we know that the response rate ranges from 26 to 50 percent, and depends on several factors.

•**Type of placebo.** In a review published in 2017 in the journal *Annual Review of Clinical Psychology,* it was shown that the more bells and whistles attached to a placebo, the higher the effect. For example, placebo acupuncture was more powerful for relieving pain than a placebo pill, and as powerful as actual acupuncture. In the review, placebo pills and injections had about a 26 percent placebo response, placebo acupuncture had a 38 percent response, and placebo surgery had a 50 percent response.

•**The condition being treated.** Placebos work best in diseases with symptoms like pain, itching, or fatigue and less well on symptoms like high blood pressure, fever, or abnormal heart rate. A placebo may not stop a tumor from growing, but it can help reduce pain and the side effects of cancer treatment. Mental health disorders respond very well to placebos, especially anxiety, panic attacks, and depression. A possible explanation is that the anticipation of an effect boosts dopamine, which can decrease depression and anxiety.

A review of 215 studies that was published in the journal *Pain* found that up to 75 percent of any pain treatment is due to the placebo effect. Getting a placebo from a trusted healthcare provider also makes any placebo more powerful.

HOW PLACEBOS WORK

The availability of brain imaging studies like MRIs and PET scans has given brain researchers a window into understanding how the placebo effect works. The current theory is that there are three important components: classic conditioning, expectations, and neurobiology.

•**Classic conditioning is the most basic component.** It is a learned, automatic reaction gained from prior experience. If a lab animal is fed every time a bell rings, it will start to salivate at the ring of the bell, whether it receives food or not.

Brain imaging shows that brain neurons that recognize an injection of morphine will become wired to brain neurons that release pain-relieving brain messengers called neurotransmitters. Over time, triggering the injection neurons will automatically trigger the pain-relieving neurotransmitters, even if the injection is just salt water, because neurons that fire together wire together.

•**Expectation is a higher brain function that involves memories, emotions, and evaluations.** Brain imaging shows that areas of the brain that are responsible for hope and belief are activated during a placebo response.

•**Neurobiology.** The placebo response can generate the same neurotransmitters that are generated by real medications or treatments. They include the neurotransmitters serotonin, dopamine, and endorphins.

PLACEBOS IN RESEARCH

The gold standard to determine the safety and effectiveness of a new treatment or medication is to use a randomized, placebo-controlled trial in which one group of volunteers is randomly assigned to a placebo group and the other is assigned to a real treatment group. Neither group knows if they are getting the treatment or the placebo. The placebo response is generated solely by the patient. Anything beyond that response is attributed to the new medication or treatment.

GROWING POWER OF PLACEBOS

New research, however, is complicated by the growing power of the placebo response. More patients in placebo groups are experiencing symptom relief than ever before, which makes the active treatments in the study appear to be less effective by comparison.

A Brief History of Placebo

Placebos have been a part of medical treatment since the time of Ancient Egypt (3100 BC to 332 BC). They became more commonplace in the 17th century, when physicians referred to them as a necessary deception for certain patients, sometimes called a "humble humbug."

In the early 1800s, physicians used metal rods (called Perkins rods) to treat painful conditions like rheumatism. It was believed that the magnetic properties of the rods could draw out pain when placed against the body. A physician named John Haygarth compared actual rods to wooden rods painted to look like the metal rods. Patients had the same response to both rods. Haygarth had the insight to conclude that both rods worked due to the "wonderful effects" of faith and hope.

In 1807, Thomas Jefferson wrote, "The most successful physicians I know use more bread pills, colored water, and powders from ashes than all their other medicines."

A study published in the journal *Pain* reported that, in 1996, clinical trial participants reported a 27 percent difference between the effectiveness of placebo and active drugs. In 2013, the difference was just 9 percent.

Interestingly, this association is seen only in the United States.

There are two possible explanations: First, American drug trials tend to be larger, longer, and have more clinical staff interacting with study participants. Both factors—complexity and relationships with health-care providers—have been shown to increase the placebo effect. In addition, the United States is the only country that allows pharmaceutical companies to market their products directly to patients, so patients may be primed by advertising to expect greater benefits.

HARNESSING PLACEBO POWER

Now that we know how powerful the placebo is, why not start using placebos as actual treatments? The main reason is ethical. Outside of a clinical trial, doctors can't give a placebo to a patient without telling them. The solution may be an open-label placebo.

Studies show that when patients are told they are getting a placebo and also told that placebos work, they still get a placebo response. In fact, open-label placebos have been used to treat cancer-related fatigue, migraine headaches, irritable bowel syndrome, chronic back pain, allergic rhinitis, and osteoarthritic knee pain with good success, according to the review published in *Pain*.

The bottom line is that the power of the placebo is within all of us. You don't need to be fooled into using it; you can just start believing in it. There is a tremendous healing power available to you when you have hope, faith, a positive attitude, and a compassionate health-care provider.

The Greek physician Hippocrates said, "The natural healing force within each one of us is the greatest force for getting well." Modern researchers are discovering he was right.

Choosing the Best Over-the-Counter Pain Reliever

Chris Iliades, M.D., retired ear, nose, throat, head, and neck surgeon, and a frequent contributor to *Bottom Line Health*.

Over-the-counter (OTC) pain and fever medications are the most common medications Americans take. Although there are many brand names, there are only four active ingredients you need to know: *acetaminophen* (Tylenol, Percogesic, and Midol), aspirin (Anacin and Bayer), *ibuprofen* (Advil and Motrin), and *naproxen* (Aleve). All four of these drugs show up in a multitude of OTC cough and cold preparations, and some products contain more than one ingredient on the list: Excedrin, for example, contains both aspirin and acetaminophen. These drugs have different side effects, and they work better for different conditions.

ACETAMINOPHEN

Acetaminophen quickly relieves both pain and fever for about four hours, but it does not reduce inflammation, as several other drugs—called nonsteroidal anti-inflammatory drugs (NSAIDs)—do. That means it can be a good choice for any painful condition that is not due to inflammation.

Acetaminophen rarely has side effects at *normal* doses. It won't cause heartburn like an NSAID might. However, an overdose can be toxic to your liver. An acetaminophen overdose can often be treated, but toxicity causes more than 50,000 emergency room visits and 500 deaths every year.

The maximum safe daily dose for an adult is 4,000 milligrams (mg). Taking just eight 500 mg pills in one day puts you right at the edge of toxicity. If you have any history of liver disease or you regularly drink alcohol, be careful with acetaminophen. A safe limit for you may be only 3,000 mg.

Remember that many OTC cough and cold preparations include acetaminophen, so taking a normal dose of Tylenol but adding an OTC combination product could put you in the danger zone.

•**Use** for pain without inflammation, fever.

•**Avoid** if you have liver disease.

ASPIRIN

Aspirin, an NSAID, comes from salicin, an ingredient found in the willow tree. In ancient Egypt, willow bark was used to treat pain and swelling. Modern aspirin as acetylsalicylic acid was developed by the Bayer Company in 1899.

Like the other NSAIDs, aspirin blocks inflammation along with reducing pain and fever. NSAIDs work by blocking the action of a fatty compound called prostaglandin that acts as a chemical messenger for your immune system. Prostaglandin helps increase blood flow and the release of white blood cells to cause inflammation. Today, aspirin is a less common pain or fever medicine because it has side effects like tinnitus at high doses, heartburn, and an increased risk of bleeding. The bleeding side effect has given aspirin new life. A study in 1974 found that a low dose of aspirin reduces the risk of a second heart attack by about 25 percent. Today, low-dose aspirin is used to reduce the risk of a blood clot leading to a stroke or heart attack for some people at high risk. Talk to your doctor before taking aspirin for this use.

•**Use** for pain, fever, and inflammation, to reduce the risk of a blood clot if your doctor advises it.

•**Avoid** if you have a bleeding disorder, a bleeding ulcer, or a history of gastrointestinal bleeding.

IBUPROFEN AND NAPROXEN

These NSAIDs are available OTC, but there are stronger prescription-strength versions, too. Like aspirin, they work by blocking prostaglandin. They reduce pain and fever quickly for about four hours, just like acetaminophen, but their anti-inflammatory effects make them a better choice for some painful conditions, such as a fracture, sprain, or a strain, a painful infection, pain from a toxin like a bee sting or poison ivy, pain from an inflammatory disease like rheumatoid arthritis or inflammatory bowel disease, pain from a burn injury, and menstrual pain, because prostaglandin causes uterine contractions.

NSAIDs cause side effects in your stomach, kidneys, and blood vessels. Prostaglandins decrease stomach acid secretions, so when they are blocked, you may get acid indigestion or heartburn. The most common dangerous side effect from NSAIDs is a bleeding ulcer. Much less commonly, NSAIDs may cause kidney damage or increase the risk of a stroke or heart attack, but these are very rare side effects and probably limited to people who already have kidney or vascular disease. If you have a history of cardiovascular disease, and you take NSAIDs for a long time, you may increase your risk of heart attack or stroke by about 0.1 to 0.2 percent.

If you have a history of ulcer, kidney disease, stroke, or heart disease, ask your doctor if NSAIDs are safe for you. You can avoid side effects by using only the recommended dose and using these drugs only as long as you need them.

•**Use** for fever, inflammation, and pain from a fracture, sprain or strain, infection, bee sting, burns, or inflammatory disease.

•**Talk to your doctor first** if you have a history of ulcer, kidney disease, stroke, or heart disease.

NSAIDS AND ACETAMINOPHEN

NSAIDs and acetaminophen work better when used together than when used separately. In fact, according to the National Safety Council, studies show that this combination may work better for pain than an opioid analgesic. You can get this benefit by alternating the two drugs or by using them at the same time, for example taking one Tylenol along with one Advil. Combination products like Advil Dual Action are now available, too.

The bottom line on OTC pain and fever medicines is that they are safe and effective if you use them as directed for the right type of pain and understand the risk profile of each drug. Other than severe acute or chronic pain, you can probably get by with acetaminophen or an NSAID. If in doubt, check with your health-care provider or pharmacist.

New Drug Regrows Hair Lost to Alopecia Areata

Emma Guttman-Yassky, M.D., Ph.D., chair of dermatology and immunology at Icahn School of Medicine at Mount Sinai in New York City. MountSinai.org

Alopecia areata is an immune system disease that causes spot baldness. About one patient in three recovers at least 80 percent of hair within 36 weeks when taking *baricitinib* (Olumiant), which recently received FDA approval.

But: Regrown hair is mostly lost if use is discontinued, and Olumiant costs about $2,500 a month, though insurance may cover it. Side effects may include increased susceptibility to herpes infections.

Adderall Is Frequently Abused

Michael Weaver, M.D., professor of psychiatry and director of the Center for Neurobehavioral Research on Addiction at UTHealth Houston.

Restrictions on prescriptions were relaxed during the pandemic so patients could keep up with their meds. That allowed unscrupulous telemedicine companies to pop up online, with physicians hastily writing prescriptions for people claiming they had ADHD. Adderall is a stimulant that can cause dangerously increased heart rate and addiction.

New Weekly Alzheimer's Patch

Stephen Salloway, M.D., professor of neurology at Brown University, Providence. Brown.edu

The FDA has approved Adlarity, a weekly *donepezil* patch for Alzheimer's dementia. Donepezil has long been available as a daily pill (Aricept) but can cause gastroin-

testinal side effects, which Adlarity makes less severe. *Rivastigmine* (Exelon), a similar drug, also has been available as a daily patch. Both drugs inhibit an enzyme that breaks down a brain chemical essential for short-term memory.

PPIs Are Overprescribed

The American Gastroenterological Association recommends that doctors prescribe prescription and OTC proton pump inhibitors (PPIs, such as *esomeprazole*/Nexium and *lansoprazole*/Prevacid) only if their use is clearly indicated such as for gastroesophageal reflux disease (GERD) and peptic ulcer disease. If you have been prescribed a PPI, discuss with your doctor whether you still need it. Do not stop taking prescribed PPIs on your own.

Laura Targownik, M.D., gastroenterologist at Mount Sinai Hospital, University of Toronto, Canada.

Antibiotic Resistance

Jamison Starbuck, ND, naturopathic physician in family practice in Missoula, Montana, and producer of *Dr. Starbuck's Health Tips for Kids*, a weekly program on Montana Public Radio, MTPR.org. She is a past president of the American Association of Naturopathic Physicians and a contributing editor to *The Alternative Advisor: The Complete Guide to Natural Therapies and Alternative Treatments*.

Antibiotic resistance is a problem for everyone. Methicillin-resistant Staphylococcus aureus (MRSA) is one of several bacteria that cause more than 2.8 million antibiotic-resistant infections in the United States every year. More than 35,000 people die each year due to these infections.

We all need to do our part to slow the further development of antibiotic resistance. Doctors are increasingly cautious not to overprescribe antibiotics. Patients can prevent infection through good hygiene and immune support, including handwashing, adequate sleep, and good nutrition. And both patients and physicians can, in many situations, use nonantibiotic alternatives, such as plant medicines, to treat infections.

Choosing an alternative to an antibiotic drug does not mean you should avoid your doctor or sidestep an accurate diagnosis. Whether it's your skin, ears, bladder, or stomach that's sick, you need your health-care provider to examine you and monitor your infection. But you can be the one to tell your doctor you'd like to avoid antibiotics, if possible, and ask if a plant medicine would be reasonable for your situation.

Here are several that I prescribe every day in my family practice…

•**Oregon grape root.** *Mahonia aquifolium* is a shrub that is native to the western United States, particularly Oregon, Washington, and northern California. The medicine comes from the root and bark, which are yellow, due in part to berberine, a plant constituent that has antimicrobial properties. Oregon grape root can be used to treat bladder, gastrointestinal, and throat infections. My typical dose is two capsules every four hours for three to five days.

•**Garlic.** *Allium sativa* is an antibacterial plant medicine I use frequently for treating ear infections. For an uncomplicated ear infection, I prescribe garlic oil directly into the infected ear. I also recommend that my patients use hydrogen peroxide in between garlic oil applications. A typical schedule is five drops of peroxide in the ear(s) in the morning, two drops of garlic oil at noon, five drops of peroxide at 5 p.m., and two drops of garlic oil into the ear(s) at bedtime. Do this for three to five days until the ear infection is gone.

•**Uva ursi.** *Arctostaphylos*, also known as Kinnikinnick or Bearberry, is my go-to herb for food poisoning, acute diarrhea, and bacterial vaginosis. A typical adult dose for infection is ⅛ teaspoon Uva ursi tincture in 2 ounces of water, away from meals, four times a day for one to five days until the infection is resolved.

•**Calendula** is my number one antibacterial plant medicine for mild skin infections such as acne and boils, or to prevent infection in cuts and scrapes. For skin infections, it's best to use a tincture applied full strength over the infected skin three times a day. To prevent infection in a cut or scrape, wash the injury with soap and water first, and then apply diluted calendula (50/50 water/tincture) twice daily for two days or until the injury is healed.

•**Echinacea** works by increasing white-blood-cell activity in the body. It's a great herb to combine with other plant medicines to boost the immune response. My typical adult dose is 60 drops of echinacea tincture, four times a day, in 2 ounces of water, taken 30 minutes away from food, in addition to any of the above prescriptions.

Alternating Antibiotics Helps Combat Resistance

In lab tests, rapidly alternating between three antibiotics killed resistant bacteria five times more efficiently than using a single antibiotic. If further testing shows this approach also works with humans, it could be a more effective way to treat drug-resistant bacterial infections.

Study by researchers at University of Kiel, Germany, reported in *New Scientist*.

New Drug May Slow ALS

Amit Sachdev, M.D., director of the division of neuromuscular medicine at Michigan State University, East Lansing. Neurology.MSU.edu

---

Preliminary results show that Relyvrio, a combination of the drugs sodium phenylbutyrate and taurursodiol, works better than other treatments for amyotrophic lateral sclerosis (ALS). Relyvrio, taken orally or by feeding tube, doesn't cure, treat underlying causes, or reverse existing symptoms. The FDA has approved Relyvrio before completion of phase 3 testing, which is expected in 2023.

Cost: $158,000 per year, at least partially covered by most insurance.

Opioids No Longer First-Line Treatment for Chronic Pain

Christopher M. Jones, PharmD, DrPH, acting director for the Centers for Disease Control and Prevention's National Center for Injury Prevention and Control in Atlanta. CDC.gov

The CDC now discourages opioids as a first-line treatment for chronic pain (lasting three months or more) or subacute pain (one to three months). These voluntary recommendations remove hard thresholds for dosage/duration of opioid pain medication prescriptions and instead recommend that prescribers personalize each patient's treatment, weighing potential risks against the benefits, and reassess over time.

COVID Rebound After Using Paxlovid

Michael Ison, M.D., professor of medicine in infectious diseases at Northwestern University Feinberg School of Medicine, Chicago, Illinois.

We know from other viruses that if you stop a medication, a virus can begin replicating again and cause symptoms in some patients. This can happen when the virus has not been fully cleared from the body. This could come from a course of therapy that is too short or the virus developing resistance to the drug.

The frequency of these rebounds with *nirmatrelvir* and *ritonavir tablets* (Paxlovid) is not completely understood. In the studies that led to the U.S. Food and Drug Administration's Use Authorization, 1 to 2 percent of patients experienced rebound.

Symptoms with viral rebound are similar to what patients had before the treatment or would have experienced without the treatment. To date, the rebound has generally been relatively mild and has not required hospitalization. Most patients need symptom management only. (Immunocompromised patients who experience rebound should talk to their doctors.)

Rebound can result in transmission to others. Affected people should quarantine until they are asymptomatic and again if symptoms recur. All patients should use masks when around others for 10 days, longer for patients who require hospitalization or who are immunocompromised.

Paxlovid has been clearly shown to decrease the risk of severe disease, hospitalization, and death and may speed recovery of symptoms. Even if rebounds occur, the patient is unlikely to progress to severe disease, hospitalization, and death.

CHAPTER 14

Men's Health

Don't Jump into Treatment for Prostate Cancer

Between 12 and 13 percent of men will be diagnosed with prostate cancer. For those with low-risk disease, the National Comprehensive Cancer Network (NCCN) says that active surveillance is preferable to surgery or radiation, but many men and their doctors are not following the NCCN guidelines.

"Studies show that the safest and best treatment for men with low-risk prostate cancer is active surveillance, but in the United States, about 50 percent of men are still being treated with surgery or radiation therapy," says Minhaj Siddiqui, M.D., associate professor of urology at the University of Maryland School of Medicine and director of urologic oncology at the Baltimore VA Medical Center.

WHAT IS LOW-RISK?

Low-risk prostate cancer grows very slowly or does not grow at all. It is the most common type of prostate cancer. Ten years after diagnosis, 99 percent of men with low-risk prostate cancer will not have died from it.

You may have low-risk cancer if...

•**The cancer is found on only one side (lobe) of your prostate.**

•**The cancer takes up less than half the lobe.**

•**The cancer cells are not aggressive,** which means they do not have a lot of cell changes seen under a microscope. This is called a low Gleason score.

•**The cancer has not spread outside of the prostate.**

Chris Iliades, M.D., a regular contributor to *Bottom Line Health*. He is a retired ear, nose, throat, head, and neck surgeon.

239

Why Not Treat the Cancer and Get It Over With?

Surgery and radiation for prostate cancer come with two frequent side effects: incontinence and erectile dysfunction. About half of men will have one of these problems. According to the Prostate Cancer Foundation, leaking urine after prostate cancer surgery occurs in almost all men, and one in five will need to wear an absorbent pad. This improves over time for most men. Erectile dysfunction (ED) occurs in about 40 percent of men. Similar risks for incontinence and ED occur with radiation therapy.

ACTIVE SURVEILLANCE

Active surveillance means keeping an eye on your cancer to make sure it does not act up. As recommended by the American Society of Clinical Oncology, surveillance may include a PSA blood test every three to six months, a digital rectal prostate exam at least once per year, and a prostate biopsy in six to 12 months followed by another biopsy every two to five years. If any of these exams suggest an increased risk, active treatment may be recommended.

A 2021 study published in *The Journal of Urology* followed close to 7,000 men who were diagnosed with prostate cancer. Sixty-eight percent were diagnosed with low-risk prostate cancer. After almost seven years of active surveillance, only one-third had converted to active treatment. The survival rate of prostate cancer is 99 percent with either active surveillance or treatment.

"The only part of surveillance that men complain about is the biopsies," explains Dr. Siddiqui. "There are ongoing studies to find out if we can reduce the frequency of biopsies."

Some surveillance programs also include occasional MRI imaging studies. After age 75, men can consider going off active surveillance if their cancer risk has remained low.

If your urologist does not offer active surveillance as the preferred choice for low-risk cancer, you should get a second opinion. "Don't be afraid to ask," says Dr. Siddiqui. "I always recommend a second opinion for any cancer diagnosis."

Pumpkin Seed Oil Is Good for Men's Health

Study of 73 men by researchers at Hamadan University of Medical Sciences, Hamadan, Iran, published in *BMC Urology*.

While claims that pumpkin seed oil can reduce male-pattern baldness are not supported by scientific evidence, pumpkin seed oil does appear to benefit men's health.

Recent finding: Taking 360 mg of pumpkin seed oil twice daily significantly reduced symptoms of enlarged prostate.

Caution: Although it is generally considered safe at dosages recommended on supplement labels, there is no established safe upper limit for pumpkin seed oil, and higher dosages have not been proved safe.

Best: Take pumpkin seed oil under the guidance of an integrative doctor.

MRI-Targeted Prostate Biopsy Reduces Overdiagnosis

Aaron Katz, M.D., chair of urology at NYU Langone Long Island in Garden City, New York, commenting on a study of 18,000 men published in *The New England Journal of Medicine*.

Men with elevated PSA scores who had MRIs of their prostates underwent fewer unnecessary tests and treatments than men who received standard biopsies. Any intermediate cancers that MRI missed could safely be managed with active surveillance.

If your annual PSA test is high: Get retested…and discuss with a urologist getting an MRI rather than a biopsy. Medicare covers it, but some insurers may push back.

All About Hair Loss

Antonella Tosti, M.D., the Fredric Brandt Endowed Professor of Dermatology and Cutaneous Surgery at the University of Miami. Dr. Tosti is past president of the American Hair Research Society, past president and founding member of the European Hair Research Society, and author of the e-book *Hair Facts: Everything You Ever Wanted to Know About Hair Loss and Hair Care.* DoctorTosti.com

Hair loss affects tens of millions of people, but not all hair loss is the same. We interviewed internationally renowned hair-disorder expert Dr. Antonella Tosti about some of the more common culprits behind thinning and shedding strands.

What is considered normal when it comes to hair loss?

It's quite normal to lose 50 to 70 hairs a day as part of the hair's natural growth cycle, which involves alternating periods of activity and rest. The hairs that fall out already have new hairs growing in to replace them. But when a person starts shedding more than 100 hairs a day, that is abnormal and suggests you may be experiencing some form of active hair loss.

It's difficult to keep track, but one method involves washing your hair in a sink—ideally one in a color that contrasts with your hair color—and counting how many hairs you see. Daily hair washers who count about 30 to 40 hairs are in good shape. (*Note:* If you have curly hair, don't tend to comb or brush daily, and shampoo only once a week, you may see 200 strands or more. This is normal.)

You can also perform what dermatologists call a pull test: Grasp small sections of hair, about 40 to 50 strands, in various locations on your scalp and give a gentle tug. If more than five hairs come out in a section, you are likely experiencing active hair loss.

How typical is age-related hair loss, and what does it look like?

It's extremely common to notice hair loss or hair thinning as one moves through their 50s, 60s, and 70s. Called *androgenetic alopecia*, it's the most common hair disorder, affecting about 80 percent of men (*male-pattern baldness*) and 50 percent of women (*female-pattern baldness*). In male-pattern baldness, the hairline starts to take on an M shape, as hair recedes at the temples. Women tend to show widening of the central parting, often more accentuated at the hairline which, if viewed from overhead, resembles a Christmas tree.

With androgenetic alopecia, the concern isn't so much that too many hairs are falling out, but rather that the hairs that replace the ones falling out are thinner and thinner. Imagine what your front lawn would look like if most of the blades of grass started losing 50 percent of their thickness. You'd start to see more and more of the earth peeking through.

Is that what's happening with the COVID patients who are losing hair after recovering from their infection?

No, that's *telogen effluvium* (TE), a condition in which multiple hair follicles enter their "rest phase" simultaneously, rather than entering it at different times as they normally would. TE is fairly common and tends to occur approximately three months after a stressful event. That can include anything from a divorce to a big move to an illness. We first saw widespread TE during the 1918 Spanish influenza pandemic, and now it's happening again with COVID. Hair falls out quickly—you'll notice it on your pillowcase, on your clothes, in the shower—as soon as a few weeks post-infection, and it affects up to half of all of the strands on your head. TE is easy to recognize because the hairs have a tiny white bulb at the root that you can see with the naked eye. TE due to COVID often appears four to six weeks after the infection and it's often accompanied by scalp pain.

Does hair lost due to TE grow back?

Yes, the shedding stops in a few months and hair begins to regrow, but it can be distressing, nonetheless. If you already had androgenetic alopecia before developing TE, the new hair will grow back thinner than before.

Are any types of hair loss reversible?

Some, like TE, reverse naturally. Others, like androgenetic alopecia, can be slowed and, in some cases, new hair growth can oc-

Frequent Washing Doesn't Cause Hair Loss

It's a myth that frequent hair washing causes hair loss. Any hairs that fall out while shampooing are already in their rest phase, whether that's because of the natural hair growth cycle or due to a health condition that's negatively impacting hair. They're destined to fall out—you can't avoid it by not touching them. In fact, frequent, thorough hair washing can often help promote hair growth, as it prevents certain diseases of the scalp, like seborrheic dermatitis, that can lead to hair loss. It also acts as a mini scalp massage, which can stimulate hair follicles in the resting phase to resume activity.

cur. There are currently two FDA-approved drugs for male-pattern hair loss and one for female. For male-pattern hair loss, there's oral *finasteride* (Propecia) and *topical minoxidil* (Rogaine). For female-pattern hair loss, topical minoxidil is approved. But many patients use different treatments off-label with their doctor's guidance, including *oral minoxidil* (both genders), *oral finasteride* (for postmenopausal women), and more. Chronic TE may respond to oral minoxidil but not topical minoxidil. There are also treatments such as topical steroids, platelet-rich plasma (PRP) injections, and hair transplants that can restore hair, and confidence, for some patients.

Hair-Loss Remedies

Ivan S. Cohen, M.D., a leader in the field of hair-transplant surgery for more than 25 years, board-certified dermatologist in private practice in Fairfield, Connecticut, and associate professor of dermatology at Yale University School of Medicine. FairfieldDerm.com

W hen topical *minoxidil* (Rogaine) was introduced in the late 1980s, it became an option for restoring thinning hair. The biggest problem was the greasy look it left, which made people reluctant to use it as often as directed. Now there are effective

options that are easy to stick with. It is important to start medical therapy early. When hair is thin but still present, hair loss is potentially reversible—but once it's gone, only transplants will work.

PRESCRIPTION MEDICATIONS

•**Oral *minoxidil* (Rogaine) is the latest breakthrough.** Its hair-thickening benefits were discovered when it was being tested for its primary purpose—controlling hard-to-treat high blood pressure. Taken orally, minoxidil works even better than its topical counterpart and, when given in a very low dose, it has very few, if any, side effects. Men can start with a 2.5-mg pill daily…women, half that amount.

Potential side effects: Heart events, notably pericardial effusion (extra fluid in the sac around the heart), are rare—but possible. Also, minoxidil at low doses rarely if ever affects blood pressure.

More common side effect: Extra facial hair—this typically happens only when there's a dramatic regrowth of hair on the scalp. Most women are willing to have unwanted facial hair waxed off in return for thicker hair on their head…or they can take a low dose of the diuretic *spironolactone* (CaroSpir and Aldactone), an androgen blocker used to treat acne that also reduces excess facial hair.

•***Finasteride* (Propecia),** a 5-alpha reductase inhibitor that treats enlarged prostate, is approved for hair loss. It blocks the hormone DHT, which causes hair to fall out. It can be taken by men and postmenopausal women (in younger women, it can cause birth defects). A young man with a family history of baldness might benefit from taking finasteride and oral minoxidil at the same time.

Potential side effects: Sexual dysfunction, which affects 2 percent to 3 percent of users… loss of concentration or mood changes…possibly depression sometimes to the point of suicidal ideation, which affects 1 percent of users. If any of these occur, stop taking it.

•***Dutasteride* (Avodart),** another 5-alpha reductase inhibitor, carries a slightly higher risk for the same side effects as finasteride and has a longer half life—five weeks versus finasteride's six hours. Because the drug stays in your system longer, side effects will take longer to go away even after you stop taking the drug. This is only for someone who doesn't respond to other medications.

•*Bimatoprost* **(Latisse)** is effective for both thinning eyebrows as well as eyelashes. This prescription ophthalmic solution should be prescribed by an eye doctor or dermatologist.

OVER-THE-COUNTER PRODUCTS

•**Nutrafol**—with curcumin, ashwagandha, saw palmetto, marine collagen peptides, and vitamins—works better for women, though is not as effective as medication. If you're averse to taking drugs or using topical minoxidil, it's worth a try.

Downside: It costs $80 a month versus $10 for oral minoxidil.

Note: Nutrafol supports the effects of hair-regrowth drugs, so you might want to ask your doctor about taking it in addition to oral minoxidil.

•**Viviscal** uses a proprietary marine collagen complex to strengthen hair. It costs about $33 a month. Beware of copycat products that lack testing.

Screening for Heart Disease in Symptom-Free Men Saves Lives

Study titled "Five-Year Outcomes of the Danish Cardiovascular Screening (DANCAVAS) Trial," by researchers at University of Southern Denmark, Odense, et al., published in *The New England Journal of Medicine.*

Cardiovascular disease, including stroke and heart disease, is the number-one cause of death in both the U.S. and Denmark. Researchers from Odense University Hospital and other Denmark hospitals wanted to see if screening a large number of men for undiagnosed cardiovascular disease—and treating those at risk—would significantly decrease their death rate over about five years. Their results were presented at the European Society of Cardiology meeting and published in *The New England Journal of Medicine.*

The Danish Cardiovascular Screening (DANCAVAS) trial follows another Danish screening trial for cardiovascular disease in older men called the Viborg Vascular trial. This trial screened men for abdominal aortic aneurism, peripheral artery disease, and hypertension. Identifying and treating these conditions reduced the five-year death rate by a significant 7 percent.

SCREENING MEN WHO ARE SYMPTOM FREE

Screening exams are diagnostic tests that look for early diseases that have not been diagnosed by signs or symptoms, called *subclinical disease.* The DANCAVAS trial included more than 45,000 Danish men ages 65 to 74. Some of these men received screening tests designed to detect subclinical cardiovascular disease. They were compared with men who did not receive screening.

The screening tests included blood testing for diabetes and high cholesterol and blood pressure measurements of the arm and ankle. The men also had an imaging study of the heart called a coronary calcium scan. This is a type of CT scan that measures the amount of calcium in the blood vessels that supply your heart. Since calcium forms in the plaques that cause coronary heart disease, a high calcium score means a high risk for a heart attack. Comparing the blood pressure in your arm to the blood pressure in your ankle is a way to measure peripheral artery disease, which is a risk factor for both heart attack and stroke.

AGE RANGE MAKES A DIFFERENCE

For all the men in the study, there was very little difference in any cause of death between five and six years after screening. Unscreened men had a five-year death rate of 13.1 percent, and the screened men had a death rate of 12.6 percent. This difference was not enough to recommend screening. However, when only men ages 65 to 69 were compared, there was a significant benefit to screening. In this subgroup of the study, men who were screened had an 11 percent lower five-year death rate, which is very significant.

243

The researchers note that men with positive screening tests were treated with medications to lower cholesterol and reduce stroke risk, which probably accounts for their improved survival due to less heart attacks and strokes. They also suspect that this benefit was found only in the younger men because they were less likely to already be on cardio-vascular disease prevention medication and they were more likely to still be smokers. Overall, more than 50 percent of men in the study were already on blood pressure medication, more than 30 precent on cholesterol medication, and more than 25 percent on blood-thinning medication.

More research is needed, and the current study group has begun enrolling men ages 60 to 64 for the DANCAVAS II trial. Researchers still need to answer additional questions, such as will this type of screening work in other countries and will it work in women as well as men. Women were not included in this study because they have a lower overall rate of heart attack and stroke than men, making mixed comparisons less reliable. Before this type of screening can be used outside a clinical trial, questions of accessibility and affordability will also need to be addressed.

Men and Body Fat

Men with More Body Fat Have Lower Bone Density

Researchers analyzed weight and bone-density data on 10,814 men and women ages 20 to 59 and found that higher fat mass (the weight of fat in the body) was related to lower bone density. High lean body mass (the weight of your body, including organs, skin, and bones, minus fat) correlated with higher bone density. The association was stronger in men than women.

Rajesh K. Jain, M.D., assistant professor of medicine, University of Chicago.

Men Are More Vulnerable to Obesity-Related Risks

According to a recent study, obese male mice develop fewer blood vessels to deliver oxygen and nutrients to fat tissue than females—creating higher heart disease and diabetes risk. Blood vessel cells in males developed damage and inflammation...in females, they did not. These biological differences help explain why females are more protected from metabolic and cardiovascular diseases than males. The findings could lead to new obesity treatments for men that target better blood vessel health.

Tara Haas, Ph.D., professor at York University, Toronto, Ontario, Canada, and lead author of a mouse study published in *iScience*.

Get a PSA Score with Annual Bloodwork

Aaron Katz, M.D., chair of urology at NYU Langone Long Island School of Medicine in Garden City, New York, commenting on a study published in *Journal of the National Cancer Institute*.

If the score rises sharply from the previous year, insist on an MRI before getting a biopsy. In 2012, the medical community recommended against using prostate-specific antigen (PSA) to screen for prostate cancer because it led to many unnecessary biopsies and treatments.

But: New data now shows a decrease in overtreatment but an increase in diagnosis of metastatic cancers. Elevated blood levels of PSA can indicate malignant cancer when it is still treatable.

Ultra-Processed Foods Increase Colon Cancer Risk in Men

Study titled "Association of Ultra-Processed Food Consumption with Colorectal Cancer Risk Among Men and Women: Results from Three Prospective U.S. Cohort Studies," led by researchers at Tufts and Harvard Universities, published in *The BMJ*.

If you're trying to eat healthy, you probably know to tread cautiously in the cookies aisle and frozen foods section at the grocery store. But food surveys show that many U.S. consumers opt for convenience when it comes to mealtime. And a recent study reveals that this big intake of fake food could be harming our colons, especially in men.

Colorectal cancer is the third most common cause of cancer and the second leading cause of death from cancer in men and women. A high-fat and low-fiber diet as well as obesity are known risk factors for this cancer. Ultra-processed foods contribute to all these risk factors, and they account for close to 60 percent of the calories in a typical American diet. To examine the link between ultra-processed foods and colorectal cancer, researchers led by Tufts and Harvard Universities in Boston (and including scientists from Brazil and Canada) used three large, long-term health studies that included both detailed diet history and cancer diagnosis.

PROCESSED VERSUS ULTRA-PROCESSED

What are "ultra-processed" foods exactly? Processed foods are a step up from the whole stuff in the produce and meats aisle: there might be some salt or preservative added to keep the product (tuna, canned beans) from going bad. Ultra-processed foods are ready-to-eat items that are made up of multiple ingredients created in laboratories and fabricated to eat right out of the box or bottle (cookies, crackers, sodas, and boxed cereals) or right out of the microwave (frozen "TV dinners"). Besides the usual salt and various sugars, ingredients in ultra-processed items can include a litany of emulsifiers, preservatives, flavors, and colors to enhance the product's flavor and convenience factor.

WHAT THE THREE STUDIES REVEALED

The three studies were the Health Professionals Follow-up Study from 1986 to 2014, the Nurses' Health Study from 1986 to 2014, and the Nurses' Health Study II from 1991 to 2015. From these studies, the research team identified approximately 160,000 women and 46,000 men who had no evidence of colorectal cancer at the start of the studies and available food questionnaires that were filled out every four years.

Using the food questionnaires, the researchers ranked diets for the amount of ultra-processed foods consumed from the lowest 20 percent to the highest 20 percent of people selected. The results of the study are published in the journal *The BMJ*. *Key results included these findings...*

•**During the 24 to 28 years of follow-up,** there were 3,216 cases of colorectal cancer.

•**Compared to men in the lowest 20 percent of ultra-processed food consumption,** the highest 20 percent of men had a 29 percent increased risk of colorectal cancer.

•**Most of these cancers in men were in the distal or last part of the colon.**

•**Foods with the highest risk for men** were ready-to-eat meat, poultry, and seafood along with sugar-sweetened beverages.

•**Women only had an increased risk for colon cancer** for certain food types: ready-to-eat, heat-mixed dishes (prepared foods that are heated in the microwave), which increased colorectal cancer risk by 17 percent.

•**Women who consumed the most yogurt and dairy-based foods** decreased their risk of colorectal cancer by 17 percent.

WHY YOUR COLON PREFERS WHOLE FOOD

There are many reasons why ultra-processed foods may increase colorectal cancer risk, according to the research team. These foods are high in fats, oils, and sugar that may change the healthy balance of microbes in the colon (the microbiome). Ultra-processed foods are typically low in fiber and increase risk of obesity. They may also have food additives and artificial sweeteners that increase cancer risk. Finally, cancer-causing chemicals may leak into foods from heat processing and plastics used in food packaging.

It's unclear why women are less at risk from these foods than men. The researchers theorize that women may consume more protective foods like yogurt and other dairy products, and they may use less salt and healthier Mediterranean-diet type foods. Another possible explanation is the female hormone estrogen, which may protect women from cancer.

Subgroups of ultra-processed foods included in the study were…

- **Fat, condiments, and sauces**
- **Packaged sweets, snacks, and desserts**
- **Artificially sweetened beverages**
- **Ready-to-eat, mixed dishes**
- **Ready-to-heat meat, poultry, and seafood products**
- **Packaged savory snacks**
- **Yogurt and dairy-based desserts**

This study adds to accumulating evidence that these pre-cooked, instant foods increase the risk of several chronic diseases, including diabetes and cancer. The researchers conclude that their findings support public health measures to limit or discourage the use of ultra-processed foods for better public health outcomes.

Low Testosterone Could Make COVID-19 Worse

Study titled "Association of Male Hypogonadism with Risk of Hospitalization for COVID-19," led by researchers at Washington University School of Medicine, St. Louis, published in *JAMA Network Open.*

Hospital records during the COVID-19 pandemic show that men are more likely to be hospitalized for severe COVID than women. Blood testing on many male patients admitted for COVID reveals that they have lower levels of testosterone than men in the healthy, general population, according to several studies. Researchers at Washington University School of Medicine in St. Louis had found that men admitted to their hospital with COVID commonly had low testosterone.

WHICH CAME FIRST? LOW TESTOSTERONE OR COVID?

Low testosterone is common in many older men because testosterone levels start to decline after age 30 and continue to drop by one to two percent every year. Testosterone levels also go down during a severe illness such as COVID, so researchers from Saint Louis University School of Medicine and Washington University School of Medicine conducted a study designed to find out which comes first, low testosterone or COVID-19.

Their study is published in the American Medical Association journal *JAMA Network Open,* and it suggests that men who have low testosterone before a COVID infection are at higher risk for COVID hospitalization than men with normal testosterone. The research team reviewed the hospital records of 723 men who tested positive for COVID, mostly in 2020. To be included in the study they had to have had testosterone levels tested before their hospital admission. The study identified and included all 723 men, who were at an average age of about 55.

Of the 723 men in the study, 116 had low testosterone before their admission and 180 had low testosterone that was being treated with testosterone replacement. The rest of the men, numbering 427, had normal testosterone. *These were the key findings…*

- **Of the 427 men with normal testosterone,** 53 (12 percent) required hospital admission for COVID.
- **Of the 116 men with low testosterone,** 52 (45 percent) required hospital admission for COVID.
- **Overall,** men with low testosterone were two to three times more likely to be admitted.
- **Men who had well-treated low testosterone** had a hospitalization rate very similar to the normal men.

The research team concludes from the study that low testosterone is a risk factor for a more severe COVID infection along with other risk factors such as older age, obesity, diabetes, hypertension, chronic lung diseases, and cardiovascular disease.

WHAT'S THE NORMAL TESTOSTERONE RANGE?

A normal range of testosterone for men is between 300 to 1,000 nanograms per deciliter (ng/dL). In their study, the investigators found that the risk of severe COVID starts with testosterone under 200 ng/dL. This risk occurs independent of other severe COVID risk factors.

Symptoms of low testosterone can include loss of sex drive, erectile dysfunction, depression, irritability, weakness, fatigue, and loss of muscle mass. These symptoms can cause a lower quality of life and can be treated with testosterone replacement therapy.

TESTOSTERONE THERAPY IS NOT RISK-FREE

The findings of the study suggest that correcting low testosterone can be a strategy for preventing severe COVID, along with vaccination. However, testosterone replacement therapy has some risks. Testosterone may increase the risk of prostate cancer or the risk from prostate cancer because testosterone speeds the growth of prostate cancer cells. Testosterone therapy has also been linked to a higher risk of heart disease in some studies, but this link is not as well established as the prostate cancer link.

Before testosterone replacement can be recommended as a risk reduction strategy for COVID, more research will need to be done. This study was an observational study, meaning it relied on a review of medical records. To prove that low testosterone is a risk factor for COVID, studies will need to compare men with low testosterone to men with normal testosterone going forward over time (a longitudinal study).

Bump on the Roof of the Mouth Common in Men

Charlie Cage, DDS, MS. DrCharlieCage.com

I see many patients with hard bumps in their mouths called tori. This is a benign bony prominence that is usually found on the roof of the mouth along the midline (a palatal tori) or the lower jaw underneath the tongue (mandibular tori). In the latter case, there are usually bumps on both sides of the mouth, but in 10 percent of cases, there may be a single torus.

This condition is quite normal. It's more common in men and appears to have a genetic component. Further, certain lifestyles can induce the production of extra bone, which is most commonly seen in the upper jaw against the checks in weightlifters or people who clench or grind their teeth.

This excess bone is harmless and does not create an issue unless someone needs dentures. It may then need to be surgically removed.

Always consult with a dentist to ensure the proper diagnosis of a tori to eliminate other serious conditions such as infections, pathology, or other medical diseases. It is routine to have this checked during a comprehensive exam that includes an oral cancer screening.

Exercise Can Fight Prostate Cancer

Study by researchers at Edith Cowan University, Joondalup, Australia, published in *Prostate Cancer and Prostatic Diseases*.

According to a recent study, a single session of intense exercise on a stationary bike boosted production of myokines, anti-cancer proteins that suppress tumor growth, for advanced-stage prostate cancer patients. In previous studies, cancer patients who exercised regularly had slower disease progression and better survival rates. Regular intense exercise may change the body's chemical environment, making it less hospitable to cancers. These results provide strong evidence for recommending that patients with prostate cancer should try to exercise at least most days.

Developing the Ideal Male Contraceptive Pill

Study titled "On-Demand Male Contraception Via Acute Inhibition of Soluble Adenylyl Cyclase," by researchers at Weill Cornell Medicine, New York City, published in *Nature Communications.*

Despite years of contraceptive development and improvements to access, almost half of all pregnancies are still unwanted, especially among adolescents. And the burden of preventing unintended pregnancies has been primarily on women.

A PILL THAT STOPS SPERM

Hormonal contraceptives are effective for women, but they must be taken regularly, and can have side effects. For men, the only options have been the condom or a vasectomy. Promising pre-clinical research from Weill Cornell Medicine is giving hope for a male contraceptive pill that only needs to be taken before sex and will prevent pregnancy by temporarily keeping sperm from being able to swim through the cervix to fertilize an egg.

This new technology has a somewhat indirect development—it's based an experimental medication that can block a cellular signaling protein found in sperm cells called soluble adenylyl cyclase (sAC). The sAC inhibitor is called TDI-11861, which has only recently been isolated by researchers at Weill Cornell Medicine Department of Pharmacology, allowing them to do studies with sAC and TRI-11861. These are preclinical studies, which are studies done in the lab or in animal models, before being tried in human trials.

The concept of blocking sAC is based on several previous discoveries. Both men and mice who are born without the gene to produce sAC are infertile, but otherwise healthy. Lab studies show that blocking sAC activity in sperm cells makes them temporarily immotile, meaning they are unable to swim through sperm fluid to reach the uterus and ovary. This effect occurs within 30 minutes to one hour, only lasts for about two to three hours, and by 24 hours, nearly all sperm have recovered normal movement. Side effects or long-term complications are less likely because the effects are time-limited and short-acting.

For their preclinical model, the research team used fertile male mice treated with TDI-11861. After treatment, the mice interacted with female mice and exhibited normal mating behavior, but after 52 different attempts, there were no pregnancies. By contrast, a group of untreated mice produced pregnancies in one-third of mating attempts.

A GAME-CHANGING CONTRACEPTION OPTION

If these results can be repeated in human trials, the research team thinks it could be a "game changer" in contraception options. The male contraceptive pill would be used on demand before sexual intercourse. The effects would not be permanent. A male contraceptive, on-demand pill could be a better option than the condom, a deterrent used for thousands of years that is far from foolproof and the vasectomy, which is usually a permanent solution.

Previous attempts to make a male contraceptive pill based on hormones or other non-hormonal treatments that block the production of sperm have been effective but limited by side effects and would require taking the pill regularly to maintain effectiveness.

The current study is published in the journal *Nature Communications.* The authors conclude that their study provides proof-of-concept to build on. The plan is to repeat pre-clinical studies in a different animal model and if successful move on to clinical trials in humans.

CHAPTER 15

Natural Remedies and Supplements

Probiotics Keep Your Gut Happy and You Healthy

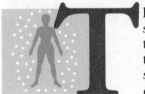

There are more than 500 species of bacteria in the human gut. This internal ecosystem, which scientists call the *gut microbiome*, contains both health-promoting and disease-inducing bacteria, and one of the keys to good health is maintaining the right balance of the two. When the gut microbiome is healthy, friendly bacteria digest milk sugar (lactose) and protein, increase the absorption of minerals, manufacture vitamins B and K, make essential and short-chain fatty acids, and prevent dysbiosis—the overgrowth of bad bacteria.

LOWER DISEASE RISK

These friendly bacteria can even lower the risk of specific diseases and disorders, like depression, autoimmune disease, heart disease, and diabetes.

•**Mental health problems.** Maintaining an optimal level of gut probiotics through a probiotic-rich diet and supplementation can reduce depression, reduce anxiety in chronic fatigue syndrome, help relieve stress-related psychological symptoms, boost mood in healthy people, and enhance memory and concentration, research shows.

That's because of the gut-brain axis—a direct link from the brain to the gut via the vagus nerve. The link is so strong that some researchers are now talking about *psychobiotics*: supplemental probiotics like *Lactobacillus helveticus* and *Bifodobacterium longum* that are uniquely effective in helping to restore and improve mental health.

•**Autoimmune disease.** There are approximately 100 different autoimmune diseases in which the immune system mistakenly attacks a

Elizabeth Lipski, Ph.D., CNS (certified nutrition specialist), professor of clinical nutrition and director of academic development for clinical nutrition programs at Maryland University of Integrative Health. She is the author of *Digestive Wellness* (5th Edition). Innovative Healing.com; DigestiveWellnessBook.com part of the body as if it were a foreign invader. They include type 1 diabetes, celiac disease, rheumatoid arthritis, Hashimoto's disease, and multiple sclerosis (MS).

Dysbiosis is a feature of most cases of autoimmune disease, and many studies suggest that correcting it with a probiotic supplement can help relieve the symptoms of autoimmunity. Researchers reported in the journal *Nutritional Neuroscience* that people with MS who took a probiotic supplement for six months had higher levels of brain-derived neurotrophic factor (a compound that helps nerve cells grow and survive), lower levels of IL-6 (an inflammatory biomarker), and less fatigue, pain, and depression (three common symptoms of MS).

In a study published in the *British Journal of Nutrition*, people with rheumatoid arthritis who took a supplement that contained both probiotics and prebiotics (nutritional factors that nourish probiotics) had less inflammation, joint stiffness, pain, and swelling, and better blood sugar control than people who took a placebo.

In Taiwan, investigators reported that people with type 1 diabetes who took a probiotic supplement had lower, healthier blood sugar

Probiotics and Cancer

A paper published in *Integrative Medicine* looked at more than 30 studies on probiotics and cancer and found that probiotics can stop cancer cells from dividing and spreading, kill existing cancer cells, and slow and reverse tumor growth in a wide range of cancers. Researchers reported in *Frontiers of Nutrition* that people who ate the most yogurt had a 13 percent lower risk of developing colon cancer. In a study of patients with bladder cancer, published in the *Nutrition Journal*, those who received the probiotic *L. casei* had an average disease-free period that was 44 percent longer than those receiving a placebo. And in a Japanese study of women with advanced cervical cancer, adding a probiotic to the treatment regimen improved the efficacy of radiation, extending survival time. The probiotics also decreased the incidence of side effects from radiation.

levels and less inflammation than those in the placebo group.

- **Cardiometabolic disorders.** This category of interrelated health problems (also called the metabolic syndrome) includes high blood pressure, high blood sugar, low HDL cholesterol, high triglycerides, and abdominal obesity (excess belly fat). Cardiometabolic conditions also include fatty liver disease, polycystic ovary syndrome, and gout.

Scientists are finding that the gut microbiome plays a role in all of these problems, probably because dysbiosis triggers chronic, low-grade inflammation and interferes with the digestion and assimilation of macronutrients (carbohydrate, fat, and protein).

Enriching the diet with probiotics through food or supplements may lower high blood pressure, high blood sugar, high LDL cholesterol, and high triglycerides, research suggests. It can trim abdominal fat, reduce body mass index, reduce fat in the liver, lower biomarkers of liver toxicity, and decrease inflammatory biomarkers.

- **Digestive diseases.** It's no surprise that friendly gut bacteria improve gut health, reducing the risk of digestive disease and helping to treat and reverse gut problems. Probiotics have been used to treat irritable bowel syndrome, stomach ulcers, ulcerative colitis (a type of inflammatory bowel disease), celiac disease, and antibiotic-induced diarrhea.

In fact, a prescription supplement called VSL#3 has been developed specifically to treat irritable bowel syndrome and ulcerative colitis. Probiotics have also been used to treat bacterial infections in the gut, such as *Helicobacter pylori* and small intestinal bacterial overgrowth.

WHAT TO EAT TO SUPPORT YOUR GUT

The best way to maintain your gut microbiome is to eat a whole-foods diet, especially foods that are rich in prebiotics. (*Probiotics* are beneficial bacteria, and *prebiotics* feed friendly bacteria.)

They consist of foods rich in soluble fiber and colors, and are found most abundantly in whole grains, beans, peas, vegetables, fruits, nuts, and seeds.

Foods that are rich in these nutritional compounds include artichokes, asparagus, avocados, bananas (under ripe), barley, beet root, bran, burdock root, chia seeds, chicory, Chinese chives, cocoa, cottage cheese, dandelion greens, eggplant, flax seeds, fruit, garlic, green tea, honey, Jerusalem artichokes, jicama, leeks, legumes, lentils, onions, peas, plantains, potatoes, radishes, root vegetables, rye, sea vegetables, soybeans, spices and herbs, sweet potatoes, tomatoes, vegetables, and yams. Eat several servings of foods from this list each day.

PROBIOTIC FOODS

You can also fill up on probiotic-rich foods...

•**Yogurt,** which typically contains several Lactobacillus species (such as *Lactobacillus acidophilus*, *Lactobacillus thermophilus*, and *Lactobacillus bulgaricus*), is a good choice. Kefir, another milk product, is even richer in probiotics than yogurt. Buttermilk and acidophilus milk also have plenty of probiotics. Among cheeses, gouda and cottage cheese are particularly rich in probiotics. If dairy doesn't agree with you, look for an oat, soy, or nut-based yogurt.

•**Try sauerkraut or kimchi.** Look for an unpasteurized variety. Fermented foods naturally contain probiotics.

•**Sour pickles** (not cured with vinegar) are packed with probiotics, as are most olives.

•**Miso soup**—which contains fermented soybean paste—is rich in probiotics. There are over 150 species of microbes in it. So is tempeh, fermented soybean patty.

•**Authentic sourdough bread** (made from a yeast-containing culture) delivers plenty of probiotics—which the latest research shows can improve the microbiome even though they've been through the baking process.

•**Unpasteurized beer and wine** are also fermented foods. But pasteurization (common in mass-produced beers) kills the friendly bacteria.

•**Raw honey** contains up to 14 species of probiotic bacteria.

•**Other foods that deliver probiotics** include coffee, chocolate, coconut, and black tea. And don't forget kombucha, a fermented, effervescent form of tea.

Slowly add more servings of probiotic-rich foods to your daily diet. If you introduce too many foods too fast, you may develop gas and bloating.

Vary Your Supplements

If you take a probiotic supplement, vary the type you take. The risk of taking the same probiotic supplement every day is that you're always ingesting the same, limited species of probiotics, and you can get overgrowth of even friendly bacteria. To vary the supplement, once you've used up the bottle, switch to another brand, taking that one until it's done. Then switch again.

Cut back on ultra-processed foods, particularly those that contain sugar and white flour, which feed bad bacteria.

PROBIOTIC SUPPLEMENTS

Despite all the research on probiotics and disease, researchers are cautious about recommending probiotic supplements for self-care. However, if you have one of the diseases or disorders that probiotics can help, taking a daily probiotic supplement might benefit you. (These conditions include the diseases and disorders discussed here as well as infections like cold and flu; skin problems like acne, eczema, and psoriasis; and genitourinary problems like vaginal infections and kidney stones.)

A Remedy for Pain, Depression, Insomnia in the Foods You Eat

Joseph Feuerstein, M.D., assistant professor of clinical medicine at Columbia University, New York City, and assistant professor at the Frank H. Netter MD School of Medicine at Quinnipiac University, North Haven, Connecticut. He specializes in family medicine, focusing on nutrition and disease prevention. Dr. Feuerstein also is certified in clinical hypnosis, clinical acupuncture and homeopathy. He is coauthor of *The Cannabinoid Cookbook: Transform Your Health Using Herbs and Spices from Your Kitchen* and author of *Dr. Joe's Man Diet*.

Don't let the word scare you off. *Cannabis sativa*—known by its more colloquial name marijuana—has come a long way since the 1960s, when it had a reputation for being a hippie counterculture drug. Thanks to research revealing the health benefits of the various non-intoxicating components of the spiky-leafed plant—and the increase in legalization across the country—more and more Americans are using cannabis to treat pain… depression and anxiety…insomnia…and more.

Cannabis is rich in naturally occurring plant compounds called *cannabinoids. Cannabidiol* (CBD, which does not produce a high) and *delta-9-tetrahydrocannabinol* (THC, which does produce a high) are just two well-known cannabinoids, but more than 100 others exist.

Recent finding: A survey of 568 adults ages 65 and older conducted by researchers at the University of California, San Diego, and published in a 2020 *Journal of the American Geriatrics Society*, found that 15 percent had used CBD or THC within the past three years… and nearly 80 percent of users reported having used it for medical purposes.

What many people don't realize is that the human body makes its own health-promoting, cannabis-like substances called *endocannabinoids*. That's right—your body naturally produces compounds that instill a feeling of calm…relieve joint pain and muscle spasms… help you drift off to sleep…and more. These cannabinoids, called *anandamide* and *2-AG*, are designed to return the body to a state of balance when something—stress, injury, trauma—pushes it out of balance. They do this by attaching to receptors in a network located throughout the brain and body called the *endocannabinoid system* (ECS). This system helps regulate bodily functions by seeking out and latching onto cannabinoids—either the endocannabinoids your body produces on its own or those found in the *Cannabis sativa* plant.

Using CBD or marijuana are among the ways to amplify your body's ECS. But you don't have to smoke or ingest CBD or marijuana to get similar benefits. Another little-known source of cannabinoids is food! *Specifically, these 11 items…*

- **Basil**
- **Black pepper**
- **Cacao**
- **Omega-3s**
- **Oregano**
- **Rosemary**
- **Cinnamon**
- **Cloves**
- **Flax**
- **Truffles**
- **Turmeric**

Consuming the foods and spices on this list stimulates the ECS…and the more you eat and the more often you eat them, the more impressive the effects. If you already regularly use CBD or THC, you can expect even more of an impact on your mood, immune system, sleep, and overall health. (In cannabis medicine, this is called an "entourage effect.")

Important: Eating these foods will not make you high or affect your results on a drug test. These 11 spices and foods fire up the ECS in different ways. *Here's how…*

- **Black pepper, basil, cinnamon, clove, oregano, and rosemary** all contain the compound *beta-caryophyllene* that directly targets the body's cannabinoid receptors, reducing inflammation and pain. (Freshly ground peppercorn's distinct peppery aroma is due in part to beta-caryophyllene.)

- **Omega-3 fatty acids** are the building blocks of anandamide and 2-AG. Oily fish, seeds, and nuts that contain omega-3s give your body what it needs to create those healthful endocannabinoids.

- **Cacao** allows anandamide levels to remain higher longer. This is one reason dark chocolate helps people feel mellow. Anandamide, sometimes called "the bliss molecule," stimulates the brain's ECS receptors similarly to THC. But our bodies also make the enzyme *fatty acid amide hydrolase* (FAAH), which helps break down anandamide—cacao helps inhibit the production of FAAH.

- **Truffles** are rich in anandamide.

Interesting fact: Anandamide attracts pigs, who eat and digest the tasty fungal fruits and then spread truffle spores in their droppings, allowing more of the tasty fungus to grow far and wide.

- **Flax** contains soluble fiber, which can lower LDL (bad) cholesterol and is an excellent plant source of omega-3 fatty acids. It contains a CBD-like compound that is thought to work on the CB receptors.

•**Turmeric,** a traditional Indian spice, contains curcumin, which has been shown to have anti-inflammatory properties. The curcumin in turmeric binds to CB receptors, which could potentially be useful to reduce appetite and help with weight loss.

Bonus: Using turmeric with black pepper can increase the absorption—and effectiveness—of this wonderful spice.

You can enjoy any of the 11 ingredients however you like—cracking black pepper and turmeric over scrambled eggs…stirring cinnamon and walnuts into oatmeal…adding cocoa powder to smoothies (make sure the label says it's 85 percent cacao or higher for maximum ECS stimulation).

Or you can try these recipes, which each contain ECS-fueling ingredients for that potent entourage effect…

FLAXSEED OIL DRESSING

This herb-infused dressing is great drizzled over salads, sautéed greens or roasted veggies. *Yield:* One-half cup.

2 tablespoons apple cider vinegar
1 tablespoon fresh chives, chopped
1 tablespoon fresh parsley, chopped
½ teaspoon dried basil
½ teaspoon dried oregano
½ teaspoon dry mustard
1 large clove garlic, chopped
3 tablespoons flaxseed oil
½ teaspoon fine sea salt
¼ teaspoon ground black pepper
⅛ teaspoon cayenne pepper

Combine the first seven ingredients in a blender, and process until smooth. Scrape down the sides, and blend again. Next, slowly stir in the flaxseed oil and blend until creamy. Add the final three ingredients, and blend once more.

Note: Flaxseed oil can be found in the refrigerated section of natural grocery stores, often near the supplements. It should be stored in the refrigerator and should not be used for cooking, as heat damages its healthful properties. (Drizzling this dressing over hot food is fine, though.)

SEASONED PUMPKIN SEEDS

Take advantage of Halloween with this fiber-filled snack. *Yield:* One cup.

1 cup pumpkin seeds
2 tablespoons coconut oil, melted
1½ teaspoons ground turmeric
1 teaspoon ground black pepper
1 teaspoon ground cayenne pepper
1 teaspoon salt

Preheat the oven to 350°F, and line a baking sheet with parchment paper. After washing and draining the pumpkin seeds, pat them dry with a dish towel or paper towels. Mix all of the ingredients except the seeds in a small bowl. Add in the seeds, and stir well to coat. Spread the mixture evenly on the parchment paper, drizzling any remaining oil over the top. Bake until lightly golden and crunchy, about 15 minutes, stirring every five minutes. Turn off the oven, and leave the seeds in the oven for five to 10 more minutes until desired doneness and crispness level is reached. Cooled seeds can be stored in an airtight container for up to two weeks.

SPICY SALMON BASIL BURGERS

Yield: Six burgers.

1¾ lbs. wild-caught salmon fillet, skin removed
3½ cups basil leaves, loosely packed
2 tablespoons lemon zest (zest of 2 lemons)
2 tablespoons fresh lemon juice
½ cup green onion, chopped
2 teaspoons sriracha hot sauce (optional)
1½ teaspoons salt
1½ teaspoons sugar
½ teaspoon black pepper
Oil for the pan (olive, grapeseed, or sunflower)
Toasted burger buns, lettuce, and tomato slices for serving

Break the salmon into large chunks, and place in a food processor along with basil. Pulse until everything is broken down into small pieces. Add the lemon zest, lemon juice, green onion, sriracha, salt, sugar, and pepper, then pulse until smooth. Divide the mixture into six portions, and shape into patties.

Heat a large nonstick skillet over medium-high heat. Coat the bottom of the pan with oil. When the oil is hot, add the burgers to the pan and cook until the bottoms are golden brown, about two to three minutes. Flip and cook on the other side until golden brown. Serve on buns with lettuce and tomato.

Medical Marijuana Goes Mainstream

Rebecca Abraham, RN, BSN, president and founder of Acute on Chronic, LLC, a full-service cannabis consulting and patient advocacy business based in Evanston, Illinois, with services available nationwide. AcuteOnChronic.com

---

Medical marijuana is now legal in most states, and older adults are reaping many of the benefits. In a survey conducted by the University of California, San Diego, 15 percent of 568 adults ages 65 and older reported having used cannabis within the past three years, mainly for chronic pain or arthritis, sleep problems, depression, or anxiety. As a critical-care nurse turned cannabis nurse and patient advocate, I spend my days teaching patients and doctors alike about this unique plant-based medicine.

A HIDDEN NETWORK IN THE BODY

Throughout the body there exists a network called the endocannabinoid system (ECS) that helps regulate dozens of bodily functions, including sleep, pain, temperature regulation, inflammation, digestion, emotional processing, and more. The ECS has one overarching goal: to keep the body functioning happily and healthfully. Special cellular receptors designed to make this happen are located in practically every square inch of the body, waiting to latch on to naturally produced neurotransmitters called *endocannabinoids*.

When something is off-balance physically or mentally due to stress, injury, or disease, the ECS triggers the release of endocannabinoids, which travel to the system in need. There, they fit into the ECS receptors like a lock and key, helping put things back on track. This might involve relieving pain, speeding up or slowing down gastrointestinal motility, boosting immune function, and more.

Possible Medical Cannabis Uses

Scientists are studying the use of cannabis for a variety of conditions, with varying levels of scientific support.

FDA Approved

- Seizures associated with Lennox-Gastaut syndrome or Dravet syndrome
- Severe nausea or vomiting caused by cancer treatment
- Appetite loss associated with HIV/AIDS

Promising clinical trials

- Chronic pain
- Multiple sclerosis

Anecdotal evidence, still being studied

- Alzheimer's disease
- Amyotrophic lateral sclerosis
- Anxiety
- Crohn's disease
- Depression
- Insomnia
- Migraine
- Post-traumatic stress disorder

But the human body isn't the only thing capable of producing cannabinoids. Cannabis is rich in them, too. Specifically, it contains *delta-9-tetrahydrocannabinol* (THC, the high-producing component of cannabis) and *cannabidiol* (CBD, which does not produce a high). More than 100 other cannabinoids exist in the plant. This is why using cannabis has long been associated with feeling relaxed, happy, sleepy, and hungry. Its cannabinoids fit into the ECS receptors, signaling the body to do what it needs to do to move towards balance and health.

When it comes to how and why medical marijuana is able to help so many different types of health issues (see sidebar), one theory is that several disease processes, including ones we don't fully understand yet, such as migraines, fibromyalgia, and irritable bowel syndrome, could be tied to a dysfunctional endocannabinoid system, one that could benefit from additional endocannabinoids beyond those produced naturally by the body. Using THC and/or CBD simply augments your body's ECS.

CONSIDER A CANNABIS CLINICIAN

But the answer isn't to ask your grandson to bring you some pot gummies the next time he comes home from college. (Believe me, this happens more often than you would believe.) Unlike Tylenol or Tums, THC is not a one-size-fits-all drug. There are dozens of different strains, some with invigorating effects and others with calming ones. Some can leave you feeling uncomfortably high, and others are known to have potentially harmful impurities.

That's why it's important to work with a cannabis clinician who can guide you on how to use medical marijuana safely and effectively. A cannabis doctor or nurse can explain the differences between smoking, eating, or even drinking THC, help you pinpoint the proper dose (including helping people avoid feeling too high), and make sure you're avoiding potential drug-drug interactions. (For example, cannabis can decrease the circulating dose of *clopidogrel* [Plavix] and may compromise the efficacy of the cancer drug tamoxifen.)

To find a local cannabis practitioner, use the Society of Cannabis Clinicians website's (CannabisClinicians.org) Find a Practitioner tool or ask friends and family for recommendations. Pick someone with medical credentials, such as an R.N., M.D., or D.O.

KEEP YOUR PHYSICIAN IN THE LOOP

Always tell your health-care provider if you start using THC or CBD. If they're unsure of how it might impact your current medication regimen, your cannabis clinician will be happy to collaborate. You may even find that, as your medical marijuana begins to work, you need less of certain prescribed drugs, such as antidepressants or pain medications.

Insurance will probably not cover cannabis clinicians, but some patients have success using their flexible spending account or health savings account. A cannabis clinician can also help you apply for a medical marijuana card, which allows you to purchase marijuana legally in most states.

Are You Getting Enough of the Sunshine Vitamin? Most of Us Aren't!

Michael F. Holick, Ph.D., M.D., former director of the Bone Health Care Clinic and the General Clinical Research Unit at Boston University. He is currently professor of medicine in the department of medicine in the section of endocrinology, diabetes, nutrition, and weight management at Boston University Chobanian and Avedisian School of Medicine. He is the country's preeminent researcher on vitamin D deficiency. BU.edu

---

Did you know that vitamin D deficiency is extremely common even in the U.S.? It is estimated that 50 percent of the world's population is vitamin D–deficient. And this deficiency is sneaky—you may not have any symptoms, but low blood levels of vitamin D (*25-hydroxyvitamin D*) can lead to low bone density, brittle bones, osteoporosis and more.

The current Recommended Dietary Allowance (RDA) for vitamin D is 600 international units (IU)* for most children and adults…800 IU after age 70. But Michael F. Holick, Ph.D., M.D., the country's preeminent researcher on vitamin D, says these amounts are just not enough. *Based on the Endocrine Society Practice Guidelines, he recommends the following to keep your D levels in the healthy zone…*

Infants: 400 IU to 1,000 IU

Children: 600 IU to 1,000 IU

Teens and adults: 1,500 IU to 2,000 IU

Note: If your body mass index (BMI) is over 30, you need two or three times this amount because vitamin D is diluted when stored in large amounts of body fat and very slow to be released.

Problem: It's very difficult to get enough vitamin D through diet and/or sun exposure—especially if you live north of Atlanta or Los Angeles, where the angle of the sun is too low

*Labels list vitamin D amounts in either international units (IU) or micrograms (mcg). 40 IU is equal to 1 mcg.

from November through March to produce vitamin D in the skin…and the temperature is too cold in the early spring and late fall for you to comfortably expose enough skin. So your first step to keeping your vitamin D levels healthy is to supplement. All adults should take a 2,000-IU vitamin D supplement every day—any national brand that contains either vitamin D-2 or D-3 will do, and it can be a tablet, liquid, or capsule, taken on an empty or full stomach.

Even better: You can help keep your vitamin D levels strong by eating the right foods. Dr. Holick explains which are the best choices to keep your vitamin D levels in the safe zone…

FOODS WITH THE MOST D

Two foods are standouts…

•**Wild-caught salmon.** The typical advice is to eat a range of oily fish, including trout, char, herring, anchovies, sardines, bluefish, mackerel, swordfish, and tuna—but of these, salmon is the best choice. While swordfish has more vitamin D in a three-ounce serving, you should eat it very infrequently—no more than once a month—because of its toxic mercury content. For the same reason, you should have tuna no more than once a week. Salmon is the closest to ideal with 446 IU of vitamin D per three-ounce serving. And because D remains stable to 200°C (about 400°F), you can cook it any way you like—poached, grilled, pan-seared, etc.

Best: Wild-caught salmon, which can be fresh, frozen or canned. Farm-raised salmon (and other farm-raised fish) have only about 10 to 25 percent of the vitamin D in wild-caught.

•**Mushrooms.** Until recently it was thought that fungi that naturally grow in sunlight, such as chanterelles and morels, have more vitamin D than mushrooms grown under other conditions.

Recent finding: Just about any type of mushroom can produce appreciable amounts of D when sun-dried or otherwise exposed to UV light. The mushrooms convert *ergosterol*, a precursor to vitamin D, into *ergocalciferol*, commonly known as vitamin D-2. While D-2 is different from the vitamin D-3 found in animal

Amount of Sun You Need for Healthy Vitamin D Levels

Only a few minutes of sun exposure a day is needed for healthy vitamin D levels, according to a recent study.

Recent finding: For white skin tones, only five minutes of unprotected midday sun exposure three or four times a week is needed…seven to eight minutes for brown and black tones. Starting in late spring through late fall is sufficient to keep levels healthy through winter.

Antony Young, Ph.D., photobiology professor at King's College London, U.K., and lead researcher of a study of ultraviolet exposure effect on skin published in *PNAS*.

products, your body still absorbs it well—an important consideration if you're vegan. You can do a Google search to find producers that expose their mushrooms to UV light. Oyster, cremini, portabella, shiitake, and ubiquitous white button mushrooms enhanced with UV light or sun-dried all are available.

FOODS WITH SOME D

Egg yolks and beef liver provide incremental amounts of vitamin D, about 40 IU per yolk or three ounces of liver.

FORTIFIED FOODS

The list of fortified foods is growing.

Example: In India, cooking oil is being fortified with vitamin D$_2$. It doesn't get destroyed with cooking and is appropriate for that country's large vegan population.

Here are the most commonly D-fortified foods in the U.S. *The amounts of D they contain are relatively small but can add to your daily intake…*

•**Milk.** While milk is not a natural source of vitamin D, it has been added in most U.S. milk products since the 1930s. An eight-ounce glass delivers between 115 IU and 125 IU.

•**Nondairy milks.** Almond, oat, and other nondairy milks usually are fortified with 100 IU of D per eight-ounce glass as well as calcium (look for at least 300 mg of calcium). Avoid blends with added sugars. In addition to soy milk, some tofu is fortified, too.

•**Yogurt.** Some brands are fortified with about 80 IU of vitamin D.

Best: Low-fat and sugar-free varieties.

•**Fortified orange juice.** You'll get an average of 100 IU in an eight-ounce glass. Look for brands with added calcium.

Caution: Avoid orange juice if blood sugar is a concern.

•**Cereals** are commonly fortified with vitamin D (as well as other nutrients), but usually a scant 40 IU per cup.

Best: Pick cereals that also have some whole grains for their fiber and that don't have (or have minimal) added sugar.

The Surprising Roles of Zinc

William W. Li, M.D., president and medical director of the Angiogenesis Foundation. His latest book is *Eat to Beat Your Diet: Burn Fat, Heal Your Metabolism, and Live Longer.* His work has led to the development of more than 30 new medical treatments and affects care for more than 70 diseases, including cancer, heart disease, and obesity.

Zinc, an essential nutrient that your body can't make by itself, is involved with many different functions of the cells in your body. It's important for your skin, your vision, your immune system, your cognition, and much more.

SHORTEN COLDS

One of the most common uses of zinc is to shorten the duration of the common cold. In clinical trials, high doses of zinc (about 70 to 80 milligrams [mg]) are proven to shorten colds by about 30 percent.

WOUND HEALING

Zinc is important for the functioning of your cells, which includes the ability to generate and grow blood vessels and nerves. That makes it a key component of wound healing.

Some of the most impressive clinical studies about zinc have been done in people with di-

abetes who have non-healing wounds in their legs and feet. Zinc can speed up healing and lead to a better quality of the healed wound.

COGNITION

Studies suggest that zinc may be beneficial for memory, too. Think about aging and the decline in cognition as a slow-motion injury to the brain. The aging brain is not repairing itself as quickly as it normally would, but zinc can improve that healing. There's still research to be done, but preliminary findings are promising.

SKIN

The skin normally stores zinc, which helps skin cells function in an optimal way and lowers inflammation. As a result, supplemental zinc may ease inflammatory conditions like acne, psoriasis, and hidradenitis suppurativa.

MACULAR DEGENERATION

The most common cause of vision loss in people over 65 is age-related macular degeneration (AMD), a common condition associated with aging where you start to lose central vision due to damage in the back of the eye. In AMD, the blood vessels that keep the retina healthy grow abnormally and start leaking. Studies done by the National Eye Institute show that a dietary supplement that contains zinc, called AREDS, can help slow down the development of AMD.

GETTING MORE ZINC

The first place to look for zinc is in your diet. You can get trace amounts from fish, shellfish, meat, legumes, lentils, chickpeas, seeds, and

---

Dosage Advice

Most of the supplements sold at the drugstore and online have low levels of zinc. While clinical studies found that 70 to 80 milligrams (mg) of zinc are effective, the typical amount you might get from a drugstore supplement is 10 mg per tablet. You'll need to take multiple tablets to attain an effective dose. Don't exceed more than 100 mg per day.

nuts. You can then top off your zinc stores with a supplement.

There are different formulations of zinc, such as zinc acetate and zinc glycinate, but all of the research that's been done in human clinical trials shows that the different types work equally well. However, many formulations you get at the drugstore, such as products like Cold-eeze, might contain much more than zinc, such as herbs or homeopathic remedies. Always read the ingredients before buying a supplement, to see what's included.

While there are no known interactions between zinc and other drugs, always talk to your physician before taking a new supplement. If zinc supplements upset your stomach, try taking them with food.

Vitamin B₃ and Healthy Aging

Charles Brenner, M.D., chair of the Department of Diabetes & Cancer Metabolism at the Beckman Research Institute of the City of Hope National Medical Center. *Disclosure:* He is a scientific advisor for a company that sells an NR supplement.

Vitamin B₃ isn't a single substance: It's a family of three *vitamers* (similar but not identical forms of a vitamin), including *nicotinamide*, *niacin*, and *nicotinamide riboside* (NR).

That last one is creating a buzz in the healthy-aging research community. Studies suggest that supplemental NR may slow cellular aging, improve metabolism, and reduce inflammation. To understand what this means in real life, we spoke with Charles Brenner, M.D., who discovered NR.

What role does NR play in healthy aging?

NR plays a role in promoting healthy aging by restoring levels of a coenzyme called nicotinamide adenine dinucleotide (NAD).

NAD is the central catalyst of our metabolism, the process that allows us to convert everything we eat into everything we are and do. As we age, a variety of stressors can reduce our NAD levels, including excessive

---

Supplement Safety

When NA is administered at a usual dosage of 2 grams per day, there are no reported adverse events in placebo-controlled trials. There are also no known interactions with drugs, but people who are taking medication should always talk to their doctors before taking any new supplements.

---

sunlight (which damages our DNA), oxidative stress, overeating, sleep deprivation, alcohol consumption, working night shift, traveling across time zones, and not exercising enough. Inflammation, infections, and diseases, such as heart failure and neurodegeneration, lower NAD levels, too.

In my research, I found that by increasing levels of NR through oral supplementation, one can safely maintain youthful levels of NAD, which is a vital component in healthy aging.

I'm excited by what we have seen in animal studies. For example, one study showed that giving NR to overfed mice improved glycemic control, protected against fatty liver, and prevented the development of diabetic and chemotherapeutic neuropathy. In another study, we found that it provided protection against heart failure and neurodegeneration. It provides more benefits to rodents who are obese, have heart failure, or neurodegeneration than it does for healthy rodents.

High NAD status isn't a panacea, but if we see NAD under attack in a disease, such as we do in heart failure or neurodegeneration, there's a good chance that boosting it will provide protection from the underlying insult.

When it comes to aging, boosting NAD through NR supplementation is just one strategy to age well. It's also important to maintaining an active lifestyle, eat and sleep well, and maintain mental activity and social connectedness.

What benefits have you seen in human studies?

In small human clinical trials, NR supplementation is associated with quicker recovery from COVID-19, improved cerebral blood flow in people with Parkinson's disease, and improved body composition in women. In a trial in which it was taken along with three other supplements, it also showed anti-inflammatory activity. It looks like it may help people with moderately high blood pressure and fatty liver disease. But more research is needed before we can make any health claims.

Anecdotally, people who take it notice that their fingernails and hair grow faster. Quite a lot of people notice that their recovery from strenuous workouts is easier and that their repair from cuts and scrapes is faster. Many people say it gives them more energy, but that hasn't been demonstrated in a placebo-controlled trial.

The Best Way to Get Your Antioxidants

Chris Iliades, a regular contributor to *Bottom Line Health*. He was an ear, nose, throat, head, and neck surgeon before becoming a full-time medical writer.

Decades of nutrition studies suggest that people who eat more fruits and vegetables live longer and have a lower risk of heart disease, cancer, stroke, cognitive decline, and eye disease associated with aging. At least part of that benefit comes from antioxidants, researchers suggest, substances that fight inflammation by reducing free radicals and oxidative stress. If antioxidant foods help you live a longer and healthier life, then high-dose supplements must be even better, right? Not so fast.

UNDERSTANDING THE TERMINOLOGY

Antioxidant supplements are purported to help you live a longer and healthier life because they fight free radicals and reduce oxidative stress. That sounds good, but what does it really mean?

When you eat, exercise, sit in the sun, or breathe polluted air, your body creates byproduct molecules called free radicals. These molecules have an uneven number of electrons, which makes them unstable. Your body can usually manage free radicals by finding an extra electron to neutralize them. Ideally, these electrons come from antioxidants—substances found in fruits and vegetables that can safely donate extra electrons—such as vitamins C and E, plant pigments beta-carotene and lycopene, the minerals zinc and selenium, and organic phenolic compounds.

If your body can't access enough antioxidants to stabilize the free radicals it creates, however, you can start to suffer cell damage and inflammation, called oxidative stress.

SCIENCE OF SUPPLEMENTS

While clinical trials show that antioxidant-rich foods are beneficial, the science is less compelling when it comes to supplements.

In June 2022, a review article in the American Medical Association's journal *JAMA* reported that there is insufficient evidence to show that antioxidant supplements have any benefit for heart disease, cancer, or longer life. Furthermore, beta carotene supplements can increase the risk of lung cancer in smokers, and vitamin E in large doses may increase the risk of bleeding into the brain.

The most likely reason that antioxidant supplements have failed is that the benefits of antioxidants come from a balance of several antioxidants with helper molecules and other nutrients in foods. It is not as simple as pulling out one antioxidant and bombarding the body with high doses. That would be like taking one instrument out of an orchestra, playing it loudly, and expecting to hear a symphony.

Another possibility is that even antioxidants in foods are not as beneficial as researchers have assumed. The nutrition studies these assumptions have been based on were observational, meaning that the researchers looked back at many diet survey questions and then compared diets and health outcomes over time. Just because people who ate more fruits and vegetables were healthier doesn't mean the diets were the cause. People who ate lots of fruits and vegetables may have also had other healthy behaviors, like not smoking, getting a lot of exercise, or avoiding junk food, that could influence health.

GET ANTIOXIDANTS FROM FOOD

The evidence linking free radicals to cancer, heart disease, cognitive decline, and vision loss is strong, so getting antioxidants from a healthy diet makes sense. *There are plenty of delicious options...*

• **Get vitamin C** from Brussels sprouts, grapefruit, leafy green vegetables, sweet potato, tomato, kiwi, lemons, oranges, and bell peppers.

• **Find vitamin E** in peanuts and almonds, avocado, red peppers, and leafy greens.

• **Load up on beta-carotene** in apricots, asparagus, beets, mangos, carrots, sweet potato, watermelon, citrus fruits, and bell peppers.

• **Get your selenium and zinc** from beef, poultry, shellfish, fish, and brown rice.

• **Find organic phenolic compounds** in red wine, tea, cocoa, berries, grapes, peanuts, and apples.

You can also avoid outside sources of free radicals by not smoking or getting a sunburn.

The Tastiest Health Tonic: A Cup of Tea

William W. Li, M.D., president of the Angiogenesis Foundation, and author of the *New York Times* bestseller *Eat to Beat Disease: The New Science of How Your Body Can Heal Itself*, and *Eat to Beat Your Diet: Burn Fat, Heal Your Metabolism, and Live Longer*. He has served on the faculties of Harvard Medical School, Tufts University, and Dartmouth Medical School. DrWilliamLi.com

---

Every day, people around the world drink an estimated 2 billion cups of tea, the beverage made from the leaves of the *Camellia sinensis* bush. Whether black, green, oolong, or white, most of those cups are downed for enjoyment or as a pick-me-up. But the many *bioactives* in tea—catechins, caffeine, chlorogenic acid, theaflavins, and more than 2,000 other natural chemicals—do more than deliver a satisfying brew.

Many of these natural chemicals are plant compounds called *polyphenols* that energize cells, improve the signaling between body systems, and rev up metabolic mechanisms like fat-burning, rejuvenating your body and reducing your risk of the chronic diseases that harm or kill millions, like cardiovascular disease, cancer, diabetes, and dementia.

In a recent 11-year study with 500,000 participants conducted by researchers at the National Institutes of Health, people who consumed two to three cups of tea a day had a 13 percent lower risk of dying from any cause, compared with people who did not drink tea. The tea drinkers also had a lower risk of dying from heart disease and stroke.

BEATING DISEASE

People who drink more tea are more likely to have better health outcomes...

• **Cardiovascular disease.** Tea helps lower the risk of cardiovascular disease in several ways. It lowers high blood pressure, a major risk factor for heart attack and stroke. It improves blood flow, protecting the heart and brain. It helps healthy gut bacteria generate more short-chain fatty acids, which reduce inflammation, a key driver of cardiovascular disease. Tea also lowers LDL cholesterol and triglycerides, and it mobilizes the body's stem cells for repair—including the repair of the lining of blood vessels.

In one study, drinking two cups of black tea daily increased endothelial stem cells by 56 percent. In another, researchers gave 20 men who had smoked for at least six years four cups of green tea every day for two weeks. Drinking green tea increased the number of circulating, reparative stem cells by 43 percent.

• **Cancer.** Your body forms microscopic cancers all the time. Most of these mini tumors are eliminated by your immune system. They only become dangerous when they hijack normal blood vessels and redirect your blood supply to feed the cancer. This process is called *tumor angiogenesis*, and extensive research shows that tea can stop these abnormal blood vessels from growing.

Cancers that have been treated by chemotherapy or surgically removed often recur because cancer stem cells remain in the body, allowing the cancer to resurrect itself. For example, between 10 to 40 percent of women who are supposedly cured of breast cancer have a recurrence.

Research shows that one of the main polyphenols in green tea, *epigallocatechin-3-gallate* (EGCG), can kill cancer stem cells. Numerous

Types of Tea

All teas are from *Camellia sinensis*, an ever-green shrub. A few times a year, the buds and the tender, young leaves at the top of the bush are picked and then dried on racks. *Some types of teas are fermented as a next step...*

• **Black tea.** Fermentation is unchecked, producing a dark, robust tea. It is the highest in caffeine.

• **Green tea.** Fermentation is immediately brought to a halt by heating. After drying, the leaves are lightly steamed or gently pan-fired in huge woks. It is the highest in catechins.

• **Oolong tea.** Fermentation is midway between black and green.

• **White tea.** Harvested before the tea buds are fully opened, this is a delicate, low-caffeine tea.

• **Matcha.** This is a green-tea powder made from tea leaves after the stem is removed. It is uniquely rich in EGCG and has been shown to kill breast-cancer stem cells.

• **Pu'er.** This highly fermented black tea has a dark, earthy, smoky taste. It delivers the probiotic *Pueribacillus*, which improves gut health and aids digestion. It also uniquely delivers strictinin, which kills cavity-causing bacteria in the mouth.

studies bear out this cellular research, with people who drink more tea having less risk of various cancers. In a meta-analysis of 43 of those studies, researchers at Harvard Medical School reported that tea reduced the risk of oral cancer by 38 percent, and also reduced the risk of breast, liver, endometrial, and biliary tract cancers.

• **Type 2 diabetes.** In a recent 10-year study reported at the European Association for the Study of Diabetes Annual Meeting, drinking at least four cups a day of black, green, or oolong tea reduced the risk of developing type 2 diabetes by 17 percent. And in a five-year study published in *BMJ Open Diabetes Research & Care*, people with type 2 diabetes who drank at least four cups of green tea had a 63 percent lower risk of death from any cause. Obesity and type 2 diabetes go hand in hand. EGCG and chloro-

genic acid (another bioactive found in green tea) have been shown to activate brown fat, a useful type of fat that helps burn white fat.

• **Dementia.** Researchers analyzed health data from more than 350,000 people ages 50 to 74 and found that those who drank three to five cups of tea daily had a 28 percent lower risk of dementia.

TIPS FOR HEALTHY TEA-DRINKING

There are many simple ways to maximize the health-giving effects of drinking tea. Choose the type you like the most, whether it's black, green, oolong, or white. All types of tea are loaded with health-giving bioactives.

• **Loose-leaf, bagged, or powdered?** If loose leaf tea is your choice, you can keep pouring water on the leaves for three brewings. After that, change the leaves.

If you choose a tea bag, dunk the tea bag up and down for a couple of minutes to shake the polyphenols out of the leaf. If you choose a powdered tea like matcha, put in as much powder as the instructions say—or as much as you want to have the most pleasurable cup of tea.

• **Temperature.** Polyphenols are present in hot and cold tea. Most laboratory-based research on tea involves first brewing tea, then refrigerating (or even freezing) it overnight, and then thawing it out for studies later. And it's still loaded with polyphenols. Steeping in hot water does not destroy healthful polyphenols like catechins, but don't drink scalding tea—it has been linked to esophageal cancer. Put very hot tea in a mug and let it cool to a drinkable temperature.

• **Added milk.** When you add milk or cream to tea, the dairy creates fatty bubbles that entrap the polyphenols, reducing their absorption by about 20 percent. If you're drinking tea for health, it's better not to use dairy. Try a plant-based milk like soy, oat, or almond, which gives the tea a rounded flavor similar to dairy but doesn't form bubbles that block polyphenols.

• **Amount.** The sweet spot for "a spot of tea" is two to three cups daily. But if you enjoy drinking more, no problem—there are no recorded cases of anybody overdosing on tea.

Supplements That Fall Short

Don't Believe Claims About Mushroom Supplements

Manufacturers say that mushroom supplements boost cognition, increase immunity, even fight cancer.

Reality: The few human studies that support these claims have small sample sizes. Some mushrooms contain antioxidants and other substances that have been shown to regulate weight, blood sugar, and carcinogens.

But: Many supplements are made from parts of the mushroom that don't contain those chemicals...and even if the correct part of the mushroom was used, the dosages contained in the supplement are just a fraction of what's been found to be effective in studies.

Best: Eat mushrooms—they do have benefits backed by solid research...and they're far cheaper than supplements.

Brian St. Pierre, RD, registered dietitian based in Portland, Maine, and nutrition advisor for Men's Health. MensHealth.com

Beta-Carotene and/or Vitamin E a No-Go for Cancer or Heart Health

Beta-carotene and/or vitamin E do not reduce risk for cancer or cardiovascular disease. A review of 84 studies concluded that these supplements don't help healthy adults reduce such risks...and beta-carotene can increase lung cancer risk. The Task Force also found insufficient evidence to recommend for or against taking multivitamins and other supplements to reduce cancer and cardiovascular disease risk.

John Wong, M.D., professor of medicine at Tufts University School of Medicine, Boston, and a member of the U.S. Preventive Services Task Force that issued the recommendations in JAMA. Tufts.edu

No Benefits from Popular Heart-Health Supplements

Study titled "Comparative Effects of Low-Dose Rosuvastatin, Placebo and Dietary Supplements on Lipids and Inflammatory Biomarkers," by researchers at the Center for Blood Pressure Disorders, the Cleveland Clinic, presented at the American Heart Association Scientific Sessions 2022 and published in the Journal of the American College of Cardiology.

Health supplements are a big industry. According to a recent market survey, Americans spend about $50 billion per year on these vitamins and minerals to pump up their nutrient needs. Many of these supplements are taken to improve heart health and lower cholesterol. Even though studies to support the advantages are scarce and inconsistent, many people believe that supplements are a better (natural, safer) choice over statins, the most common cholesterol-lowering drugs.

WHAT WAS TESTED...

To learn more about the possible benefits of supplements for heart health, researchers from the Cleveland Clinic Center for Blood Pressure Disorders tested six popular supplements against a commonly used statin drug to see how much each of these would lower cholesterol numbers over 28 days. The supplements tested were fish oil, cinnamon, garlic, turmeric curcumin, plant sterols and red yeast rice. The study results were presented at the 2022 American Heart Association's Scientific Sessions and published in the *Journal of the American College of Cardiology*.

The study included 190 people ages 40 to 75 without any history of heart disease. The primary aim of the study was to see how the supplements compared to a statin in lowering low-density lipoprotein (LDL or "bad") cholesterol. LDL is the cholesterol that is linked closely to the risk of death from heart disease and stroke because it deposits fats inside your arteries. Since 2020, deaths linked to LDL cholesterol have gone up nearly 20 percent. The study also looked at the effect on high-density lipoprotein (HDL or "good") cholesterol and triglycerides, which are fats also linked to stroke and heart attack.

At the start of the study, LDL cholesterol levels in the study group ranged from 70 to 189 milligrams per deciliter (mg/dL). The optimal range for LDL cholesterol is less than 100 mg/dL in adults. People in the study were randomly assigned to a supplement, statin, or placebo group.

People in the supplement groups were given the usual recommended dose. People in the statin group were given a low dose of the statin *rosuvastatin* (Crestor). The placebo group was given an inactive pill and served as the control group. *These were the key findings after 28 days...*

•**The statin group averaged nearly a 40 percent reduction in LDL cholesterol** and a nearly 20 percent reduction in triglycerides. There were no significant side effects.

•**None of the supplement groups had a significant reduction in LDL cholesterol or triglycerides.** Their results were similar to the placebo group.

•**The garlic group had a notable increase in LDL.**

•**The plant sterol group had a notable decrease in HDL cholesterol.**

SUPPLEMENTS MIGHT TAKE MORE TIME... BUT LISTEN TO YOUR DOCTOR

The researchers conclude that none of the supplements tested had a beneficial effect on cholesterol or triglycerides and would be unlikely to reduce the risk of heart disease or stroke. Based on the results of their study, they strongly advise against substituting a supplement for a statin when a statin is indicated. They note that other supplements may have better results and that their study was limited to 28 days, so it is not known if supplements taken for longer periods might have some benefit.

6 Stress-Busting Herbs to Try Today

Jessica Arconti Fleming, DO, RH, osteopathic doctor in Roanoke, Virginia, a Registered Herbalist (RH) with the American Herbalist Guild, and a certified nutritionist.

Herbs are powerful medicines. In fact, an estimated 50 percent of all modern medicines are derived from herbs, including aspirin (*acetylsalicylic acid*) from the salicin in willow bark, morphine from the opium in the poppy plant, and *paclitaxel* (Taxol), a chemotherapeutic agent, from the taxanes in the yew tree. Among the most powerful and wide-acting herbs are a class called adaptogens.

ADAPTING TO STRESS

Adaptogens help your body *adapt* to stress. Research shows that prolonged, nonstop stress can drive you into chronic disorders and diseases, such as high blood pressure, heart disease, high blood sugar, diabetes, overweight, digestive problems, and more. Stress is so destructive to physical, mental, and emotional well-being that it can worsen any health condition.

Along with their ability to counter stress and thereby aid in the prevention and treatment of ill health, adaptogens can also restore and rejuvenate your cells, tissues, and organs (including the brain) to improve mood, increase focus, and boost physical energy. In my clinical practice, I have found six adaptogens that are uniquely effective.

SIBERIAN GINSENG

This Asian herb, also called eleuthero, can improve mental function, strengthen memory, and clear up brain fog. Researchers reported in *Nutrients* that people who took eleuthero for three months saw improvements in memory, thinking ability, and resistance to stress. It is excellent to take right before a presentation, test, or other challenging mental task. It is also good for banishing fatigue, according to a study published in the *Journal of Ethnopharmacology*.

This is my favorite adaptogen. I used it myself during medical school and residency for improved stamina, concentration, and better mood, and to relieve exhaustion.

Dosage: Take 2 to 3 grams of dried root daily or 2 to 4 milliliters (mL) of a tincture two to three times daily.

Warnings: In high doses, Siberian ginseng may increase blood pressure.

RHODIOLA ROSEA

This herb is rich in rosavins, salidrosides, and other compounds that help control stress. It is excellent for boosting cognitive function. In a scientific paper published in the *International Journal of Psychiatry in Clinical Practice*, researchers reported that the herb can relieve feelings of stress, anxiety, anger, confusion, and depression in people under severe stress; reduce fatigue in doctors on night shifts; and improve concentration, work speed, and quality.

Dosage: Look for a product standardized to contain 2 to 3 percent rosavin and 0.8 percent salidroside rhodiola. Take 200 to 400 milligrams (mg) daily, ideally in a formula that combines rhodiola and eleuthero.

Warnings: Because it is mentally stimulating, rhodiola rosea is contraindicated for people with bipolar disorder. It can lower blood sugar levels and blood pressure. Rhodiola can stimulate the immune system, which can worsen autoimmune diseases. Like grapefruit, it can affect how the body processes medications that are broken down by the liver.

ASHWAGANDHA

This gentle, balancing adaptogen—from Ayurveda, the ancient system of natural healing in India—can lower levels of the stress hormone cortisol, researchers reported in the *Indian Journal of Psychological Medicine*. As a result, it may help with stress, insomnia, and mild anxiety.

Dosage: Take 1 dropperful of a tincture (about 40 drops or one teaspoon) three times a day in a shot of water. (Tinctures taken directly can irritate the mucosa in the mouth and digestive tract.) Or take a 500 mg capsule twice daily. You can also add it to tea, soups, or bone broth. Because it is a non-stimulating adaptogen, you can take ashwagandha long-term.

Warnings: If you are allergic to nightshades, like white potatoes, tomatoes, bell peppers, and eggplants, do not take ashwagandha. Also avoid it if you have hormone-sensitive prostate cancer or if you take benzodiazepines, anticonvulsants, or barbiturates.

TULSI

Also known as holy basil, tulsi is another gentle adaptogen that you can take long-term. And like many adaptogens, tulsi is useful for insomnia and mild anxiety, according to a study in *Evidence-Based Complementary and Alternative Medicine*. There, researchers also cited evidence that it can help lower artery-damaging blood fats like LDL cholesterol and triglycerides.

If you're considering quitting smoking, consider tulsi: According to the experience of many herbalists and their clients, it helps re-

---

How Adaptogens Work

Adaptogens improve health and healing in several ways (although, like many medications, their exact mechanism of action isn't fully understood). First, they balance the body's hormone-generating endocrine system, particularly the hypothalamic-pituitary-adrenal (HPA) axis, which controls your body's response to stress. In many people, constant, daily stress puts the HPA axis into overdrive, generating high levels of hormones like adrenaline that are helpful in small, occasional doses but destructive in large, constant amounts.

Adaptogens also regulate the immune system, reducing chronic low-grade inflammation, a leading cause of chronic disease. They are also antioxidants, so they cut the rampant oxidation that damages cells. And they can help regulate the levels of many other key biochemicals, including glucose (blood sugar), plasma lipids (like cholesterol and triglycerides), nitric oxide (for circulatory health), and liver enzymes, according to a scientific review published in the medical journal *Nutrients* in 2021.

Patience Pays Off

Adaptogens tend to act more slowly than medications because they work to rebalance and regenerate many core processes of the body. Stay on the herb or formula for at least one month, at which time you should reevaluate its use with your health professional. During that month, try to implement other stress-reducing lifestyle changes, such as establishing set hours for going to bed and getting up (which helps reduce insomnia), not drinking caffeine in the afternoon or evening, exercising regularly, and practicing a stress-reduction technique, such as deep breathing or mindfulness-based stress reduction, for a few minutes a day.

duce the symptoms of nicotine withdrawal. It can also elevate mood in people with mild depression, according to a study from researchers in India.

Dosage: Take 1 to 2 tablespoons of tulsi tincture in a 12-ounce cup of water.

Warnings: Don't take tulsi for two weeks before or after surgery because it can slow blood clotting.

MACA

Maca is a cruciferous vegetable similar to broccoli, native to the Andes mountains of Peru (and purportedly used by Mayan warriors for strength and stamina). It's a great alternative to caffeine to boost energy, mood, and perhaps libido, according to a report in *Food & Function*. And a study published in the *Journal of Ethnopharmacology* shows it can also boost athletic performance and sexual desire.

Dosage: Add a tablespoon or so of the dried or powdered root to a daily smoothie. (Maca is more like a food than an herb and doesn't dissolve well in water.)

Warnings: Maca is contraindicated in Hashimoto's disease (autoimmune disease of the thyroid). Extracts from maca might act like estrogen. If you have any condition that might be made worse by estrogen, do not use these extracts.

SHATAVARI

This adaptogen—the primary tonic for women in Ayurvedic medicine—can improve symptoms associated with menopause, like hot flashes and insomnia, according to a study in the *Journal of Research into Traditional Medicines*. Shatavari also stimulates the digestive tract, helping relieve constipation, according to a study in the *International Journal of Ayurvedic Medicine*.

Dosage: Take 30 to 90 drops of tincture, two to three times daily.

Warnings: Because it is rich in phytoestrogens, do not take shatavari if you have a history of estrogenreceptor-positive breast or ovarian cancer.

TAKING ADAPTOGENS

When choosing an adaptogen, discuss the herb with your doctor or another qualified health professional familiar with nondrug treatments. Although adaptogens are generally safe, there can be contraindications. For example, many adaptogens are contraindicated if you are taking medications to inhibit the immune system or to thin the blood.

For anyone with a complex, chronic disease, such as heart disease or type 2 diabetes, discuss an herbal supplement with a medical professional before taking it.

Considering CBD? It Can Ease Pain, Anxiety, and Inflammation

Dustin Sulak, DO, one of the first physicians in Maine to incorporate the legal use of cannabis as a medicine in 2009. He is the founder of Integr8 Health, a private practice in Falmouth, Maine, that specializes in medical cannabis, and the author of *Handbook for Cannabis for Clinicians: Principles and Practice*.

One-third of Americans have tried cannabidiol (CBD), a once obscure medicinal extract from the cannabis plant, hoping for relief from pain, anxiety, insomnia, and other ills. But even though many of us are purchasing CBD—in oils, gummies, pills, tinctures, so-called "edibles," and topical creams, lotions, and salves—that doesn't mean we feel confident about using the products we're buying.

FAKE PRODUCTS ABOUND

There are good reasons why we feel confused about CBD. In a new study published in *JAMA Network Open*, researchers from Johns Hopkins Medicine tested 89 products and found that only 24 percent were accurately labeled. Along with being mislabeled, it's possible that products are contaminated with toxins. And clear directions about how to use CBD—the right frequency and optimal dose for your problem—are hard to come by. But it's possible to choose and use the right product, and get the best possible results. The first steps are knowing what CBD is, how it works, and what it can do for you.

CBD IS NOT MARIJUANA

CBD is one of dozens of cannabinoids in the cannabis plant, a single species with several subtypes: Type 1 produces the psychoactive cannabinoid that triggers the high of marijuana (*tetrahydrocannabinol* [THC]). Type 2 is a combination of THC and CBD. Type 3, which has been bred since around 2009, mainly produces CBD.

Federal regulations state that if a cannabis plant produces less than 0.3 percent THC by weight, the plant is hemp, not marijuana, and it can be legally used for CBD extracts.

MANY BENEFITS

In my practice, I have treated thousands of patients with cannabinoids. I find daily use of CBD extracts can help promote alertness and clear thinking, relieve chronic pain and inflammation, ease anxiety, help with occasional sleeplessness, improve mood, increase resilience to stress, relieve irritability, and enhance performance and recovery from exercise (including post-exercise soreness). I've seen that low or moderate doses of CBD help many patients with autism spectrum disorders and attention deficit/hyperactivity disorder. It also reduces anxiety and agitation in people with dementia.

HOW CBD WORKS

How can one compound have such diverse benefits? One way CBD works is by enhancing the activity of the endocannabinoid system (ECS), an inner network of receptors that are distributed in every tissue and organ throughout the body. The ECS is responsible for maintaining a stable internal environment (called homeostasis) despite stressors from the external environment, like infections, toxins, and injuries. Those internal environments include the immune, cardiovascular, gastrointestinal, musculoskeletal, and nervous systems. This broad, homeostatic action likely accounts for some of CBD's ability to help you stay healthy, resist stress, and heal from illness and injury.

CBD also acts on a variety of cellular receptors in the body…

- **Adenosine A1,** which is involved in anti-inflammatory, neuroprotective, and neuro-regulatory autonomic regulatory effects
- **The dopamine D2 receptor in the brain,** which probably accounts for CBD's anti-psychotic effects
- **The 5-HT1A receptor for the neurotransmitter serotonin,** which could explain CBD's benefits on mood, anxiety, and nausea
- **The TRPV1 receptor,** which influences pain transmission and inflammation.

In fact, laboratory studies have identified 65 distinct pharmacological targets in the body for CBD.

CHOOSING A CBD PRODUCT

CBD products fall into two main categories: broad or full-spectrum products and isolates.

- **Broad or full-spectrum products** contain some of the naturally occurring compounds from the hemp plant, including legally allowed trace amounts of THC.

When possible, choose a full spectrum product, because animal and human studies show that the full range of constituents in hemp products work together synergistically, outperforming isolated CBD.

- **Isolates** contain CBD and no other cannabis plant compounds. They are good for people who can't have any THC in their system, like those who are subject to drug tests in states where cannabis is not legal for medical use. (Even though CBD does not create a "high" like marijuana, it can show up in drug tests.)

Look for a product that has a third-party certificate of analysis. This certificate helps guarantee that the product is pure (free of pesticides, heavy metals, solvents, yeast, mold, and toxins) and that the labeling is accurate. Use organically grown CBD products to further ensure safety and quality.

Look for a product with labeling that shows how much CBD it contains—not just in the whole bottle, but in each drop, gummy, pill, or portion. For tinctures, this is milligrams per milliliter (mg/mL); for gummies and pills, it is milligrams (mg).

FIND THE BEST DOSE

For most people, I recommend starting at 5 mg per dose, once or twice daily. If needed, increase your dose by 5 mg every two days until you start to feel beneficial effects. At that point, stop increasing and try staying at the same dose for the next week. For many people, the amount that provides only modest benefits in the first couple of days will, after consistent use, provide more benefit over time. You can resume increasing by 5 mg per dose every other day until you find that a dose increase does not provide any additional benefit. After you find the amount that works for you, if you notice the effects wear off too early in the day, add more doses per day. Two to three daily doses may be ideal. The optimal amount for most people is 5 to 30 mg per use, one to three times daily. If you're still not getting results with CBD, you may want to add CBDA to your regimen.

Take each dose with a meal. Studies show that CBD is absorbed up to five times better when taken with food that contains fat or oil. If you're using CBD drops, place them under your tongue or between your cheek and gums and hold for one to two minutes before swallowing to improve absorption.

If you want to try CBD for sleep, increase your bedtime dosage by two to four times the amount you typically take. For example, if you're taking 25 mg twice a day, at breakfast and lunch, take a 50-mg dose at bedtime.

CBDA—Even More Powerful Than CBD?

The hemp plant doesn't directly produce CBD: It produces cannabidiolic acid (CBDA), which converts to CBD. CBDA targets enzymes (called *cyclooxygenase isoenzymes*) that are linked to inflammation. Animal research and clinical observation suggest that it may have benefits similar to over-the-counter anti-inflammatory pain medicines, without the side effects on digestive and heart health. It may be even more potent than CBD at preventing seizures, fighting inflammatory pain, relieving nausea, and easing anxiety.

CAUTIONS

CBD uses the same detoxification pathway in the liver as some medications, which means taking CBD could inhibit the breakdown of a drug, making blood levels higher. Ask your doctor to use a drug interaction checker to see if CBD is interacting with a drug you're taking. If it is, ask your doctor if a lower dose would be safe for you.

Another caution: There have been infrequent reports of elevated liver enzymes, a sign of liver irritation, in people taking CBD. If you're taking more than 100 mg daily, have your liver enzymes checked when you start taking CBD and after one month.

Natural Medicine Travel Kit

Jamison Starbuck, ND, naturopathic physician in family practice in Missoula, Montana, and producer of *Dr. Starbuck's Health Tips for Kids*, a weekly program on Montana Public Radio, MTPR.org. She is a past president of the American Association of Naturopathic Physicians and a contributing editor to *The Alternative Advisor: The Complete Guide to Natural Therapies and Alternative Treatments.*

I love my natural medicine travel kit and firmly believe that no family should be without one. Use it to augment your conventional first-aid travel kit, which should be stocked with bandages, topical antibiotic creams, and pain medications. Here are some ideas of what to put in your natural kit so you're ready to travel.

FOR DIARRHEA, GAS, AND CRAMPING

•**Activated charcoal (AC).** Several studies show that AC reduces excessive intestinal gas accumulation, according to the European Food and Safety Authority. It also appears to have an anti-diarrheal effect. In 2018, researchers reported in *Current Medical Research and Opinion* that it is a suitable treatment that offers fewer side effects than other anti-diarrheal medications. For an acute bout of painful gas or diarrhea, take three to four 250-milligram (mg) charcoal capsules with an 8-ounce glass of water. Repeat in 30 minutes or after every bowel movement as needed for up to 24 hours. Do not use charcoal daily because it can interfere with the absorption of nutrients and medications. Don't take it within two hours of taking medication, as it may make some medications ineffective.

•**Peppermint tea.** Drink 4 ounces of strong, hot, unsweetened peppermint leaf tea every few hours.

If you have a fever or diarrhea for more than 24 hours, seek medical attention.

FOR CUTS OR INSECT BITES

•**Calendula tincture.** Wash the wound or bite with soap and water, and then apply calendula tincture, full strength, directly as an antiseptic and to help skin heal. For open wounds, dilute with water (one part water to two parts calendula) before use. A study published in *Wound Repair and Regeneration* reported that calendula leads to faster resolution of the inflammation phase of wound healing.

FOR SPRAINS AND STRAINS

•**Arnica gel or a combination product** such as T-Relief is excellent first aid medicine. Made from the *Arnica montana* plant, homeopathic arnica lotion or gel applied topically quickly helps with bruising and swelling. A study published in the journal *Medicines* noted that arnica extract relieves pain as well. Apply

three times a day directly to the skin. Do not put arnica on any open cuts or wounds.

FOR MOTION SICKNESS NAUSEA, VOMITING, OR DIZZINESS

•**Ginger** is a well-studied anti-nausea remedy. A study in the journal *Pharmacology* notes: "The efficacy of ginger rhizome for the prevention of nausea, dizziness and vomiting … has been well documented and proved beyond a doubt in numerous high-quality clinical studies." Put 45 drops of a ginger tincture in two ounces of warm water and sip as often as needed.

A one-ounce bottle of each of the tinctures is usually enough for one travel-related ailment. Tinctures, homeopathic remedies, and activated charcoal have very long shelf lives, retaining effectiveness and safety for at least five years. They are stable at high and low temperatures, though you should protect all of them from temperature extremes. Don't store them in a car.

Sleep on Your Left Side to Reduce Reflux

A study showed that people who sleep on their left side have less stomach acid in the esophagus than those who sleep on their right side or back. That's because most of the stomach is on the left side of the upper abdomen. When you sleep on your left side, gravity pulls the contents of your stomach lower than your esophagus, which runs down the center of the body.

American Journal of Gastroenterology.

Understanding Anemia and Iron Deficiency

Michael Auerbach, M.D., a clinical professor of medicine at Georgetown University School of Medicine, Washington, D.C., and a hematologist/oncologist at Auerbach Hematology and Oncology Associates.

There are many kinds of anemia. Some are rare genetic conditions. Others are caused by vitamin deficiencies, cancers that affect the bone marrow, or chronic conditions, such as kidney disease. The most common kind, however, is caused by iron deficiency. Iron-deficiency anemia is serious business. Whether it's discovered because of routine blood tests or because you go to your doctor feeling unwell, it's important to find out exactly what's causing it.

GETTING A DIAGNOSIS

When you see your doctor for a checkup or an illness, you often get blood tests that are part of what's called a *complete blood count* (CBC). Anemia is diagnosed when these tests show low levels of red blood cells, abnormal red blood cells, or low levels of hemoglobin, a molecule that contains iron and carries oxygen to all the tissues in your body.

Your doctor may suspect you have iron-deficiency anemia, rather than some rarer condition, based on your blood counts and medical history.

You might have no symptoms, but if you do, they could include tiredness, shortness of breath, brittle nails, or a sore tongue. Iron deficiency is also associated with cravings for chewing on ice (called *pagophagia*) or dirt (a condition known as pica). Scientists don't yet know why.

Every case of iron deficiency needs to be explained because the possible underlying causes include some serious conditions. These causes fall into three main categories: blood loss, low iron intake, and poor iron absorption owing to conditions such as kidney disease, inflammatory bowel disease, and the after-effects of weight-loss surgery. Blood loss is the most common cause, followed by poor absorption. If there is no obvious cause, expect more tests. These could include a colonoscopy or an upper endoscopy to detect bleeding and pick up cancers, ulcers, and other problems that cause bleeding. You also might get blood tests to check for conditions such as celiac disease and infection with *Helicobacter pylori*, a bacterium that causes stomach ulcers.

WHAT'S NEXT?

Once you have iron deficiency, you can't reverse it by dietary changes alone: You

---

How to Take Iron Supplements

• **Take a pill every other day instead of daily to absorb more iron.**

• **If you can tolerate it, take your iron pills without food.** If you can't, take them with food, but avoid pairing them with coffee, tea, cereal, eggs, milk, calcium, or fiber supplements.

• **Avoid enteric-coated iron tablets.** They interfere with absorption.

• **Take your iron pills at least two hours before or four hours after any antacids.**

• **If you struggle with side effects,** ask for a smaller dose, a different formulation, a liquid version, or a switch to intravenous iron.

• **Don't worry about dark greenish stool while taking iron.** It's normal.

Note: Children are at high risk of iron poisoning, so always store pills out of their reach.

---

need much higher doses than food can provide. Most people will be prescribed oral iron supplements. These pills are safe, inexpensive, and effective, but they do come with side effects, such as metallic taste, nausea, constipation, and vomiting, which bother some people enough that they stop taking their pills. (See the above sidebar.)

If you can't tolerate the side effects of iron supplements or have a condition that limits the absorption of iron by your digestive tract, you should be offered intravenous iron supplementation. To get this treatment, you go to a doctors' office or hospital, where an iron solution is infused into a vein. One or two treatments usually restore iron levels, making this an excellent option for people with persistent iron deficiency or supplement intolerance.

Older versions of intravenous iron carried a higher risk of a severe allergic reaction than today's versions, which cause minor reactions in fewer than 1 percent of patients. Most of the time, the reactions cause passing side effects, such as flushing and back pain, during the infusion. Some people may need a steroid to lower risks before the infusion.

Don't take an iron supplement without checking with your health-care provider. People who don't need the extra iron could end up with excess iron, which can cause health problems

---

The Science of Meditation

Yi-Yuan Tang, Ph.D., professor of neuroscience, health science, and prevention science in the College of Health Solutions at Arizona State University. Dr. Tang created the Integrative Body-Mind Training (IBMT) technique.

According to the most recent statistics from the U.S. Centers for Disease Control and Prevention, 14 percent of Americans meditate, making it the most popular mind/body practice in the United States besides yoga. We know that meditation is incredibly effective at lowering stress, bolstering the immune system, and improving cognition and focus. But did you know that meditation actually changes your brain and body, paving the way for those sought-after improvements?

When you meditate, you are literally strengthening parts of the brain that control memory, emotions, problem-solving, and more. Perhaps even more intriguing is the fact that you don't need to practice all that much to enjoy the rewards.

As recently as a decade ago, some researchers believed that 1,000 to 10,000 hours' worth of meditation was needed to reap the benefits, but we now know that just five to 10 sessions can be enough to create change that is significant enough to be seen on a brain scan.

HOW TO MEDITATE

One of the more researched and more popular types of meditation is mindfulness meditation (MM). *Here's how to do it…*

•**Settle into a comfortable position.** You can recline, sit in a chair or on the floor, walk, or do a gentle exercise such as tai chi.

•**Focus your attention on something happening in the present moment,** such as your breath, a word, or a mental image.

•**As you focus, notice any new sensations or thoughts that arise.** Notice them but don't judge them.

•**If your mind wanders, don't chastise yourself** ("Stop daydreaming! You aren't doing this right!") and instead gently bring your mind back to the present. ("Oh, your mind wandered a bit. Time to refocus on your breath.")

STRESS REDUCTION

That emphasis on nonjudgment plays a role in stress reduction. Every time you bring your focus back to the meditation, it's like exercising a calming muscle that strengthens with use, during meditation as well as in everyday life. This translates to reduced reactivity to stressful thoughts, emotions, and events, almost like a higher baseline for stress tolerance.

Mindfulness-based practices reduce activity in the amygdala, an area of the brain that governs the fight-or-flight stress response, fear, and emotion. This reduction helps people to be less reactive to upsetting situations and to recover more quickly after a stressful event occurs.

Research my colleagues and I conducted showed that just five to seven sessions of a form of MM called *integrative body-mind training* (IBMT) was enough to increase positive affect and reduce negative affect.

Positive affect is the extent to which a person feels happy or is able to experience other positive emotions, such as joy, calmness, and contentment. It is tied to multiple desirable health outcomes, including reduced rates of heart disease, a reduced risk of catching a cold or the flu, and a reduced risk of frailty as one ages.

SHARPER FOCUS AND COGNITION

Our brain's default mode can be described as "mind-wandering," meaning that, for most of us, even when we're doing nothing, our brain is highly active. Work projects, to-do lists, worrying about finances: This feels like the norm for many of us, but it's quite taxing for the brain.

A specific area of the brain called the *default network* manages all that mind-wandering, and it requires energy and resources that are also needed for memory and cognition.

Over time, the more energy and resources that go to the default network, the fewer you have available for paying attention and remembering other things.

When my colleagues and I trained college students in IBMT, we were curious to see what effects a short-term practice might have on mind-wandering. We found that just five 20-minute sessions of IBMT were enough to significantly reduce activity in the default network when subjects were at rest.

This preserves resources in the short term, assisting with focus and clearheadedness, but it's reasonable to believe that it may also offer protection against age-related cognitive decline when sustained for years and decades.

Other research of ours shows that 10 sessions of IBMT create changes in the white matter of the brain, particularly in the self-control and reward networks that support learning and information processing. That means MM can impact how quickly and easily you absorb and retain new information.

STICK TO NEW HABITS

White matter also plays an important role in executive functioning, a set of mental skills that allows us to focus and remember the thousands of steps required to go about our day and to help us set goals and cement new habits into place.

If MM strengthens the white matter in the brain in self-control-related areas, and we know that it does because we can see these changes on brain scans, it's reasonable to think that it also helps people adopt and stick to healthy new habits such as trying a new exercise routine or eating more plant-based foods.

In fact, some people spontaneously change their lifestyle after meditating, showing new interest in health and wellness. This may be a direct result of insights that can happen during MM that motivate us to make changes for the better.

Bug Bites: Prevention and Treatment

Jamison Starbuck, ND, naturopathic physician in family practice in Missoula, Montana, and producer of *Dr. Starbuck's Health Tips for Kids*, a weekly program on Montana Public Radio, MTPR.org. She is a past president of the American Association of Naturopathic Physicians and a contributing editor to *The Alternative Advisor: The Complete Guide to Natural Therapies and Alternative Treatments.*

When summer rolls around, many of my patients ask how to prevent bug bites. Some folks claim that eating a lot of garlic, taking high doses of B vitamins, or avoiding sugar and beer works to keep insects at bay. I haven't found these strategies to be universally effective, though they do work for some people.

Essential oils can do a good job of repelling insects, particularly citronella, an oil derived from the Cymbopogon plant, and the oil of lemon eucalyptus. Both are available in skin sprays and lotions, candles, and insect-repelling incense. These must be reapplied every 60 minutes to be effective, and they generally don't work well against ticks, wasps, or bees. Additionally, some people are allergic to essential-oil preparations, making these repellents even more unpleasant than a mosquito bite.

My favorite suggestion surprises some of my patients: In my view, the most reliable repellent is to be mentally a few steps ahead of the insects. For example, investigate your hedge before trimming it. As I learned the hard way, many years ago, failing to check on insect habitats can end up in a disaster. I got 15 stings on my face and head seconds after slicing through a hornet nest hidden just inside the hedge with my first enthusiastic swipe with the electric hedge trimmer.

Reliable bug repellents are wearing long-sleeved shirts and pants when walking through moist areas where mosquitoes live, checking overhangs and gutters before painting or washing your house, and looking for bees or spiders in the coupler of a trailer or under the shady roof of a doghouse before you move them.

If you do have the misfortune of being bitten by a summertime insect, a few natural medicines work well to relieve the pain and speed healing. My immediate, go-to remedy for any kind of bite is T Relief lotion. This homeopathic preparation is available online and over the counter in most natural food stores. Apply a small amount directly to the bite several times a day until the bite injury is healed.

If the insect bite is pink, hot, and puffy, apply ice and take homeopathic Apis 30 C for relief. The dose is two pellets under the tongue, away from meals, twice daily for one to three days.

Warning: Apis is made from bee venom, so do not use it if you are allergic to bees.

Spider bites carry a greater risk of local infection than other insect bites, so I prescribe Echinacea tincture applied full strength directly to spider bites several times a day and taken internally to boost your immune response. The typical adult internal dose of echinacea tincture is 60 drops in 2 ounces of water, away from food, four times a day for up to a week.

With all insect bites use common sense, not only in prevention but also in treatment. If a bite is very painful, if you develop a fever, or if the bite or surrounding tissue appears infected, see your doctor.

CHAPTER 16

Pain and Autoimmune Disease

You May Be Treating Your Pain Wrong

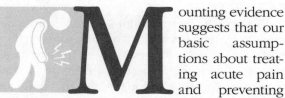 **M**ounting evidence suggests that our basic assumptions about treating acute pain and preventing chronic pain may be wrong. While it is disconcerting when new research turns a previously held idea on its head, in this case, it's good news. Learning more about what we are doing wrong—and what we should be doing instead—can help us promote healing and prevent injuries from turning into chronic pain. *We asked regenerative pain specialist Thomas Buchheit, M.D., to set us straight…*

THE OLD MODEL

For decades, the prevailing approach to treating pain from sprains, strains, or muscle injuries has been to aggressively suppress all forms of inflammation.

It is easy to see how we got here. We know that chronic inflammation and inflammatory changes are destructive. Even a casual reader of medical reporting knows that inflammation is implicated in a host of diseases and conditions.

Examples: The cumulative effect of decades of gut inflammation is associated with a variety of conditions…and conditions such as rheumatoid arthritis are the result of the chronic inflammatory processes damaging joints. By extension, we have powerful medications, such as steroids, cytokine inhibitors and other disease-modifying agents that improve the lives of patients suffering from these chronic inflammatory conditions.

So it is only natural that we reach for *nonsteroidal anti-inflammatory drugs* (NSAIDs) such as *ibuprofen* and *naproxen* when we sprain an ankle playing with our grandkids or strain our back working in the garden. We

---

Thomas Buchheit, M.D., director of the Regenerative Pain Therapies Program at Duke University, Durham, North Carolina. Duke.edu

believe that reducing the inflammation will make the pain go away.

What we've gotten wrong: The medical community has extrapolated our understanding of the danger of chronic inflammation into a general "inflammation bad" assumption. We have assumed that because chronic inflammatory change is damaging, all inflammatory change—including that associated with acute injury—is harmful. But, in fact, when it comes to acute pain, inflammation actually might be good for us.

How inflammation might help: When we are injured, our bodies go into healing mode. Our immune system produces a sequence of biological responses—the *healing cascade*. Inflammation is not only an early part of that, but it stimulates components of the sequence that follow.

The idea that inflammation plays this role in healing is not new. Several established therapies consist of a controlled introduction of inflammation to stimulate the healing cascade. In a procedure called microfracture surgery, a surgeon pokes holes in bones of the knee so that the resulting inflammation will spur growth of healthy cartilage to replace damaged cartilage. For the same reason, micro-injuries sometimes are introduced to damaged tendons to promote healing. And platelet-rich blood plasma, teeming with inflammation-causing white blood cells, often is injected at an injury site. All these therapies embrace inflammation as a kick-starter of the healing cascade.

WHAT NEW RESEARCH TELLS US

Despite our understanding of its role in healing, the bias against inflammation persists. But recently, we've seen the most compelling evidence to date to bolster the argument that blanket suppression of the immune response using steroids or NSAIDs for an acute injury is not only counterproductive but also potentially harmful. In early 2022, researchers at Montreal's McGill University investigated the healing response in mice and humans. When they gave anti-inflammatories to mice with acute sciatic back pain, the mice were more likely to still be in pain 115 days later…while untreated mice started feeling better in just a few days.

And when the researchers looked at data on more than 2,000 humans with acute back pain, they found that those who took NSAIDs were far likelier to still have a back-pain complaint up to a decade later.

Conclusion: While suppressing the immune response is analgesic—it reduces your pain—it may convert your pain from acute to chronic because you've disrupted the healing cascade.

WHAT TO DO INSTEAD

•**Change your mindset.** Rather than over-relying on anti-inflammatories when you're in acute pain, shift your thinking to promoting healing. The medical specialty "regenerative pain medicine" promotes restoration of healthy tissue. Practitioners suggest several ways patients can jump-start healing while forgoing anti-inflammatories. Physicians from multiple specialties offer regenerative medicine options. Look for one who uses more than just injections to treat the problem. Search for board certification in a related specialty, such as orthopedic surgery, pain management/anesthesiology or physical medicine and rehabilitation…training and experience…as well as hands-on formal residency training and extensive experience (not just a weekend course) for any procedures they perform.

•**Exercise.** Your tough-as-nails grandparents were right—working through minor aches and pains may be the best way to resolve these issues. Obviously, if there is a fracture, a ligament tear, or other serious injury, this may not be possible. If in doubt, make sure a physician and physical therapist guide your exercise routine. Using an injured body part can get it working again and pain-free.

•**Physical therapy.** For a tendon or muscle partial tear or other serious injury that could become chronic, find a good physical therapist. Ask your physician for recommendations. Also find a therapist who analyzes your body mechanics and tailors the treatment to your needs. He/she will know just which movements are most beneficial and will motivate you to perform them.

•**Stretching and motion strengthening.** Tendons heal when they're put under strain.

Eccentric exercises—where the tendon is under strain for various amounts of time, depending on the injury—are especially effective for rotator cuff issues and other tendinopathies. The most reliable remedies for acute back pain are stretching and strengthening, which prevent muscle atrophy, shore up the structure of the spine, and spur healing.

•**Acupuncture.** This ancient Eastern practice promotes tissue restoration and reduces pain without suppressing the immune response.

•**Local anesthesia for surgical procedures.** Applying a local anesthesia in addition to, and sometimes instead of, general anesthesia for surgery reduces acute pain without disrupting the inflammatory response.

NUANCE MATTERS

Just as we once erred in the oversimplification "inflammation bad," we should avoid a whole-hog embrace of "inflammation good." There is a sweet spot when it comes to the amount of inflammation that's beneficial for an acute injury. Anti-inflammatory medications could help you get through the first few days after an accident to reduce your pain so that you can begin using the injured body part—stretching, exercising, doing physical therapy, etc. Just don't keep using anti-inflammatories beyond that initial acute phase or what's needed to start functioning. The optimal duration of anti-inflammatories will likely be days, not weeks or months.

Most of us can tell if we are pushing too hard and causing damage. If you struggle with that, a physical therapist can help.

New Treatment to Reduce Migraine Frequency

Roger Cady, M.D., board-certified headache medicine specialist and CEO of RK Consulting in Ozark, Missouri, commenting on a study of 865 migraine sufferers published in Lancet Neurology.

An infusion of 100 mg or 300 mg of the monoclonal drug *eptinezumab* (Vyepti) cut 4.8 and 5.3 monthly headache days, respectively, and reduced headache severity for sufferers who had tried at least two other treatments. Efficacy continued for 12 weeks. Serious side effects—anaphylactic reactions among two participants in the 300-mg group—were uncommon and resolved with treatment.

Natural Ways to Beat Migraine

Alexander Mauskop, M.D., founder and director of the New York Headache Center in New York City, and professor of clinical neurology at SUNY, Downstate Health Sciences University. He is the author of The End of Migraines: 150 Ways to Stop Your Pain. *NYHeadache.com*

Up to 40 million Americans, 75 percent of them women, suffer from migraine headaches. Symptoms can include throbbing head pain, nausea, vomiting, sensitivity to light and sound, fatigue, and dizziness. According to the World Health Organization, migraine is the second-leading cause of disability, with only back pain causing more downtime.

To prevent or relieve migraines, which can strike as often as every couple of days, doctors prescribe two types of drugs: *preventive*, to stop attacks before they start, and *abortive*, to stop attacks once they've started. But preventive drugs also can deliver debilitating side effects—memory loss, hair loss, bone loss, and much more. Because of the drugs' downsides, only 20 percent of people with migraines (migraineurs) stick with these drugs long-term. In contrast, abortive drugs are mostly safe and reasonably effective: 30 percent of migraineurs who try them get good results, with few side effects. But if drugs don't work, or if they cause troublesome side effects, there's another option for migraine sufferers: *non-drug* treatments. Non-drug treatments are safe and inexpensive. And the best of them have scientific evidence to support their effectiveness.

Based on scientific research and decades of clinical experience, here are what I consider to be the eight best non-drug therapies to prevent and treat migraine...

1. Aerobic exercise. Strong scientific evidence shows that aerobic exercise can improve migraines. A Swedish study of 91 migraineurs found that exercising for 40 minutes, three times a week, was as effective as *topiramate* (Topamax), a preventive migraine drug—with topiramate causing significant side effects in the study. And in a study by Swiss researchers, both high-intensity interval training and moderate-intensity exercise decreased the number of migraine headache days per month. This is the best non-drug way to prevent migraines, so try to follow the government's official recommendation for regular exercise: a minimum of 30 minutes of moderate-intensity exercise (like brisk walking), at least five days a week.

2. Meditation. Researchers from Wake Forest School of Medicine in Winston-Salem, North Carolina, conducted a study on meditation with 19 migraineurs: 10 learned mindfulness-based stress reduction (MBSR) and nine received standard migraine care. Those practicing MBSR—meditating, on average, 20 minutes a day—had 1.4 fewer migraines per month, and the migraines were generally less severe and shorter.

There are several ways to learn meditation. You can listen to free podcasts by a wonderful meditation expert and psychologist, Tara Brach, PhD. An excellent book to learn meditation is *Mindfulness in Plain English*, by Bhanta Gunaratana. There are also apps for meditation, such as Headspace.com and Calm.com. You can also find local meditation courses offered by churches, community centers, and gyms.

3. Magnesium. Up to one-half of migraine sufferers are deficient in the mineral magnesium. I have conducted and published research on the positive role of magnesium in migraines—including a review paper in the *Expert Review of Neurotherapeutics*—and have seen dramatic improvement from magnesium in many of my patients. Ideally, you should obtain the mineral from magnesium-rich foods, such as whole grains, dark leafy vegetables, avocados, and legumes. But making sure you eat these foods on a regularly basis is not easy, and sometimes it's not sufficient to raise magnesium levels. I strongly feel that every person with migraine headaches should try taking 400 milligrams (mg) of magnesium glycinate daily. For maximum absorption, take magnesium with a meal.

4. Coenzyme Q10 (COQ10). After magnesium, a deficiency of coenzyme Q10—a necessary ingredient for the production of energy in every cell in the body—is the most common nutritional deficiency in migraineurs. In one study published in the journal *Neurology*, 48 percent of patients who were taking CoQ10 had a 50 percent decrease in migraines, compared with 14 percent who took a placebo. The study dose was 100 mg three times daily.

5. Cognitive-behavioral therapy (CBT). This psychological therapy focuses on changing unhelpful ways of thinking and feeling and changing learned patterns of unhelpful behavior. For migraineurs, the main focus is on coping with and reducing the pain of headaches—such as learning how not to panic and become emotionally paralyzed by migraine headaches—and learning how to inform and interact with family, friends, and employers, who can be understanding and perhaps even helpful.

Therapy usually involves eight to 12 structured sessions. They may include an introduction to the CBT model involving thoughts, feelings, and behaviors; pain monitoring; relaxation training; avoiding migraine triggers; and how to pace daily activity. CBT is usually conducted by a social worker or psychologist. Group sessions are also effective. Online, web-based CBT is another good alternative. Two excellent sites that offer free CBT are ThisWayUp.org.au and MoodGym.anu.edu.au.

6. Acupuncture. This modality from traditional Chinese medicine uses tiny needles to stimulate specific acupuncture points, balancing the flow of energy (*qi*, pronounced "chee") within the body. There is a large body of scientific literature on the use of acupuncture for migraine, including studies that show acupuncture is more effective than standard pharmacological treatments. In an editorial published in *Cephalagia*, the journal of the International Headache Society, the author wrote, "…acupuncture should be offered to patients who do not respond to prophylactic [preventive] treatment with drugs, terminate drug treatment because of adverse events, or have contraindications to drug treatment."

Acupuncture does have drawbacks, however. It is time-consuming, relatively expensive when compared with generic prescription drugs, and temporary. You need to continue having it done every week or two.

To locate a licensed acupuncturist in your area, consult the practitioner directory of the National Certification Commission for Acupuncture & Oriental Medicine (NCCAOM), NCCAOM.org/find-a-practitioner-directory.

7. Transcutaneous nerve stimulation (TENS). In this migraine therapy, you attach electrodes to the skin. The electrodes are connected to a small, battery-operated device that delivers alternating current. *Two types of TENS devices are particularly effective for migraine…*

•*Cefaly* is a TENS device that is applied to the forehead. It's approved by the FDA for the acute and preventive treatment of migraines. Some of my patients find it particularly effective for the acute treatment of migraine attacks. The cost of a unit is approximately $400. (A basic TENS unit costs as little as $50, but is awkward to apply to the forehead.)

•*Nerivio* is another device approved by the FDA for the acute treatment of migraine attacks. Unlike other TENS units, it involves stimulation of a remote site—the upper arm—to produce effects in the brain. The frequency of stimulation fluctuates through the session. Nerivio is controlled by a smartphone app. In a study published in the journal *Headache*, participants used it for 45 minutes at the beginning of an attack. Over two hours, it was more effective than non-stimulation for pain relief. Users achieved a pain-free state and relief of bothersome symptoms like nausea and sensitivity to light and noise. Insurance may cover the device. Without it, prescription-only Nerivio costs $599 for 12 treatments.

8. Riboflavin (vitamin B₂). This nutrient stimulates the production of energy in cells. In a three-month study published in the journal *Neurology*, 55 migraine patients received either a daily dose of 400 mg of riboflavin or a placebo. Fifty-nine percent of those taking the riboflavin improved by at least 50 percent,

---

What Works for Me

I'm a neurologist who specializes in headaches, but I'm also one of the millions of Americans with migraines. Preventively, what has made the biggest difference for me is meditating for 30 minutes every day and exercising at least three times a week. Avoiding my two biggest migraine triggers—alcohol and lack of sleep—has helped, as well.

---

compared with 15 percent of those taking the placebo. However, the improvement occurred only in the third month, which means you need to give riboflavin plenty of time to work. Riboflavin has a fluorescent, yellow hue, and your urine may become bright yellow when you take the vitamin, but this is harmless. There are no serious side effects from taking 400 mg daily. (Despite its apparent safety, pregnant women should not take a 400 mg dose.)

Do You Get a Pain in Your Ear While Chewing?

Jonathan Wanagat, M.D., Ph.D., assistant professor, division of geriatrics, UCLA

Pain in the ear while chewing suggests a disorder of the temporomandibular joint. In the medical world, problems with the jaw and muscles of the face that involve this joint are referred to as temporomandibular disorders (TMDs). In lay terms, the condition is often called TMJ.

The temporomandibular joint connects the jaw to the temporal bones of the skull, which are in front of each ear. A major nerve is near the jawbone, and when it's irritated, the pain can radiate back to the ear.

Conditions that can lead to a TMD include recent dental work, arthritis that has reduced the cartilage around the jaw joint, and teeth grinding/clenching. Stress, which makes some people grind and clench their teeth and/or tighten facial muscles, is a common cause of a TMD. A December 2020 American Dental Association poll showed that incidences of teeth grinding and clenching increased by 71 percent in the early days of the pandemic. Jaw pain jumped by 62 percent.

Resting the jaw, reducing stress, and taking a short course of anti-inflammatory medications can help resolve TMD pain. Dentists treat TMDs with custom bite guards. It's important to address this issue because grinding and clenching place excessive force upon the teeth and can lead to cracks, fractures, and even broken teeth. Dentists reported more of those incidences during the pandemic as well.

Another reason for ear pain while chewing could be from a swollen and/or infected ear canal. See your physician if the pain is frequent, doesn't subside in a few days, or gets worse.

Put Your Best Foot Forward: Strong Feet Keep You Free from Pain

Erin Futrell, Ph.D., assistant professor of physical therapy at Springfield College, Springfield, Massachusetts. Dr. Futrell is a board-certified specialist in orthopedic physical therapy. Her research focuses on gait retraining in runners and on intrinsic foot muscle strengthening in runners and non-runners.

When you think about exercising your core, you probably think about planks, crunches, and other moves aimed at strengthening your abdomen, back, and pelvic area. But your body has another set of core muscles that help keep you upright, mobile, and free of pain: the core muscles of your feet. Exercising these muscles might have benefits for everyone from runners who want to prevent injuries to frail older adults who want to prevent falls. If you've never thought about your foot muscles, it's time to start.

BENEFITS OF TRAINING YOUR FEET

There's good reason to believe that a foot-strengthening routine might keep all sorts of feet healthier and less prone to pain and deformity. Even common conditions such as bunions and hammertoes might be prevented

Foot Muscle Basics

Health professionals call the muscles that make up the core of your foot intrinsic foot muscles. Intrinsic means that these muscles begin and end in your feet, unlike the extrinsic muscles that run through your ankles, connecting your feet to your lower legs. A couple of intrinsic muscles cross the top of each foot.

Several layers of intrinsic muscle are in the soles of each foot. These lower layers contain multiple muscles with specific functions. For example, there's one called the abductor hallucis that helps to move your big toe and maintain your arch, and there's one called the abductor digiti minimi that moves your pinky toe. Every time you take a step, these muscles are at work, making adjustments as your feet make their way over floors, up staircases, or across grass, pavement, and other surfaces. Even when you are just standing in place, these muscles are active, constantly working, along with your nervous system, to keep you balanced and to maintain your awareness of the ground beneath your feet.

or limited by keeping feet in better working condition from childhood onward.

Older adults, whose foot muscles typically become weaker with age, might see particular benefits. A recent research review of nine studies conducted in adults ages 65 and older found that those who did intrinsic foot-strengthening exercises saw increases in strength, balance, and mobility. Some people also reported less pain in their feet and joints.

Because the studies included other interventions, including additional exercises and, in some cases, minimalist shoes, researchers cannot yet say which approaches helped most. Foot strengthening may even reduce the risk of falling because it improves sensation and what's known as *proprioception*, the body's ability to sense movement and location.

Exercises for core foot strength appear to be very safe. They also are easy to learn, though some people may need help to get the hang of certain moves. Physical therapists can help if needed.

SAMPLE FOOT WORKOUT

Sit with one foot crossed over the other and point your toes, foot, and ankle down, gently pulling on your toes with one hand. Hold for five seconds and repeat five times. Switch feet and repeat. In the same position, flex the toes, foot, and ankle up, and then gently pull with your hand five times for five seconds. Switch feet and repeat.

Next, work the core muscles of your feet.

Once you master each of the following moves, try repeating them several times over three to five minutes, several times a day. Work with one foot at a time.

Implications for Runners

Strengthening intrinsic foot muscles (muscles that begin and end in your feet) can help runners prevent problems such as plantar fasciitis, a common condition that causes a stabbing pain in the heel. The condition involves inflammation of the plantar fascia, a band of tissue that supports the arch of the foot and absorbs shock when you walk or run. When foot muscles are weak, this band takes a harder beating. Having stronger foot muscles might also prevent injuries beyond the feet, such as shin splints, and improve runners' gaits in ways that help them run more efficiently and protect their knees and other joints.

Some runners have tried "minimalist shoes," which have little or no cushioning and support. The theory is that such shoes build foot strength by letting foot muscles work more naturally. But many runners have learned that throwing out their cushioned shoes without first building up their foot muscles and gradually introducing new footwear is a recipe for injury. Introduced gradually, minimalist shoes can work well for some people. When people take the idea to the extreme and try running barefoot, most find it too hard on their feet.

•**Toe lifts** (also known as toe yoga). Sit in a chair, with your bare feet flat on the floor. Lift your big toe while keeping the other toes down. Now press the big toe down while lifting the other toes. Press the big toe down while lifting the other toes. Then press your pinky toe down.

•**Toe spread.** Sit in a chair, with your bare feet flat on the floor. Try to spread all your toes apart from each other. Try not to curl your toes. Then gently press all your toes together without curling them.

•**Doming** (also called foot shortening). While standing or seated, stiffen your toes and press them into the ground. Squeeze the arch, drawing the ball of the foot towards the heel, creating a higher arch. Hold for 10 seconds, then release.

•**Towel curls.** Sit or stand on a smooth surface, with your foot on a towel. Curl your toes and attempt to grab and pull the end of the towel toward you.

To work on a wider range of foot and ankle muscles, add these moves (if your physical condition and sense of balance allows you to do so safely)…

•**Active standing.** Stand with your toes pointing forward or slightly out. Dome both feet. Unlock your knees slightly and squeeze your buttocks. Tip your pelvis into a neutral position, pull your navel toward your spine, pull your shoulders down and back, and draw your chin in. Practice this posture repeatedly throughout the day.

•**Double leg heel raises** (on a level surface). Standing on level ground, rise on the balls of both feet. Go as high as you can, applying most of the pressure behind your big and second toes. Return to the starting position and repeat.

•**Double leg heel raises** (on a step, holding railing). Stand on the edge of a step and let your heels rest below the level of the step. Rise on the balls of both feet. Go as high as you can, putting most of the pressure behind your big and second toes. Return to the starting position and repeat.

Pain in the Backside

Krina Vyas, M.D., physiatrist with the Hospital for Special Surgery and assistant professor of clinical rehabilitation medicine at Weill Cornell Medical College, New York.

Sciatica is surprisingly common. According to a study published in 2020 in the *Journal of the AAOS* (the American Academy of Orthopaedic Surgeons), one-quarter of people on Medicare have been diagnosed with it. The condition isn't limited to people over 65: It can happen at any age. Just what is sciatica and what can be done to ease its painful symptoms?

WHAT'S GOING ON

You have two sciatic nerves that run down either side of the lower half of your body, through your buttocks to your feet. Each is formed from a group of nerves that branch out on either side of the lower spine and come together to form two thick, long nerves.

When people experience sciatica, they may feel back pain accompanied by leg pain. The pain might feel dull, achy, shooting, or burning. You might also feel some numbness or a "pins and needles" tingling sensation. Usually only one side of the body is affected.

While the name sciatica means irritation of a sciatic nerve, the pain rarely starts with the sciatic nerve itself, but rather with one of the nerves from which it is formed. Typically, the cause is a pinched nerve or what's called *nerve root entrapment*. The true medical term for sciatica is *lumbar radiculopathy*. It's often called sciatica because the pain radiates along the sciatic nerve.

Depending on the location of the pinched nerve, you may feel pain only during certain activities or when you're in certain positions— when you sit or stand, bend over, lift objects, or simply cough or sneeze. The degree of pain depends on the degree to which the nerve is being pinched.

If you have feelings of muscle weakness or numbness, especially severe numbness in the groin, along with bladder dysfunction or incontinence, seek emergency help right away. It could be a serious condition called *cauda equina syndrome*, which typically requires immediate surgery.

HOW IT HAPPENS

One of the chief causes of sciatica is having a herniated ("slipped") disc. Discs are the cushions that sit between each of the vertebrae. An injury or bad body mechanics can lead to a tear in the outer ring of a disc, allowing its gel-like center to protrude and put pressure on the adjacent nerve root. A herniated disc can occur over time from wear and tear, or very suddenly as a result of a movement such as bending over the wrong way.

As you age, it's also possible to experience spinal stenosis, a narrowing of the canal that houses the spinal nerves. This puts pressure on them and causes pain. While spinal stenosis can happen anywhere along the spine, the lumbar area is a common place.

SOOTHING SCIATICA

Mild sciatica may go away on its own with self-care, such as resting, applying heat or cold packs, and taking over-the-counter medications such as a nonsteroidal anti-inflammatory drug or acetaminophen.

If you don't get relief within a couple of days, it's a good idea to see a physiatrist, a doctor who specializes in musculoskeletal problems, or an orthopedist.

Many people muddle through their first bout of sciatica and wait to see a doctor until it happens again or becomes persistent. But over time, untreated sciatica can lead to poor sleep, being afraid to exercise, and even depression. There's no reason to delay. By seeing a doctor, you'll get relief as well as modifications in body mechanics that can help prevent a recurrence.

•**Physical therapy.** A physiatrist or orthopedist will likely start with a conservative approach to treatment, such as physical therapy (PT). A course of six to eight weeks of therapeutic exercises, including ones you'll do at home between PT sessions, is crucial to recovery. The goal is to strengthen your core and back muscles to improve mobility in your low back, hips, and legs. Keep in mind that, although you may have some pain, moving through PT exercises won't damage you physically.

Another important part of this therapy is learning better ergonomics. Your therapist can show you ways to move with greater ease and to prevent the repetitive motions that may have led to the problem. These include how to bend and lift properly, such as using the hip hinge when picking something up from the floor. You may also be shown how to modify movements to ease discomfort.

•**Complementary therapies can also help.** Pilates is excellent because it focuses on developing core strength. Yoga improves stiffness and increases flexibility. A research analysis published in *Evidence-Based Complementary and Alternative Medicine* found that acupuncture may help ease sciatica pain because it has an analgesic effect, similar to pain-relief medication.

If these steps aren't helpful enough, your doctor is likely to order an MRI to better identify the source of the problem and create a different game plan. *Options include…*

•**Injections.** Epidural steroid injections may provide the relief you need. Some people respond to a single injection, while others need more than one to get through an episode of sciatica. Doctors must be well trained in administering these injections and proceed with caution because repeated use of steroids can cause tissue degeneration. It is recommended not to have more than three injections within a 12-month period.

•**Surgery.** This is an option when all other treatments fail to relieve the pain from a disc herniation or stenosis, and when the pain is eroding your quality of life. There are various types of what's called spinal decompression surgery available, depending on which nerve roots are affected. They can be helpful in easing refractory back and leg symptoms that have not responded to conservative management. But it's important to have a candid conversation with an orthopedic surgeon to understand the benefits and the risks.

Best Medication for Low Back Pain

Study titled "Nonopioid Pharmacological Management of Acute Low Back Pain: A Level I of Evidence Systematic Review," by researchers at the Department of Orthopaedic, Trauma, and Reconstructive Surgery, RWTH University Hospital, Aachen, Germany, et al., published in the *Journal of Orthopaedic Research*.

If you've ever overdid it with lifting, or slipped on ice, or simply turned funny, there's a good chance you've experienced debilitating back pain. According to an international team of researchers, acute low back pain, which is intense and usually lasts less than 12 weeks, is common and the leading cause of temporary disability worldwide. Despite the impact of this condition, research-based evidence on the best medication for treatment is limited and conflicting.

The team, which included medical university centers in Germany, Italy, New Zealand, and the U.K., have published a systematic review of studies on medications for low back pain to investigate which medications effectively reduce both pain and disability. Their findings are published in the *Journal of Orthopaedic Research*.

STEROIDS NOT INCLUDED

The team looked at studies through 2022 that were randomized controlled studies. These are studies that compare one treatment against another or to a placebo, and they are considered the "gold standard" for drug studies. The team limited the medications to non-steroidal anti-inflammatory drugs (NAIDS), paracetamol, muscle relaxants, and a placebo. NSAIDS are drugs such as Motrin, Advil, or Aleve. Paracetamol is the European name for *acetaminophen*, most commonly known as Tylenol in the United States.

Because acute low back pain usually goes away without treatment, the study did not include drugs such as antidepressants, opioids, or injection drugs such as steroids that may be used for chronic back pain. These medications are not recommended for acute back pain. The team selected 18 studies that included 3,478 people over age 18 with low back pain for less than 12 weeks. The mean age was 42, and 54 percent were female. The mean time suffering from back pain before receiving study medication or placebo was about 15 days, and the follow-up period was about eight days. People with back trauma or muscle damage were not included.

WHAT WORKS FOR BACK PAIN

To judge the effects of treatment on pain and disability, all the participants in these studies had self-reported their level of pain and disability before treatment. Pain was measured by using the numeric rating system (NRS). NRS asks a person to rate their pain using multiple scales from 0 to 10 (with 0 being no pain, 5 being moderate pain, and 10 being worst severe pain), 0 to 20, or 0 to 100 (if that better fits the intensity of their pain). Disability was measured by the Roland Morris Questionnaire (RMQ). The RMQ rates disability from 0 to 24, asking questions such as, "Does pain interfere with your sleep?" After about one week of treatment, the people in these studies repeated the NRS and RMQ.

These were the key results of the review...

•**Placebo had no significant effect on NRS or RMQ**

•**Acetaminophen alone had no significant effect on NRS or RMQ**

•**Muscle relaxants reduced NRS by 2.5 points and RMQ by 4.8 points**

•**NSAID alone reduced NRS by 5 points and RMQ by 10.2 points**

•**A combination of acetaminophen and an NSAID reduced NRS by 5.8 and RMQ by 10.3**

The review supports the combination of acetaminophen and an NSAID as the best treatment. This finding supports other recent research that this combination works better than each drug alone. It is also important to note that most people do not seek medical care for acute low back pain. An over-the-counter combination of acetaminophen and an NSAID is a viable option, since there are no muscle relaxants available in the U.S. without a prescription.

In the United States, 25 percent of people report having low back pain in the past three months. People at higher risk are usually over age 30, overweight, in poor physical shape, especially with weak back and stomach muscles. Smoking, drinking alcohol, and having a job that requires bending or lifting are other risk factors. Although most people can manage acute low back pain at home, medical care is advised if pain lasts for more than one week, or if there is tingling or numbness in the buttocks or legs.

Diet Can Help Stop Recurrent Kidney Stone Pain

Andrew Rule, M.D., professor, nephrology and hypertension, Mayo Clinic, Rochester, Minnesota.

Enriching your diet with foods high in calcium and potassium may prevent kidney stones. His team at the Mayo Clinic found that low dietary calcium and potassium are a more important predictor of recurrent kidney stone formation than fluid intake is. Diets with a daily intake of 1,200 milligrams of calcium may help prevent first-time and recurrent kidney stones. While higher potassium intake is recommended, the study didn't recommend a specific level. High-potassium foods include bananas, oranges, grapefruits, cantaloupes, honeydew melons, apricots, potatoes, mushrooms, peas, cucumbers, and zucchini.

Avoiding Ankle Accidents

Frank DiLiberto PT, Ph.D., associate professor of physical therapy and director of the Physical Therapy Movement Analysis Laboratory at Rosalind Franklin University of Medicine & Science, North Chicago, Illinois.

Ankle rolls and sprains are unwelcome surprises: You step off an unexpected curb, have an unsteady moment on a hiking trail, or move the wrong way during a sporting activity and are suddenly hobbled. Under the surface, the ligaments that connect the bones of your ankle, leg, and foot have been stretched beyond their limits or even torn.

Your throbbing ankle may bother you for a few minutes to days in the case of a minor roll, or for weeks or months in the case of a sprain that causes more severe stretching or tearing. Worse, your injury may leave your ankle chronically unstable, making you vulnerable to more unpleasant surprises and a less active future.

PREVENTION

The good news is that you can take steps to prevent these common injuries. Prevention is especially crucial for people who have rolled or sprained their ankles in the past. The American Physical Therapy Association estimates that about three-quarters of people who injure their ankle once will do it again. Prevention includes taping the ankle or wearing a brace when you exercise, especially soon after a sprain. Proper footwear, such as hiking boots for challenging trails and well-designed walking and running shoes, also can make a difference.

But the key to prevention is developing your balance along with strength and flexibility in your feet and ankles. That way you will be more likely to keep your footing when you encounter that next twisting trail or ill-placed curb.

If your ankles have become unstable and injury-prone, or even if your initial injury isn't improved in a few days, ask your primary care physician to refer you to a physical therapist (PT), or seek one out directly if your insurance doesn't require a referral. *A PT can help you develop an individual rehabilitation and* *prevention program, sometimes in just a few visits. In the meantime, here are a few exercises anyone can try...*

•**Single-foot stand.** Stand on one foot and lift the other behind you, trying to maintain your balance. If needed, hold on to a counter or chair back for support. See if you can balance for a few seconds, and then build your way toward 30 seconds and one minute. Once you gain some mastery, try the same exercise with your eyes closed: It's much harder without visual cues.

What to Do Immediately After a Sprain

Ankle sprains make themselves known immediately: First, you feel pain right where the ligament has torn or stretched, usually on the outside of your ankle. Next, the ankle may start to swell and bruise. It may feel tender to the touch and hurt when you move it. It may also feel stiff, weak, or unstable.

If you have a good deal of pain at rest or otherwise, or can't put weight on your affected foot, seek medical attention. You should get a physical exam and may get an X-ray to evaluate the injury severity. Your health-care provider may suggest you wear a brace for some activities and may refer you to a physical therapist for exercises and hands-on therapy to help you recover.

For any sprain, it's a good idea to apply ice to the area for 15 to 20 minutes every two hours for the first one to two days. Contrary to popular belief, you don't want to stay off your injured ankle too long: Instead, you should walk on the affected foot as soon as you can in a progressive fashion (start small and see how your ankle responds) without making the pain or swelling worse. You can use crutches or other walking aids if needed to alleviate pain and support your balance.

Many sprains heal in one to two weeks, but a severe sprain can take a few months.

•**Pillow balance.** Do the same single-foot balancing exercise while standing on a pillow, keeping a counter or chair back nearby for support. Expect your foot to wobble as you try to correct your balance and build up your time on one foot. If you can get up to one minute with your eyes open, try it with your eyes closed.

•**Single-leg half-circle taps.** Place six dots (stickers, coins, or pieces of paper) in a half-circle 30 inches from the center of your standing point. Now stand on one leg and slowly touch each dot with the other foot. Repeat on the opposite side. To increase the difficulty, do the exercise while standing on a pillow. Work on the exercise for 30 to 60 seconds, once or twice a day.

•**Standing calf stretch.** Stand facing a wall, countertop, or sturdy chair back. Put your hands on the surface in front of you for support. Place one ankle about one step back and the other foot forward. Keeping your back heel flat on the floor, slowly bend the knee of your front leg until you feel a mild to moderate stretch in the back calf. This should not create discomfort in the front of your ankle. Repeat three times, holding for 30 seconds. Switch legs and repeat the exercise.

•**Heel raise.** Once again, stand with your hands resting against a wall, a countertop, or a chair back for support. With your feet shoulder-width apart, slowly rise on your toes and come back down. Start with about 10 repetitions, increasing the number as the exercise gets easier. Aim to do 3 sets of 10 to 15 repetitions every few days as long as the exercise is pain-free.

Vitamin D and Fish Oil May Lower Risk for Autoimmune Diseases

BMJ.

Vitamin D and omega-3 fatty acid (fish oil) supplements were shown to reduce the risk of developing autoimmune diseases, including rheumatoid arthritis, thyroid disease, and psoriasis, in a new study of 25,871 adults

(mean age 67). People who took vitamin D (2,000 international units per day) for five years had a 22 percent lower risk of developing an autoimmune disease than people in a placebo group. Supplementation with 1,000 daily milligrams of an omega-3 fatty acid (fish oil) supplement reduced risk by 15 percent. Taking both supplements lowered risk by 31 percent.

Beat Autoimmune Disease with This Short-Term Diet

Jennifer Roelands, M.D., an OB/GYN trained in integrative medicine who works with women who have autoimmune disorders.

We all know that good food is medicine and that cleaning up our diets is often a key component of improving health. But it's not only about adding healthy foods. For people with an autoimmune disease, like rheumatoid arthritis, celiac disease, or multiple sclerosis, seemingly healthy foods can trigger an inflammatory cascade. Enter the autoimmune protocol, an elimination diet that can tease out which foods are problems for you (and which you can eat freely).

THE THEORY BEHIND THE DIET

In autoimmune diseases, the body confuses healthy cells and foreign invaders, causing the immune system to attack and damage normal cells. The exact cause of these disorders is unclear, but one prevailing theory is that of the leaky gut.

A normal, healthy gut is somewhat permeable: It lets water and nutrients travel from the gut to the bloodstream but keeps harmful substances from passing through the same way. Some people, however, have too much permeability, so toxins and other substances can slip through and cause bodywide inflammation and an autoimmune response.

Certain foods are believed to increase the gut's permeability. The AIP diet eliminates those foods (temporarily) to give the gut a chance to heal and tighten up the weak spots that allow the toxins through.

Autoimmune diseases that may respond to the AIP include adrenal fatigue, ankylosing spondylitis, celiac disease, Hashimoto's disease, lupus, multiple sclerosis, polycystic ovarian syndrome, psoriatic arthritis, rheumatoid arthritis, narcolepsy, lyme disease, type 1 diabetes, fibromyalgia, psoriasis, Crohn's disease, and Graves' disease.

It's done in two phases: Elimination and reintroduction.

ELIMINATION

The first step is to eliminate foods and medications that cause gut inflammation and permeability for about 30 days. (That's how long it takes for the gut to heal.) In that time, you'll want to avoid a variety of potential problem foods.

- **Additives and preservatives** in store-frozen or packaged foods
- **Alcohol:** Beer, liquor, wine
- **Coffee**
- **Dairy:** Milk, eggs, yogurt, cheese, cream, butter, ice cream
- **Gluten:** Bread, baked goods, crackers, cereals, pasta
- **Grains:** Rice, rye, quinoa, corn, oats, wheat, barley
- **Legumes:** Black beans, pinto beans, lima beans, peanuts, soy, cocoa, lentils
- **Nightshades:** Bell peppers, eggplants, tomatoes, potatoes, cherries, red spices, goji berries, and tomatillos
- **Non-steroidal anti-inflammatory drugs (NSAIDs):** ibuprofen, naproxen, diclofenac, and aspirin
- **Nuts and seeds:** Almonds, chia, cashews, pecans, pistachios, walnuts
- **Select spices:** Allspice, anise, pepper, poppy seeds, celery seed, cumin, caraway, mustard, nutmeg, and fennel seed
- **Sugars:** molasses, brown sugar, regular sugar, and any foods containing sugar
- **Tobacco.**

Some people eliminate all of these foods at once, while others prefer a more gradual

---

Safe Snacks During Elimination

Oven-Dried Broccoli Bites

Ingredients...

Broccoli florets
Salt and herbs to taste

Directions...

Preheat oven to the lowest setting. Lightly season the broccoli with salt and herbs. Gently dry broccoli florets on baking racks set over cookie sheets. This process is slow, but worth the effort for a crispy, slightly chewy snack that is great with almost any dip. Alternatively, use a dehydrator at 105 degrees for six hours to get the same texture.

Sweet Dip

Ingredients...

Can of coconut milk
Tbsp. applesauce or two dates

Directions...

For a sweet dipping treat, take the thick cream layer from a can of coconut milk and puree it with a spoonful of applesauce and one or two de-pitted dates for sweetness. Dip fresh berries or apple chips in this mix for a treat, or top it with berries and toasted coconut flakes for something a bit nutty.

Guacamole and Chips

Ingredients...

2 avocados
Sea salt
Lime juice
Garlic powder

Directions...

Mash two avocados with some sea salt, lemon/lime juice, and garlic powder to create a simple guacamole. Add one-quarter cup of minced red onion and one-quarter cup of minced cilantro for more flavor. Enjoy with plantain chips.

Source: 32 Fabulous AIP Snacks (HealthyAutoimmune.com); WellWomanMD.com

| Meal Ideas During the Elimination Phase | | |
BREAKFAST	LUNCH	DINNER
• Fruit salad with bananas, strawberries, and blueberries • Sweet potato hash with steak • Sautéed ham and spinach • Mushroom and onion mix with pork loin • Chicken livers and spinach	• Salmon with lemon slices over a bed of arugula • Turkey breast and avocado • Turkey burgers • Grilled chicken breast and asparagus • Tuna	• Ground beef patties • Chicken thighs and asparagus • Bunless mushroom burger • Roasted broccoli and grilled tilapia • Roasted duck and Brussel sprouts • Shrimp over zucchini pasta

approach and cut one food group at a time. Ultimately, the clock starts once all of the foods are out of your diet. It's a good idea to keep a journal to track how you feel as your body heals.

WHAT YOU CAN EAT

During the elimination phase of the AIP, stock up on anti-inflammatory foods…

•Fats: avocado oil, olive oil, coconut oil, beef tallow, chicken fat

•Fermented foods: sauerkraut, kimchi, kombucha

•Fruits: apples, bananas, berries, pears, peaches, mangos, and all other fruits, one to two servings per day

•Flavoring: salt, cilantro, thyme, dill, cinnamon, basil, mint, rosemary, and most cooking herbs and spices, apple cider vinegar, coconut sugar, honey, coconut flour, maple syrup, or blackstrap molasses

•Proteins: beef, lamb, chicken, pork, fish, turkey

•Vegetables: yams, broccoli, cauliflower, carrots, cabbage, lettuce, mushrooms, onion, kale, arugula, cucumber, and all other leafy greens and organic vegetables (excluding nightshades).

•Herbal teas not derived from seeds.

REINTRODUCTION

After three weeks, choose one food to reintroduce. The most common triggers are gluten and dairy, so they're a good place to start. Don't start a reintroduction during times of stress, after a poor night's sleep, or when sick, as all of those factors can affect your results.

Eat a small amount of the food and wait 15 minutes to see if you have a reaction. If you don't have symptoms, eat a larger portion and monitor how you feel for two to three hours. If you still have no reaction, eat a normal-sized portion of the food. Monitor any reaction to that food for one to two weeks. If you experience symptoms, like joint pain or fatigue at any time, end the test and note that the food is an irritant. If not, you can add the food to your safe list. Then choose the next food item on the list to add. Test one food at a time until you've worked though the list.

MOVING FORWARD

The elimination phase of the AIP is short. You don't have to live without everything on that list for the rest of your life, but you're likely to find a few things you'd do best to avoid long-term. One study showed that the AIP reduces inflammation and encouraged remission in 78 percent of the study participants. Decreasing inflammation is a key factor in healing with an autoimmune disorder. Remember, 70 percent of your immune system is located in your gut.

Rheumatoid Arthritis Treatment Update

Vasileios Kyttaris, M.D., assistant professor of medicine at the Harvard Medical School and a board-certified rheumatologist at the Beth Israel Deaconess Medical Center Division of Rheumatology, Boston.

Rheumatoid arthritis affects about 3 to 4 percent of women and 1 to 2 percent of men. RA is an autoimmune disease. That means your body's defense system—your immune system—attacks normal tissues instead of foreign invaders like germs.

The method of attack is inflammation, which causes the swelling, pain, and gradual erosion of joint tissue.

The American College of Rheumatology issues new treatment guidelines based on new drugs and clinical studies every few years. In the latest guidelines, the disease-modifying antirheumatic drug (DMARD) methotrexate is still the gold standard, but new biologic and targeted synthetic DMARDs have become an important part of the treatment landscape.

•**Biologics** are genetically engineered antibodies that block specific steps in the immune system path to inflammation. The first biologic approved for RA blocked a type of cytokine called tumor necrosis factor. Cytokines are proteins the immune system needs to cause inflammation. These biologics are called tumor necrosis factor (TNF) inhibitors. There are now several other classes of biologics that block different pathways.

Targeted synthetic DMARDs are the latest addition to the treatment arsenal. The most common one for RA is called a Janus kinase (JAK) inhibitor. JAK inhibitors, unlike TNF inhibitors, block multiple cytokines that immune cells need to increase inflammation. *All these drugs have their own risks and benefits...*

•The old, conventional synthetic DMARDS tend to be safe, effective, inexpensive, and can usually be taken in pill form.

•Biologics need to be given by injection or infusion and may increase the risk of serious infections, but they may be stronger than the conventional synthetic DMARDs.

•Targeted synthetic DMARDs have similar risks and efficacy as the biologics, but have the advantage of being taken orally.

TREATMENT GUIDELINES

If you have been recently diagnosed with RA, the first step is for your health-care provider to determine your level of disease activity, which could be low, moderate, or high. The next step is to set a target or treatment goal you want to reach in six months. Although about one-third of patients may be able to reach symptom-free remission, in most cases, the target is low disease activity.

There are three steps to treatment, depending on your disease activity...

***STEP 1:* For low disease activity, you may start with a single conventional synthetic DMARD.** Hydroxychloroquine may be the first choice, since it is well tolerated by most people. Hydroxychloroquine and sulfasalazine do not suppress your immune system, so they may be favored over methotrexate for mild disease, or when there is a history of an immune-sensitive cancer like melanoma. Less aggressive disease may be predicted in people who do not have RA antibodies on a blood test, a scenario called *seronegative RA*. Hydroxychloroquine or sulfasalazine may be a good choice for these people.

***STEP 2:* If low disease activity is not maintained after six months,** or your disease activity starts as moderate to high, methotrexate single treatment (*monotherapy*) is recommended. About 50 percent of people reach their target on methotrexate monotherapy. Methotrexate is recommended over biologic monotherapy because it is almost as effective, easy to take, and much less expensive. If your target is not reached, you may be switched from oral methotrexate to subcutaneous injections. If you still don't reach your target, step three is the addition of other DMARDs.

***STEP 3:* For patients who do not reach their goals on methotrexate alone,** there are two options recommended. One is triple therapy, which is methotrexate, hydroxychloroquine, and sulfasalazine. The other is methotrexate plus a biologic (usually a TNF inhibitor) or targeted synthetic DMARD (a JAK inhibitor). TNF inhibitors generally have a better safety profile. Patients who still need more help to stay on target can switch to a different biologic or targeted synthentic DMARD. Choosing which is the best is hit or miss, since there is not enough research available yet to guide the choice.

Patients often ask why they can't start with biologic monotherapy instead of methotrexate. The reason is that some studies find a biologic to be more effective and others don't. The results are not consistent.

At one time, there was a fear that biologics increased the risk of white blood cell cancer,

Walk to Ward Off Knee Pain

According to a recent study, older adults with knee osteoarthritis who walked for exercise had 40 percent less chance of experiencing new frequent knee pain compared with people with arthritis who did not walk.

Good news: Walking also was found to be effective at slowing joint damage… and is especially beneficial for people who are bow-legged and also have knee osteoarthritis.

Study of 1,212 people aged 50 and older with knee osteoarthritis by researchers at Baylor College of Medicine, Houston, published in *Arthritis & Rheumatology.*

but that has not been supported by more recent research. However, biologics still increase your risk of some rare but serious infections, and they are still very expensive. So for the time being, they are not used as initial therapy.

TAPERING TREATMENT

For patients on multiple drugs who have sustained remission or low disease activity for at least six months, the doses of drugs can be lowered and some drugs may be gradually discontinued, but stopping therapy completely is not recommended, due to the risk of a flare.

For patients who are doing well on a TNF inhibitor, tapering off the drug has been associated with a 30 to 50 percent relapse rate. With other biologics, tapering down to monotherapy with methotrexate is possible. For people on triple therapy, sulfasalazine should be the first drug removed; the next drug would be hydroxychloroquine.

LIFESTYLE GUIDELINES

A Mediterranean-style diet reduces the risk of heart disease, which is more common in RA. Exercise and strength training are important for maintaining a heathy weight and to strengthen muscles that support joints. Obesity makes RA worse, and so does smoking. If you are on methotrexate, you should avoid alcohol because of an increased risk of liver damage.

The American College of Rheumatology has been changing the treatment guidelines for RA whenever new research or new drugs become available. This type of evidence-based research has been very successful. In 1950, the life expectancy of a person with RA was about 67 years. Today it is 80.

Living with RA is also much different. With proper treatment and care, most people with RA can now have a good quality of life, continue to work, and enjoy physical and social activities.

Rheumatoid Arthritis Linked to Intestinal Microbiome

Arthritis & Rheumatology.

Antibodies to a common intestinal bacterium, *Prevotella copri*, are elevated in people with rheumatoid arthritis (RA). While this link was seen a decade ago, a new study shows that the antibodies can be found in the earliest stages of the disease, including what might be termed "pre-RA." The investigators hypothesized that the antibodies might cross-react with synovial tissue proteins in the joints to trigger chronic inflammation.

Exercise Is Good for Arthritic Joints

Recommendations from the National Institute for Health and Care Excellence, which publishes guidelines based on evidence-based recommendations, London, U.K.. NICE.org.uk

While exercise may be painful at first, over time, it can ease pain, help patients maintain a healthy weight and improve overall health and quality of life.

Best exercises: Low impact such as walking, cycling, and exercising in water…strengthening exercises such as leg raises to build muscle… stretching and balancing exercises…aerobic to help your heart and lungs. Discuss with your doctor what exercise regimen—and pain relief, if needed—is appropriate for you.

Meniscus Implants Are Better Than Nonsurgical Care

Research from two clinical trials presented at a combined annual meeting of the American Orthopedic Medicine Society–Arthroscopy Association of North America, reported in UCLA Health. UCLAHealth.org

According to a recent finding, a synthetic meniscus implant after surgery to repair a meniscal tear offered 63 percent better post-surgery relief from knee pain compared with nonsurgical care, which offered only 28 percent improvement in pain. Patients enrolled in the studies had one or more partial meniscectomies at least six months before the study and were followed for two years.

Meditations for Arthritis Pain

Arthritis Advisor. Arthritis-Advisor.com

Breath meditation—inhale through your nose, expanding your belly with each breath, and exhale through your mouth. As thoughts intrude, let them go and refocus on the experience of your breath. When you feel pain during the day, tap into this meditation with a few deep breaths. *Mindful meditation* (5,4,3,2,1)—look around for five things you wouldn't normally notice…touch four things you wouldn't normally touch…hear three ambient sounds…acknowledge two background smells…and savor one taste, such as a sip of water. *Progressive relaxation*—tensing then releasing muscle groups from your toes to your head helps counter your nervous system's stress response to pain. *Body scan*—starting at your feet and working upward, mentally scan each body part, noting its sensation, bringing your attention to areas that are tight or achy

and releasing them. *Autogenic training*—with each breath, focus on a different body part while mentally repeating a descriptive phrase.

Examples: "My legs are comfortably heavy" or, "My heart beats quietly."

Exercise Options If You Have Osteoarthritis

William Harvey, M.D., professor, Kinesiology and Physical Education, McGill University, Montreal, Canada.

In the summer, I swim to exercise without aggravating the osteoarthritis in my hip, but my gym doesn't have an indoor pool. What are some safe but effective alternatives?

Good for you for recognizing the importance of keeping moving. If you don't exercise, your muscles will get weaker, your arthritis symptoms will worsen, and you will lose vital strength and mobility. Walking, yoga, and tai chi are three activity options that won't stress your joints, don't require a pool, and can be done at home or close to home.

•**Walking.** You may worry that walking will cause your arthritic hip to deteriorate faster, but research suggests you can walk for at least 10,000 steps each day without doing additional damage to your arthritic hip joint. If you want some "virtual" company or need support or direction, follow this link https://bit.ly/30ieJfG to learn about the Arthritis Foundation's Walk with Ease program.

•**Yoga.** People with arthritis who practice yoga regularly can reduce joint pain, improve joint flexibility and function, and lower stress and tension.

Iyengar yoga is often recommended to people who have arthritis because it can be adapted for limited mobility. Assistive props, such as ropes and foam blocks, can be used during challenging poses. For example, if you have a hard time bending over and touching your toes, you can place a foam block on the floor and reach for that instead.

•**Floor stretches are another great way to gain the benefits of yoga without inflict-**

ing undue stress on your joints. Follow this link https://tinyurl.com/22vka39k to learn how to do a dynamic reclined hip stretch sequence that can help you gently release tension around your hip joint and hamstrings.

•**Tai chi.** With its gentle, fluid movements, tai chi is gaining popularity as a way to fight off arthritis pain and increase flexibility and strength without straining joints. Recent studies have found that the slow, graceful exercise, which originated centuries ago as a martial art, can improve balance, reduce stress, and offer pain relief. For more info, follow this link https://bit.ly/3ikGudL to watch—or participate in—a tutorial on tai chi stretches for arthritis.

Steroid Injections Can Worsen Knee Osteoarthritis

"Medial Joint Space Narrowing and Kellgren-Lawrence Progression Following Intraarticular Corticosteroid Injections Compared to Hyaluronic Acid Injections and Nontreated Patients," by researchers from the University of California, San Francisco and "Impact of Intra-Articular Knee Injections on the Progression of Knee Osteoarthritis: Data From the Osteoarthritis Initiative (OAI) Cohort," by researchers from the Chicago Medical School of Rosalind Franklin University of Medicine and Science, presented at the Radiological Society of North America Annual Meeting, November 2022.

Osteoarthritis (OA) is a chronic disease that becomes progressively worse over time. There is no cure for OA, and about 10 percent of people with OA of the knees are treated with a knee injection to relieve symptoms such as pain, stiffness, and swelling. Two types of OA knee injections are corticosteroid and hyaluronic acid. Corticosteroids are medications similar to hormones produced by the body that block swelling. Hyaluronic acid is a substance similar to joint fluid that lubricates and cushions the knee joint. Injections of these medications are often used when oral drugs and other therapies have failed to relieve the pain.

TWO INDEPENDENT STUDIES FAVOR HYALURONIC ACID

Two studies comparing hyaluronic acid and corticosteroids were presented at a meeting of the Radiological Society of North America. The results of both studies favored hyaluronic acid as the safer choice. Previous studies have shown that corticosteroids may reduce knee pain in OA for four to eight months, and hyaluronic acid may relieve pain longer. A 2017 study found that corticosteroid injections did not work any better than sterile salt water (saline) injections based on a two-year span.

The two studies were independent from each other, but both used data from a 14-year, ongoing observational trial by the National Institutes of Health called the Osteoarthritis Initiative. In this trial, about 5,000 people with OA have been followed at multiple sites over 14 years. These patients have been diagnosed with imaging studies and had their treatments recorded. One of the new studies was done by the University of California, San Francisco. In this trial, 210 patients from the Osteoarthritis Initiative were included. Seventy patients had been treated with injections, 44 with corticosteroid, and 26 with hyaluronic acid. For comparison, 140 patients who did not have injections were included as a control group.

This study looked at magnetic resonance imaging (MRI) done two years before the study, at the beginning of the study, and two years after the study. After matching patients for age, sex, weight, and severity of OA, the imaging studies were compared. The result was a significant progression of OA in the knees of patients injected with corticosteroids as compared to the control group and the hyaluronic acid group. In addition, the hyaluronic acid group had less OA progression compared to the control group.

The second study was done by researchers at the Chicago Medical School. In this study, 50 patients received corticosteroid injections, 50 patients received hyaluronic acid injections, and 50 patients were given no injections. As in the other study, patients were matched by age, sex, weight, and severity. Knee X-rays were compared from the beginning of the study to X-rays done two years later. In this study, patients in the corticosteroid group also had more OA progression than the hyaluronic acid and no injection groups.

KNEE INJECTIONS SHOULD BE A LAST RESORT

Although they caution that these types of observational studies are not as reliable as a real time, randomized, and controlled clinical trial, both study groups conclude that corticosteroid injections should be used with more caution, and hyaluronic acid injections should be studied further. Both groups also suggest that joint injections should only be considered after other therapies such as oral pain medications, physical therapy, exercise, and weight loss have been tried first.

Green Glasses May Ease Chronic Pain

American Society of Anesthesiologists.

In a small study, people with fibromyalgia who wore green-tinted glasses for four hours per day for two weeks used fewer opioids than people who wore blue or clear glasses. The research suggests that some wavelengths of green light stimulate the brain pathways that help manage pain. The glasses also reduced fear-based anxiety. Another study linked green LED exposure with fewer episodic and chronic migraine headaches.

How Do I Beat Bunion Pain?

Samuel K. K. Ling, assistant professor, department of orthopaedics and traumatology, faculty of medicine, the Chinese University of Hong Kong. Dr. Ling developed a type of minimally invasive bunion surgery that has provided pain relief for up to 10 years in his patients.

A bunion is a deformity of the metatarsophalangeal joint that causes a large bump on the outside of the big toe. *The*

first step to treating pain is always conservative management…

- **Wear well-fitting, comfortable shoes** with ample space for your toes and the widest part of your foot.
- **Use over-the-counter arch supports** or prescription orthotic devices to help position the foot correctly.
- **Avoid walking barefoot.**
- **Use warm soaks and ice packs for pain relief.**
- **Take nonsteroidal anti-inflammatory drugs if needed.**
- **Maintain a healthy weight.**

If these strategies aren't enough, you may want to consider surgery. Traditionally, surgery has been considered a last resort because it has a two- to three-month recovery time, and most patients aren't happy with surgical results for about six months. But new minimally invasive (MI) techniques aim to shorten that recovery time and make bunion surgery an option for people in earlier stages of the disorder. (See page 220 for more information on advances in bunion surgery.)

In a minimally invasive procedure, instead of fully opening the skin to access the bones, the surgeon will use several small incisions and special instruments to see and work inside the foot. Evidence suggests that MI techniques may offer shorter healing times and less pain without sacrificing effectiveness. MI surgery can be tricky for surgeons to master, so look for an experienced doctor for a consultation.

Battling Bunions

Jamison Starbuck, ND, a naturopathic physician in family practice in Missoula, Montana, and producer of *Dr. Starbuck's Health Tips for Kids,* a weekly program on Montana Public Radio, MTPR.org.

A slightly goofy word that connotes pain and deformity, *bunion* is derived from the Greek word for turnip. It's a bony bump growing out from the side of one's big toe. Bunions happen at the *metatarsophalangeal* joint, where the first long bone of the foot meets the first bone of the big toe.

Bunions are common: Approximately 30 percent of people ages 18 to 65 have them, and the prevalence increases with age. More than 70 percent of the elderly have them. They are more common in women than in men.

The primary cause of bunions seems to be genetics. Secondary factors, such as frequently wearing tight-fitting or high-heeled shoes; injuries to the feet, ankles and knees that change your stride; and inflammatory ailments, like rheumatoid arthritis, also contribute to the development of bunions. But we inherit the shape and structure of our feet from our biological parents. If your mom or dad has bunions, especially bunions bad enough to require surgery, you may also eventually develop them.

Bunions typically develop slowly, and not all of them require surgery. Your best bet in preventing a bunion from becoming so painful that surgery is necessary is to pay attention to your feet. Wear comfortable shoes that have good arch support, low or no heels, and a wide toe box that gives your toes lots of wiggle room. If you notice your feet changing or your shoes fitting differently, see a podiatrist or an orthopedic doctor who specializes in feet. These specialists can help you manage bunions with foot pads, inserts, or individualized orthotics. Early treatment won't take away a bunion, but it can prevent the bunion from worsening and causing you pain.

If, despite your best efforts, a bunion causes pain and limits your activity, it's time to consider surgery. Be prepared for a short surgery and a long recovery time. Full recovery from bunion surgery, reaching the point where you are glad you did it, can take up to a year.

When my patients need bunion surgery, I recommend the following to ensure the best outcome and swiftest recovery…

•**Take a single dose** (2 pellets under the tongue 15 minutes away from food) of homeopathic arnica 30 c or 200 c in the morning of surgery and again in the evening after surgery.

•**To reduce inflammation and speed bone healing,** take the herbal medicines boswellia (300 milligrams [mg]), turmeric (100 mg), and ashwagandha (100 mg) four times per day for six weeks after surgery. Be sure to tell your surgeon in advance that you plan to take these herbs to help with your recovery.

•**Avoid caffeine and alcohol during the first three weeks after surgery,** as both can increase inflammation and pain.

•**Follow all surgical instructions and postsurgery physical therapy recommendations thoroughly.** Don't rush the process or skimp on your prescribed exercises. Treat yourself well and you'll be back on your feet in a few months' time.

Adrenaline Could Be the Key to Pain Relief Without Addiction

Prof. Dr. Peter Gmeiner, Ph.D., chair of pharmaceutical chemistry, Friedrich-Alexander-Universität Erlangen-Nürnberg, Bavaria, Germany.

New substances that activate adrenaline receptors alleviate pain in a way that's similar to opiates but without side effects such as respiratory depression and addiction. There are already some analgesics that target the alpha 2A adrenergic receptor, such as brimonidine, clonidine, and dexmedetomidine, but they can have a strong sedative effect. The separation of analgesic properties and sedation is a milestone in the development of non-opioid pain medication. These drugs are in the basic research phase and not yet available to patients.

Compression Garments Don't Help Muscle Recovery

Meta analysis of 19 randomized controlled trials led by researchers at Tohoku University, Sendai, Japan, published in *Sports Medicine*.

It has become popular, especially among athletes, to wear tight-fitting elastic sleeves on arms or legs during or after exercise in the belief that doing so helps muscles recover faster.

Recent finding: Regardless of the type of exercise or how compression garments are worn, no such benefit has been found.

High-Tech Solution for Chronic Pain

Cory Gloeckner, Ph.D., assistant professor at John Carroll University in University Heights, Ohio, and lead author of a University of Minnesota study published in *Journal of Neural Engineering.*

Chronic pain may be reduced by broadband sound plus electrical stimulation.

Recent finding: In guinea pigs, this combination activated neurons in a way that suggests it could be an effective non-opioid option for chronic pain control. Human trials will begin soon. Broadband audio files (white noise is one kind) are free online and "TENS" units, which deliver electrical stimulation, are available for under $50. Precise timing, intensity, and location of electrical stimulation matter—treatment requires a consultation with a health-care provider.

New Hope for Lupus

Nature Medicine.

Autologous chimeric antigen receptor (CAR) T-cell therapy shows promise as a treatment for lupus. In a study of five people, a single dose of the treatment induced remission in all patients within three months. They remained in remission for an average of eight months after treatment. The first person to receive CAR-T treatment as part of the study was still in remission more than a year later.

Hidden Celiac Disease

Amy Burkhart, M.D., RD, one of only two physicians in the United States who is also a registered dietitian and trained in integrative medicine. She is a specialist in celiac disease and gluten/wheat-related disorders, as well as a celiac disease patient herself. TheCeliacMD.com

For the one in 100 Americans who have celiac disease (CD), a gluten-free diet is much more than a fad. It's critical to maintaining health and avoiding severe nutritional deficiencies. When people with CD consume gluten, their body initiates an immune response that attacks the villi—the tiny, finger-like projections lining the small intestine that help absorb nutrients.

People with CD are four times more likely to develop small bowel cancer in the first year after diagnosis (unless they follow a gluten-free diet), twice as likely to develop coronary heart disease, and often live with other autoimmune conditions such as diabetes or multiple sclerosis. Unfortunately, CD remains vastly undiagnosed: About 80 percent of people living with CD have no idea they have it.

DIFFERENT SYMPTOMS IN SENIORS

Chances are you've heard of CD and associate it with the diarrhea, painful cramps, constipation, and bloating that strike children and young adults. But for the 20 to 40 percent of patients who are diagnosed over age 50, gastrointestinal symptoms are often more subtle or even nonexistent. *Older people with CD tend to experience different symptoms…*

- **Fatigue**
- **Brain fog/difficulty concentrating**
- **Anemia** (due to an inability to properly absorb iron and other micronutrient deficiencies)
- **Anxiety or depression**
- **Joint pain**
- **Osteoporosis** (due to an inability to properly absorb calcium)
- **Canker sores, loose-fitting dentures, and other dental problems**
- **Hair thinning or loss**
- **Headaches**
- **Skin rashes.**

Screening for Celiac

A simple blood test can help screen for CD. If the test detects noteworthy levels of certain antibodies and other markers indicative of CD, your doctor may order an upper endoscopy (a procedure during which a long, flexible tube with a miniature camera at the end explores your upper digestive system) along with an intestinal biopsy to confirm the diagnosis. You must be eating gluten at the time these tests are done for the results to be accurate.

Many of these symptoms are often chalked up to aging, so millions of people in their 50s, 60s, and above never seek out CD testing. It's likely nowhere on their radar. Furthermore, doctors who completed their training more than 15 years ago likely learned very little about CD, as research regarding CD and gluten sensitivity is quickly evolving. Most doctors still think a patient needs to have diarrhea and bloating in order to be screened, or they think, "If she's made it to 65 and never been diagnosed, she doesn't have it." The average time to diagnosis for older patients with symptoms is about 15 or 16 years.

RISK FACTORS

If you have a first-degree relative (parent, child, brother, or sister) with CD, you have a one in 22 chance of developing the disease yourself, versus the general population's one-in-100 risk. Have a second-degree relative with CD, such as an aunt, uncle, niece, nephew, grandparent, or grandchild? Your risk is one in 39. Women are at higher risk compared with men, and it affects individuals of all races and ethnicities.

TREATMENT

There's only one treatment for CD: strict avoidance of gluten, which is easier said than done. It may seem simple to stop eating obvious sources of gluten, such as traditional breads, cakes, and pastas, but gluten hides in all sorts of products, including oats, soy sauce, BBQ sauce, and marinades, crisp rice cereal, beer, sliced deli meat and vegan "meats," and more.

Gluten can also sneak into otherwise gluten-free food during manufacturing or cooking, so people with CD need to become meticulous label readers. Label-reading can be difficult for those with vision issues as the print is often very tiny and the wording can be confusing.

For instance, rice, which is naturally free of gluten, may say "Made on shared equipment with wheat-containing foods," which means it is likely unsafe for someone with CD.

When dining out, people with CD must ask restaurants if they use separate toasters, deep-fryers, and utensils when preparing food. French fries, for instance, are naturally gluten-free, but if they're fried in oil also used to prepare breaded chicken nuggets, they can easily pick up some gluten and cause intestinal damage.

You should also speak with your health-care provider about the need for supplementation. People with CD are often low or deficient in iron and other nutrients.

Being diagnosed with CD can feel scary, but it's also a blessing in disguise, as you can expect to feel better and live a longer, healthier life once you're on a gluten-free diet. And thanks to the general uptick in interest in the gluten-free lifestyle, it's easier than ever to thrive with this condition.

CHAPTER 17

Respiratory Health and Allergies

7 Surprising Asthma Triggers

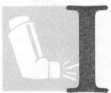

If you have asthma, you already know that things like cigarette smoke, animal dander, and dust can trigger a dangerous attack. But there are many other—often unexpected—triggers of asthma flares.

1. THUNDERSTORMS

During a thunderstorm, rain and lightning split pollen grains open and expose the peptides inside. Winds and downdrafts then spread those tiny particles widely. Normal, intact pollen grains measure 20 to 100 microns and settle to the ground, but these fragments, at less than 2.5 microns, remain in the air, where they can easily be inhaled deeply into the lungs.

In 2016, Melbourne, Australia, witnessed the world's most extreme case of thunderstorm asthma. Within 30 hours, more than 3,000 people went to emergency rooms for asthma attacks, 35 were admitted to intensive care units, and 10 died. Researchers note that as global temperatures rise, thunderstorms are expected to become more common, making this a more widespread trigger.

2. FOOD ADDITIVES

When nitrites, nitrates, and sulfites are used as added food preservatives, sensitive people can experience worsening respiratory symptoms. (Foods that contain these compounds naturally generally do not trigger asthma.)

Common culprits include sauerkraut, deli and cured meats, wine, beer, cider, dried fruits and vegetables, packaged potatoes, bottled lime and lemon juice, and pickled foods.

3. VOLCANOES

If you're planning a trip to Hawaii or any other place with active volcanoes, pack extra

Jeffrey G. Demain, M.D., FAAP, FACAAI, FAAAAI, founder, Allergy Asthma & Immunology Center of Alaska, Clinical Professor, Department of Pediatrics, University of Washington, Affiliate Professor, WWAMI School of Medical Education, University of Alaska, Anchorage.

medication and have a rescue plan in place. Volcanic ash releases sulfur dioxide, which can cause significant injury to the lungs when inhaled and trigger an asthma attack. Some people may also be sensitive to the sulfur dioxide released from natural hot springs.

4. NSAIDS

Nonsteroidal anti-inflammatory drugs, like aspirin, ibuprofen, and naproxen, worsen asthma symptoms in about one in five people with asthma. If you notice symptoms after taking any of these drugs, opt for *acetaminophen* (Tylenol) instead.

5. HOUSE PLANTS

Asthma attacks can be caused by mold spores that are often found in the soil of many household plants. Minimize indoor plants and keep them out of rooms in which you spend a lot of time. English ivy, a peace lily, or a rubber plant are safer options, but keep them out of the reach of children and pets.

6. CLEANING PRODUCTS

Cleaning away dust and dirt can hurt asthma more than help it if you use certain products. Avoid cleaners that contain peroxyacetic acid, peracetic acid, and fragrances (including candles and air fresheners).

Don't use bleach (sodium hypochlorite) or quaternary ammonium compounds in enclosed spaces. Instead, opt for soap and water, vinegar, lemon, hydrogen peroxide (no stronger than 3 percent), ethanol (ethyl alcohol), or premade products certified by the EPA Safer Choice Program.

7. LIVING NEAR A MAJOR ROAD

People who live, work, or go to school near a major road have higher rates of asthma and more symptoms. The closer to the road, the stronger the effect.

A study published in the *American Journal of Respiratory and Critical Care Medicine* reported that long-term exposure to traffic air pollution also may increase the risk of developing chronic obstructive pulmonary disease—especially among people who had asthma or diabetes, and researchers reported in *Environmental Health Perspectives* that

Warming Cities

Heat, ozone, pollen levels, and carbon dioxide levels are all higher in cities—and that has real effects on people with asthma and allergies. A team of researchers planted ragweed in urban, suburban, and rural areas. They found that in the urban areas, which had 30 percent higher levels of carbon dioxide, pollen rates were twice as high. As the world gets warmer, pollen levels are rising every year, and the pollen season is getting longer. Spring is now starting up to 30 days earlier, and the transition from summer to fall is occurring later, especially in northern states, a team of researchers reported. Climate change is also leaving more asthma attacks in the wake of receding glaciers in places like Alaska, Washington, Oregon, California, Montana, Wyoming, Colorado, and Nevada. As glaciers recede, they leave behind tiny particles of crushed rock that can be inhaled deep in the lungs.

traffic-related pollution decreased lung function in urban women.

REDUCE RISK WITH GOOD CONTROL

While you can't avoid things like thunderstorms, you can protect yourself by working with your physician to make sure your asthma is well controlled. If you're using a rescue inhaler, such as albuterol, more than a few times a week, talk to your doctor about your medication regimen.

Many new medications can reach deeper into the lungs and treat your symptoms using different mechanisms.

It's also important to have a spirometry test at least once per year to measure and monitor your lung function and capacity. If your family doctor doesn't offer spirometry, make an appointment with an allergist or pulmonologist to supplement your asthma care team.

Vaping Is Not a Gateway to Cigarettes

Study of 37,105 young adults by researchers at University College London, U.K., published in *Addiction*.

Rates of vaping over the past 11 years among young people in England climbed to 5 percent—yet smoking rates for that period dropped from 30 percent to 25 percent.

Sleep Apnea: Bad for Your Brain

Chris Iliades, M.D., retired surgeon and regular *Bottom Line Health* contributor.

According to the American Heart Association and the American Academy of Neurology, obstructive sleep apnea (OSA) is bad for brain health. Studies show that OSA causes cognitive impairment, which is the loss of your brain's ability to remember, think, concentrate, learn, and make decisions.

WHAT HAPPENS DURING OSA?

In people with OSA, the oral or nasal airway collapses during sleep and breathing stops for a short period. This is called apnea. Blood oxygen levels decrease and carbon dioxide levels increase. Rising carbon dioxide triggers your brain to wake you up enough to breathe. Almost everyone with OSA snores, usually loudly, so a sleeping partner may hear loud snoring followed by quiet, and then sudden gasping for air. In mild-to-moderate OSA, there may be between five and 30 episodes per hour. In severe OSA, these instances can occur more than 30 times per hour.

A 2021 study reported at the American Academy of Neurology annual meeting showed that people with OSA were 60 percent more likely to score in a lower range on cognitive testing than people without it. The worse the OSA, the worse the cognitive decline. The average age of study participants was about 70.

Further, OSA increases the risk of heart attack, stroke, heart arrhythmia, high blood pressure, and type 2 diabetes.

ARE YOU AT RISK?

The American Heart Association estimates that OSA may affect close to 40 percent of U.S. adults and up to 80 percent of people with cardiovascular disease. It is more common in men and in people who are overweight. You could be at higher risk if you have a family history of OSA. Other risk factors include smoking, drinking alcohol, taking sleeping pills, and having any type of narrowing of the nasal or oral airway, like a deviated nasal septum or large tonsils or adenoids.

REDUCE RISK, IMPROVE HEALTH

Lowering risk can be as simple as exercising. An important study presented at the 2021 meeting of the American Heart Association showed that exercise reduces the risk of both OSA and cognitive decline.

In the study, 47 patients with varying degrees of cognitive loss were tested for a cognition score. Half of the patients were given a six-month-long supervised exercise program. After six months, the exercise group had fewer OSA episodes, a 32 percent improvement in their cognitive scores, *and* better glucose metabolism in the brain.

In addition to exercise, lifestyle changes that reduce the risk or improve symptoms of OSA include not drinking, not smoking, and losing weight. Sleeping on your side and propping up your upper body during sleep may also reduce OSA. In some cases, surgery can be used to correct a deviated septum or remove tonsils and adenoids if they are contributing to OSA.

DIAGNOSIS

Mark Twain said, "There ain't no way to know why a man can't hear himself snore," but there is a way to find out if you have sleep apnea. If your sleeping partner describes periods of snoring and apnea, or you wake up

When OSA Is Deadly

In rare cases, OSA can be deadly: It was the cause of death for Supreme Court Justice Antonin Scalia. In fact, before the invention of continuous positive airway pressure (CPAP) technology, many people with severe OSA were treated with a permanent breathing hole in their neck, called a tracheostomy, to prevent death during sleep.

groggy with a headache and feel sleepy all day, you should have a sleep study.

During the sleep study, you spend a night in a sleep lab, where specialists called polysomnographers document sleep apnea and grade the severity. Sleep study kits you can use at home are now available, so you may not need to spend the night sleeping in a laboratory.

TREATMENT

For mild sleep apnea, lifestyle changes, sleeping position, and sometimes an oral appliance that keeps your tongue from blocking your oral airway may be all you need. For more severe OSA, the treatment of choice is CPAP. During CPAP treatment, you wear a mask while you sleep that provides humidified oxygen through your nose to force open your airway. It is very effective but takes some getting used to, and you may need to experiment with different types of masks, levels of air pressure, and humidification devices to find the most comfortable option.

A new technology called hypoglossal nerve stimulation may eliminate the need for CPAP for some people who can't tolerate it. With this treatment, a pacemaker implanted in the chest stimulates the hypoglossal nerve to open the back of the throat.

OSA is that it is both common and dangerous. If you have the symptoms, tell your doctor and get OSA under control now. Your brain and your sleeping partner will thank you.

CPAP Reduces the Risk of Cardiovascular Rehospitalization

Journal of Clinical Sleep Medicine.

People with cardiovascular disease (CVD) and newly diagnosed obstructive sleep apnea who consistently use a continuous positive airway pressure (CPAP) treatment device have a lower likelihood of rehospitalization for CVD, according to a new study of 1,301 Medicare recipients. CPAP therapy delivers a stream of air through a mask to help keep the airway open during sleep. Over a two-year follow-up, the 30-day readmission rate in those who had high adherence to CPAP use was 60 percent lower than for those with low adherence. The study did not investigate the cause of the initial or subsequent hospitalizations.

Sleep Testing at Home

Northwestern Medicine.

A new home sleep test can diagnose moderate-to-severe obstructive sleep apnea (OSA) with 95 percent accuracy, researchers from Northwestern Medicine have found. Anne Sleep is the first wearable system that has been cleared by the U.S. Food and Drug Administration as a sleep diagnostic platform and a general patient monitor. A demo of the system can be accessed at Sibelhealth.com (but be sure to work with your doctor, since the system is available through prescription only). OSA is a condition in which the airway closes up to 30 or more times every hour during sleep. It can lead to severe daytime fatigue, stroke, hypertension, diabetes, depression, and motor vehicle accidents. The home device could help diagnose more patients to prevent and improve the adverse effects of sleep apnea on cardiovascular, metabolic, and brain health.

Let's Talk Voice Disorders

Norman D. Hogikyan, M.D., FACS, director of the Michigan Medicine Vocal Health Center, a subspecialist in laryngology and clinical medical ethics, and professor and associate chairman of Otolaryngology-Head and Neck Surgery in the University of Michigan Medical School in Ann Arbor.

Almost everyone has experienced a bout of hoarseness after singing along at a concert or cheering on a favorite sports team. It's also not uncommon to get hoarse from a garden-variety case of laryngitis—inflammation of the larynx (or voice box)—brought on by infections that are typically viral, such as the common cold. These conditions are usually self-limiting and improve with rest and plenty of fluids. But there is a surprising array of other health issues that can cause voice problems.

•**Gastroesophageal reflux.** Stomach acids that back up all the way to the larynx can affect your voice. Symptoms include a husky-sounding voice, noticeable phlegm, and frequent throat clearing, and are often worse earlier in the day. Treating reflux should resolve voice issues.

The problem is that many people and primary care doctors alike are too quick to attribute hoarseness to reflux. If hoarseness doesn't improve after a few weeks of taking reflux medication, it's time to consider other possible causes.

•**Vocal fold lesions.** Various types of growths or lesions can develop on the vocal folds (also called vocal cords). *Nodules* can form at points on the folds that experience the most wear and tear when you use your voice, particularly with repetitive voice overuse or misuse.

Polyps are benign masses that can occur following a vocal fold mucosal injury, and cysts can form within the vocal folds underneath their lining. Papilloma are human papillomavirus-related lesions that also can occur in the larynx. Early signs of a lesion include persistent hoarseness, vocal fatigue, limitation of upper vocal range, and increased effort to speak.

•**Dysphonias.** *Dysphonia* is the general medical term for hoarseness and can be applied broadly to many types of voice problems. It is also part of the name of some voice disorders. *Muscle tension dysphonia* refers to voice problems due to excessive laryngeal muscle tension and suboptimal vocal biomechanics. *Spasmodic dysphonia* is a neurological condition characterized by involuntary spasmodic movements of vocal fold muscles. *Functional dysphonia* refers to dysphonia caused by disordered use of voice structures that are otherwise normal, and may be related to traumatic events, stress, or exposure to an irritant.

•**Vocal fold paralysis.** Affecting one or both vocal folds, paralysis indicates vocal fold immobility. If one is affected, then the voice is typically breathy, weak, or airy, and this is sometimes accompanied by trouble swallowing (*dysphagia*). Paralysis of both vocal folds often causes breathing problems due to narrowing of the airway. Causes of paralysis include accidental damage to the nerve supply to the vocal folds during surgery on nearby structures, or a tumor or other growth along one of those nerves. Some people recover on their own, while others require active treatment.

•**Larynx cancer.** A malignant lesion or cancer in the larynx can cause hoarseness and breathing or swallowing problems. Some other symptoms include pain when swallowing, ear pain, or coughing up blood-tinged secretions.

•**Neurological diseases.** A wide range of neurological disorders, such as Parkinson's disease, amyotrophic lateral sclerosis (ALS), or tremor, can affect the voice. Reduced voice strength and projection, abnormal articulation, or a shaky voice are possible symptoms.

WHEN TO SEE A DOCTOR

A voice disorder that persists for two to four weeks or gets progressively worse needs to be evaluated—particularly in a smoker or someone who has some of the associated symptoms discussed above. The specialists who diagnose voice disorders are otolaryngologists, also called ear, nose, and throat (ENT) doctors, and laryngologists, subspecialists who focus on the larynx and associated structures.

TREATMENT

Treatment depends on the nature of the problem and your vocal goals and needs. Voice disorders due to a typical viral laryngitis will usually resolve with supportive measures such as rest and fluids. Other types of infections or inflammation should improve with the appropriate medication prescribed or recommended by a doctor.

Vocal fold mucosal lesions, such as nodules, are believed to be rooted in voice behaviors, and are treated primarily with voice therapy by a speech pathologist. Voice therapy includes a variety of techniques that will be tailored to an individual patient and may include learning better voice hygiene and vocal mechanics—how to warm up, cool down, and use your voice in a biomechanically favorable way—to help heal the voice and vocal folds.

In fact, voice therapy is part of many treatment plans, especially when the voice disorder stems from how and how much you use your voice. A team approach to treatment that includes a speech pathologist with experience in the vocal arts can be particularly helpful when caring for a singer or other occupational or professional voice user. Because the principles of healthy voice use for singing can apply to speaking too, a care team with diverse voice-related backgrounds can help many types of patients.

Surgery is also used to treat some types of voice problems, alone or in conjunction with voice therapy or other medical treatments. Laryngeal surgery can be performed endoscopically, often incorporating an operating microscope and surgical laser. Some laryngeal surgical procedures can also be performed under local anesthesia using flexible endoscopes in the outpatient clinic. Open surgery through the neck is indicated for some laryngeal problems.

PREVENTION TIPS

With its beauty, strength, and ability to evoke and demonstrate emotion, your voice is part of your unique personality. Here's how to protect it.

•**Don't smoke.** Apart from all its other ills, smoking is the worst thing possible for your voice and the number-one risk factor for developing larynx cancer. Though the risks of vaping are still being investigated, my advice is also not to vape.

•**Use, don't abuse, your voice.** If you're a screamer or a yeller, you're putting a lot of strain on your voice-producing structures. The same is true if you continue to use your voice when it's already hoarse.

•**Hydrate.** Drinking water and noncaffeinated, nonalcoholic beverages is beneficial for your voice.

•**Use amplification.** For any type of public speaking, such as in an outdoor setting, auditorium, or in a gym where you will be inclined to push your voice, use a headset microphone so you can talk with a conversational intensity (without shouting) and yet reach your audience. A headset is ergonomically better than leaning over a microphone. Amplification devices and speakers built into classrooms (often

---

The Voice Box

The larynx is often called the voice box, a reference to what most people think of as its main purpose. *But it has three main functions, thanks to where it sits at the crossroads of your respiratory and digestive tracts…*

•**It prevents aspiration of food into your airway.**

•**It's the doorway to your trachea,** or windpipe, so it's involved in breathing.

•**Its two vocal folds (what many call the vocal cords) vibrate to create phonation, or voice production.**

Understandably, any problems with the larynx can affect the voice, breathing, and swallowing. Voice disorders can stem from a problem within the tissue structures themselves, but a voice disorder can also be a consequence of a medical condition elsewhere in the body.

---

with students in mind) are also very helpful for teachers.

•**Listen to your voice if it is complaining to you.** Just as a sore knee is a warning to back off on a running regimen, hoarseness is a sign that something is wrong, and your voice needs a break. If hoarseness persists, get evaluated by a specialist.

Possible Cause of Swallowing Difficulties

Brijen J. Shah, M.D., gastroenterologist, Mount Sinai Beth Israel Hospital, New York City.

Zenker's *diverticulum*—when the esophagus develops a pouch where it joins the pharynx (back of the throat) that traps bits of food during swallowing. In addition to problems with swallowing and the feeling that food is stuck in the throat, symptoms include choking, coughing, bad breath, and excessive throat-clearing after eating. Another danger is that trapped food released after eating can become aspirated into the lungs and cause pneumonia. Zenker's diverticulum is relatively uncommon and usually occurs in older people. It is diagnosed by endoscopy or X-ray and can be treated with minimally invasive surgery... or for people who are not good candidates for surgery, the condition can be managed by eating puréed foods slowly.

Stop the Drip of Postnasal Drip

Neil L. Kao, M.D., board-certified internist, allergist, and immunologist practicing in Greenville, South Carolina.

You might be surprised to know that we all have some degree of postnasal drip all the time—mucus dripping down the back of the nose into the throat. Your nose makes about a quart of the thick, wet substance a day to help trap and destroy bacteria and viruses before they cause infection. Under normal circumstances, it is barely noticeable.

But: It becomes a problem when there's too much mucus. Mucus is made up of protein and other chemicals that can irritate the tissues lining the nose and throat. It can collect in places below the throat, such as the esophagus and trachea...and it is particularly annoying when it pools next to your voicebox, causing you to feel like there is a lump in your throat and making your voice scratchy.

WHAT CAUSES MUCUS OVERLOAD

Sometimes extra mucus is a temporary reaction to eating a hot food or a spicy meal or when you exert yourself physically...or longer lasting when you have a cold.

Other causes are long-standing—you may have allergies or constantly breathe in dust if you work in construction, for instance. A bacterial infection and acid reflux or GERD also can lead to postnasal drip and should be treated appropriately. Unfortunately, sometimes just getting older is the cause.

SOLVING POSTNASAL DRIP

Trying to clear out mucus on your own can be challenging, but there are options. *You can try all of these at the same time or one at a time to see what works...*

•**Saline nasal rinses and sprays.** Products such as the NeilMed sinus-rinse kit and Navage for nasal lavage use water to wash out your nose.

How they work: With your head over a sink, water is poured in one nostril and drips out the other, clearing irritants.

Important: These products should be used with distilled or filtered water or saline solution, which some people find more soothing. A saline nasal spray such as Ayr also can help clear mucus by moistening the lining of the nose.

•**Mucus-thinning agents.** Mucinex oral tablets or liquid and other mucus-thinning products make mucus easier to clear, especially when you suction it out with a bulb syringe.

•**Gargling with very warm water** can help loosen mucus caught in the throat.

•**Other over-the-counter medications** to reduce secretions are helpful when allergies are the cause, specifically…

•Steroid nasal sprays, including Flonase, decrease inflammation and the allergic response.

•Antihistamines, such as Claritin, Benadryl, Allegra, Zyrtec, and Xyzal, work systemically. The "D" versions, such as Claritin-D and Allegra-D, include a decongestant, which reduces the amount of effort needed to inhale air through the nose. Always follow package directions to avoid overreliance.

Caution: Physicians do not recommend using OTC nasal decongestant sprays such as Afrin because of the high risk for addiction and rebound nasal congestion when the medicine wears off.

If you don't get relief within a few days, see a doctor—an ear, nose, and throat (ENT) specialist, allergist, or speech therapist can determine the true culprit and find a solution.

Caring for Chronic Sinusitis

Ahmad Sedaghat, M.D., associate professor of otolaryngology-head and neck surgery at the University of Cincinnati.

C hronic sinusitis is a common condition that affects up to one in 20 people in the United States. Yet many people who have it never get properly diagnosed because they blame their symptoms on something else—usually allergies. Getting an accurate diagnosis and the right treatments could help a lot of people breathe easier.

SIMILAR TO ASTHMA

Chronic sinusitis (or, more accurately, *rhinosinusitis*) is an inflammation of the nasal passages and sinuses that lasts for at least three months. The typical symptoms include facial pain or pressure, a congested or dripping nose, and a diminished sense of smell. Many people with chronic sinusitis also have nasal allergies, which can make symptoms worse. But the allergies aren't the underlying cause.

Unlike the acute attack of sinusitis you might get after a cold, chronic sinusitis isn't usually caused by infection. While people with chronic sinusitis can get sinus infections, their symptoms persist even when the infections are gone.

In fact, chronic sinusitis is a condition much like asthma. People with asthma have inflamed airways in their lungs that swell and produce excess mucus in response to a variety of triggers. People with chronic sinusitis have tissues in their nose and sinuses that overreact in much the same ways. Pollen, viruses, bacteria, or fungi might trigger the inflammation, but so might cigarette smoke or other forms of air pollution. And what causes problems in one person may not in someone else.

GETTING A DIAGNOSIS

If you feel like you have endless allergies or a cold that never quits, you might have chronic sinusitis. *The big tip-off is having at least two of these symptoms for at least three months…*

•**Facial pain or pressure.** Your sinuses are air-filled spaces in your forehead, cheeks, between your eyes, and deeper within your head. When the tissue lining those spaces swells and fills with mucus, pain and pressure can result, even if no infection is present.

•**Nasal congestion.** While congestion from a cold typically goes away in a few days and congestion from allergies often comes and goes with the seasons or other changes in your environment, this congestion persists.

•**A nose that drips,** either through your nostrils or down the back of your throat (post-nasal drip). In most cases, the mucus is not colored. If you do see green or yellow discharge, it's more likely you have a bacterial infection.

•**A weak sense of smell.** This also happens to people with some respiratory infections, including COVID-19. Whatever the cause, a lingering loss of smell can be a big deal, making your food less enjoyable and creating safety issues, since you might not smell smoke, hazardous fumes, or spoiled food.

In addition to these primary symptoms, some people with chronic sinusitis may cough because of post-nasal drip and feel pressure in their ears. Many people report poor sleep and fatigue or "brain fog."

WHAT TO EXPECT FROM THE DOCTOR

If your doctor suspects chronic sinusitis, you will need a test to confirm or rule out the diagnosis. One possibility is a CT scan, which can produce images of the inside of your head. The pictures can show any swelling inside your sinuses and whether you have polyps, noncancerous growths that can develop in inflamed sinuses and nasal passages. Not everyone with chronic sinusitis has polyps.

If you see an ear, nose, and throat doctor, you will likely get a different test: a nasal endoscopy. For this procedure, done in the doctor's office, a lighted scope will be passed up your nose so the doctor can get a good look at the nasal lining. Unless you've had sinus surgery, the scope won't fit through the narrow slits inside your nose that lead to your sinuses, but the doctor will be able to look for signs of inflammation, including thick mucus and any polyps in the area where the sinuses drain into the nose.

Also, the doctor will consider whether you might have other conditions linked with sinusitis. For example, some people with immune deficiencies are prone to sinusitis. So are people with forms of vasculitis, rarer conditions involving blood vessel inflammation.

GET RELIEF

If you do have chronic sinusitis, there are two easy things you can try that make most people feel better...

•**A nasal rinse, at least once a day.** Rinsing the nasal passages with a saltwater solution (see sidebar) has been shown in multiple studies to help relieve symptoms. The rinses help to clear mucus and may also reduce inflammation by removing irritants, such as pollen and dust, from the nose.

•**A corticosteroid nasal spray.** You can choose any brand or generic version sold over the counter, such as *fluticasone propionate* (Flonase), *triamcinolone* (Nasacort), or *budesonide* (Rhinocort). These sprays, which also treat allergies, help lower inflammation and reduce congestion and runny nose. (To

---

How to Rinse Your Nose

Nasal rinses are an effective treatment for chronic sinusitis, if you do them correctly. *A few guidelines...*

•**A little spritz from a tiny spray bottle is not enough.** Use at least a cup of fluid in a large squeeze bottle, bulb syringe, or a neti pot.

•**Most doctors recommend an *isotonic* saline solution,** which has the same salt concentration as your body. A *hypertonic* solution, which is saltier, may be more effective, but also more irritating. Recipes (combining iodine-free salt and baking soda) are easy to find, but it's worth buying premixed packets to make sure you get the right concentration. Add the mixes to distilled or boiled and cooled water.

•**Whether you use a bottle, syringe, or a pot,** bend over the sink (or in the shower) and gently squirt or pour the solution into one nostril at a time. Don't worry about whether the fluid comes out the opposite nostril; that's not possible for some people with blocked nasal passages.

---

increase effectiveness, lean forward so that you are looking toward the floor; then aim the spray up and slightly to the side, away from the center of the nose, and sniff lightly).

An increasingly used alternative: With a doctor's prescription, you can get a liquid corticosteroid that can be added to your saline rinse. This combo may help the steroid reach deeper into the affected sinuses.

Additional drugs might be used in some situations...

•**Corticosteroid pills, such as prednisone.** These might be used if you have polyps and severe symptoms. Because a steroid that affects your whole body can cause side effects such as sleeplessness and mood swings, they typically aren't prescribed for more than three weeks at a time.

•**Antibiotics.** If you have a flare-up caused by a bacterial infection, you might get a short course of antibiotics. In some cases, doctors

Pet Allergies May Worsen After a Vacation

If you leave your pet at home while traveling, you may experience a surge in allergy symptoms when you return. The so-called Thanksgiving Effect can cause you to develop a severe allergy to a family pet that you hadn't been allergic to before. To get back to normal, see an allergist to develop a treatment plan.

American Academy of Asthma, Allergy and Immunology.

prescribe a certain type, called *macrolide* antibiotics, for a longer time, not to fight infection but to control inflammation.

•**Biologics.** Several newer injected drugs that target parts of the immune system involved in inflammation have been approved for people who have chronic sinusitis with polyps. While the drugs can be effective, they are extremely expensive. Right now, they are used sparingly.

If you don't get relief from nasal rinses and medications, you might consider surgery. Using a scope inserted in your nose, a surgeon will remove any polyps and widen the openings of your sinuses to improve drainage and allow medications to better reach inflamed tissues. Surgery helps many people, but it's not a cure, so you should expect to continue medications and nasal rinses after your procedure.

Hay Fever Season May Get Worse

Study by researchers at University of Michigan, Ann Arbor, published in *Nature Communications*.

Predictions based on current trends of rising global temperatures and carbon dioxide levels show pollen season starting 40 days earlier…ending 19 days later…and being more intense by the end of this century. Annual pollen emissions could increase by as much as 40 percent.

Exercise and Summer Allergies

Melanie Carver, chief mission officer, Asthma and Allergy Foundation of America, Arlington, Virginia, quoted at AOL.com.

Avoid exercising in the early morning—that's when pollen counts generally are highest. Late afternoon and evening are better. *Watch the weather*—high heat and humidity can increase mold…and wind, humidity, and lightning during thunderstorms can break pollen into tiny particles that are easier to inhale. *Dress to fight allergies*—wear sunglasses and a hair covering to reduce the amount of pollen that gets into your hair and eyes…when you get back inside, remove all clothing and wash it…shower to rinse off any pollen lingering on your skin or hair.

Gas Ranges Can Be Bad for Your Health

Consumer Reports. ConsumerReports.org

Gas ranges emit nitrogen oxides inside homes at more than double the Environmental Protection Agency standard for outdoor air. Pollutants typically associated with power plants, cars, and trucks, nitrogen oxides can increase asthma risk in children and worsen lung diseases. Electric and induction ranges do not have harmful emissions.

If you already have a gas range: Create as much ventilation as possible—preferably with a range hood that you turn on every time you use the appliance. If you don't have a range hood, open windows and doors and use a fan to help clear the gases.

CHAPTER 18

Sleep and Restorative Health

Rise and Shine! Wake Up Feeling Energized

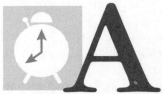

Are you getting enough sleep at night yet find yourself dragging the next afternoon or, worse, as you get out of bed in the morning? Getting restorative sleep revolves around being true to your chronotype, whether you're a morning person, a night owl or somewhere in between. And being energized revolves around your body type so you know when to move, when to rest, when to eat and how to boost your mood in ways that match your metabolism. We asked sleep expert Dr. Michael J. Breus how we can wake up energized. His most recent book, *Energize!*, is based on data from 5,000 people who served as part of his research.

DETERMINE YOUR CHRONOTYPE

The number-one cause of exhaustion is going against your chronotype.

Example: Forcing yourself to stay up late when your body really wants you in bed at 9 p.m. Ignoring your chronotype can cause a cascade of negative events, including sleep deprivation, chronic stress, mood disorders, and compromised health.

In addition to practicing good sleep hygiene—consistent sleep and wake-up times (even on weekends)…unplugging from blue-light–emitting devices an hour or two before bed…and stopping any alcohol three hours before bed—you should identify your chronotype and set your sleep schedule accordingly. Which chronotype do you fit into?

•**Lions are early risers—5:30 to 6 a.m.** Your body starts secreting the sleep-promoting hormone *melatonin* in mid-evening, which explains why you crave a 9 p.m. bedtime. Ideally you want at least seven-and-a-half hours of sleep.

Michael J. Breus, Ph.D., clinical psychologist in Los Angeles and sleep expert whose latest book is *Energize! Go from Dragging Ass to Kicking It in 30 Days*, coauthored with Stacey Griffith. TheSleepDoctor.com

Also: Lions tend to be introverts, so if you're exhausted by social situations, schedule alone time to recharge.

If you enjoy naps: 1 p.m. is the optimal nap time for you, and no more than 20 minutes.

•**Bears are in-betweeners.** Your wake-up time is about 7 a.m. Your body starts secreting melatonin around 10 p.m., so you're ready to sleep at 11 p.m. Aim for at least seven-and-a-half hours of sleep. Bears gain energy in social situations, so schedule three fun interactions each week. Keep naps under 20 minutes, starting at 2 pm.

•**Wolves are up at 8 a.m.** and don't climb into bed until 12:30 a.m. for their seven-hour sleep minimum. Self-care—being active and adequately rested—will help you stay on an even keel. Nap only if you can keep it between 10 and 20 minutes—and only before 2:15 p.m.

•**Dolphins are insomniacs, often up at 7 a.m.** Put off getting into bed until midnight and only if you're sleepy. If you're wired when you go to bed, you could set off an anxiety/insomnia cycle that will keep you up all night. Naps are counterproductive for dolphins, no matter how sleepy you feel during the day.

DETERMINE YOUR BODY TYPE

Your body shape is a good indicator of your metabolic rate and helps you schedule when to exercise and eat.

•**Endomorphs** are pear-shaped or curvy and have a slow metabolism. You tire quickly, so an effective exercise and weight-loss strategy is to do spurts of activity rather than long workouts.

Before You Start

Keep an energy journal for a week for self-discovery. Note how you feel when you wake up and go through the day, when you feel energized and when you're dragging. You'll pinpoint times of low energy and the circumstances—maybe it happens when you skip a meal or sit at your desk for too long…things you can then avoid.

•**Mesomorphs** are athletic and muscular with a medium metabolism. You gain energy when you push your limits but experience burnout or injury if you work too hard. Your best weight-loss strategy is to do a combination of cardio and strength training.

•**Ectomorphs** are lanky with a fast metabolism. You don't usually need a weight-loss strategy, but focus on building muscle for better endurance.

If you're not sure about your chronograph and body type, get help at MyEnergyQuiz.com.

YOUR POWER PROFILE

Add your metabolic speed—slow, medium, or fast—to your chronotype to get your "power profile," a portrait of your body, habits, and personality. Once you know if you're a Slow Lion or a Fast Wolf, for instance, you can follow your "power protocol"—a schedule that includes optimal times to eat, exercise, and sleep.

When to move—the daily 5×5: To create flexibility, stamina, strength, and balance, everyone benefits from five different kinds of movement for five minutes each at a particular time during the day—upon waking, mid-morning, afternoon, mid-evening, and before bed.

•**Stretch** when you wake up to lift your mood, improve brain function, and increase energy.

•**Shake,** with movements such as neck stretches, arm circles, leg swings, and trunk twists.

•**Bounce** with jumping jacks, burpees (an exercise that uses body weight for resistance), and skipping for a jolt of the feel-good hormones *dopamine* and *serotonin* and energizing *adrenaline*.

•**Build** to grow muscle for faster calorie burn and reduce risk for injury and age-related diseases. You can go equipment-free with squats, crunches, dips, kicks, and wall sits.

•**Balance** for improved coordination. Paired with deep breathing, you'll also get a calming effect from yoga moves such as tree pose and dancer—but avoid an inversion pose before bed because it will raise your heart rate.

How timing varies: Stretching in the morning and balance exercises before bed bookend the day for all chronotypes, but when to shake, bounce, and build varies by power profile...

- **Lions,** who are laser-focused early in the day, should shake it out midmorning...build in the afternoon...and bounce into a second wind when energy falls off in the evening.

- **Bears** should shake it out midmorning... bounce to reset in the afternoon...and build muscle in the evening.

- **Wolves** should bounce midmorning to clear away any brain fog...shake in the afternoon (usually after forgetting to move for hours)... and build in the evening when they are most energetic.

- **Dolphins** can bounce midmorning to wake the half of the brain that's still sleeping... build during peak energy in the afternoon... and shake off an evening spike in nervous energy.

Best times if you do set workouts...

Lions: 6 a.m., when your adrenaline is flowing...or wait until 5 p.m.

Bears: Before lunch or dinner to burn calories and prevent post-meal snacking.

Wolves: Before dinner—your peak performance time is 6 p.m.

Dolphins: 7 a.m. for a wake-up jolt. To improve sleep, weight train at 5 p.m. or do restorative yoga at 10 p.m.

WHEN AND WHAT TO EAT

Limiting the number of hours during which you eat—known as *intermittent fasting*—can make a difference in both energy levels and weight loss. Your body type determines your best fasting time frame—in all cases, stop eating at least three hours before lights out.

Ectomorph: Eat for 12 hours, and fast for 12 hours for optimal energy.

Mesomorph: Eat for 10 hours, and fast for 14 hours to be thinner and trimmer.

Endomorph: Eat for eight hours, and fast for 16 hours to help lose the pounds you're struggling with.

Caution: Anyone with an eating disorder should never practice intermittent fasting...and everyone else should check with their doctors before starting.

What you eat also influences sleep and energy...

Sleep-promoting foods: High-fiber vegetables, such as kale and broccoli, are great sources of *tryptophan*, a chemical that helps regulate *melatonin*. Mushrooms are rich in vitamin D as well as the B vitamins riboflavin and niacin. Leafy greens, fatty fish, quinoa, buckwheat, flax, chia and pumpkin seeds, legumes, nuts, avocado, and dark chocolate all have magnesium to help you maintain healthy levels of GABA, a neurotransmitter that promotes better sleep.

Sleep-disrupting foods: Beware of sugar—high intake is linked to lighter, less restorative sleep. The more sugar you eat, the more you crave, especially at night, and you'll wake up ravenous because poor sleep sends the hunger hormone *ghrelin* into overdrive.

Water–coffee conundrum: We lose about a liter of water every night while sleeping (more if you snore and have sleep apnea) as fluid is expelled with every breath. Start each day by drinking 16 ounces of water. Avoid anything with caffeine—tea or coffee—for the first 90 minutes after waking. Even decaf coffee and tea should be avoided. One or two cups of coffee a day, timed correctly, won't impact your sleep. But wait 90 minutes after waking—your *cortisol* and *adrenaline* levels are ramping up after you get up, and having caffeine immediately will make you jittery. Cut off caffeine after 3 p.m. so your body has time to clear it by evening.

YOUR EMOTIONAL ENERGY

Don't overlook drags on your emotional energy. Grappling with difficult people or situations or trying to force a feeling on yourself is draining.

Instead: Try to go with life's emotional ebbs and flows. Accepting your emotional fluctuations and those of others helps you gain energy from relationships. Do uplifting activities—laugh, listen to music, etc.

Music Before Bed Helps You Sleep Better

Study of 62 young adults by researchers at Singapore Management University, published in *Psychomusicology: Music, Mind, and Brain.*

According to a recent study, participants who listened for five days to happy music…five days to sad music… and five days to pink noise before bed found that both types of music improved sleep quality and feelings of well-being the next morning. Listening to pink noise did not show the same result.

Sleep Well for Good Health

Candice Seti, PsyD, clinical psychologist in private practice in San Diego, California. Visit her website at TheInsomniaTherapist.com

Most of us think of sleep as necessary for everyday refreshment and regeneration: If we don't get enough, we're tired the next day. But sleep does much more than recharge the body for daily activity: It protects health, too.

In a recent 10-year sleep study published in *Neurology*, researchers analyzed health data from nearly 500,000 people with an average age of 51. They found that those who had three symptoms of insomnia—trouble falling asleep or staying asleep, waking up too early in the morning, or trouble staying focused during the day due to poor sleep—were 18 percent more likely to have had a heart attack or stroke. *In fact, having even a single one of these three symptoms was associated with a higher risk…*

•**Trouble staying focused during the day increased risk by 13 percent.**

•**Trouble falling or staying asleep increased risk by 9 percent.**

•**Waking up too early in the morning and not getting back to sleep increased risk by 7 percent.**

Another study, published in the March 2020 issue of the *Journal of Neurology, Neurosurgery and Psychiatry*, analyzed data from more than 50 studies on sleep and cognition and found a significant link between poor sleep and a higher risk of cognitive decline and dementia.

GETTING A GOOD NIGHT'S SLEEP

Fortunately, there's a simple, straightforward, science-proven way to restore good sleep: cognitive behavioral therapy for insomnia (CBTI). Hundreds of scientific studies show that CBTI is effective in overcoming poor sleep by teaching you to change your thinking and your actions. Here are essential strategies from CBTI that you can use if you're sleeping poorly.

NEGATIVE SLEEP THOUGHTS

Acute insomnia is sleeping poorly for a night or two. Common causes include traveling, consuming caffeine late in the day, or a disruption to your regular sleep schedule. Whatever the cause, if you begin to believe you won't fall asleep quickly because you haven't slept well for a night or two—your negative sleep thoughts can turn acute insomnia into chronic insomnia. *Negative sleep thoughts come in many forms…*

•**I'm tired now, but I'm going to be wide awake in bed.**

•**I can't fall asleep unless I take a sleeping pill.**

•**I must get eight hours of sleep, or I won't be able to function tomorrow.**

•**I'm never going to fall asleep.**

Instead of believing these negative sleep thoughts, substitute thoughts that promote a rational sleep perspective…

•**Any sleep I get is better than none.**

•**If I stop checking the clock and relax instead, it's going to be better and I'll fall asleep faster.**

•**If I don't sleep well tonight, it's very likely I'll sleep well tomorrow.**

•**I've gotten a poor night's sleep before, and I've gotten through the next day.** I'll be fine.

SLEEP SCHEDULE

The body thrives on routine. Do the same relaxing thing every night at bedtime, whether it's reading, watching TV, listening to music, or taking a hot bath. Your body will associate those activities with falling asleep.

To sleep well, establish a sleep schedule: Go to bed and get up at the same time every day. If you sleep seven hours a night, the schedule could be 10 p.m. to 5 a.m., midnight to 7 a.m., or 2 a.m. to 9 a.m.—whatever works best for you.

Many people struggle to maintain a sleep schedule on the weekends, when they go to bed late and sleep in. This creates the common phenomenon of Sunday Night Insomnia. You've gotten up later than you usually do on Saturday and Sunday, so when you're trying to go to sleep at your scheduled time on Sunday night, your body isn't ready. That's because the neurotransmitter adenosine builds up in the brain every hour you're awake. As it rises, you experience drowsiness, heavy eyelids, and bodily warmth to help you sleep. When you get up later than usual, you don't have enough adenosine in your system at your scheduled bedtime.

The solution: Do your best to stick to your sleep schedule over the weekends, too.

Short naps are restorative, but naps longer than 30 minutes can impair your ability to sleep at night. And don't nap after 2 p.m., which can interfere with nighttime sleep.

BED IS FOR BEDTIME

Your brain associates certain spaces with certain activities. When you're in your office, it's time to work. When you're in your kitchen, it's time to eat. When you're in your bed, it's time to sleep. But if you use your bed to work, watch TV, talk on the phone, or play with your dog, your brain does not associate your bed with sleep—making it harder to fall asleep when you get in bed.

To optimize your bed as a sleep cue, get in bed only to go to sleep and get out of bed when you wake up. (Sex is the exception.) This will improve your sleep efficiency score—the percentage of time you sleep when you're in bed. Aim to be asleep for 90 percent of the time you're in bed.

Poor Sleep, Poor Health

Lack of sleep is punishing to the heart and brain because sufficient sleep—six to eight hours a night, with seven hours being the sweet spot for most people—is uniquely restorative, allowing the resting body to strengthen and repair. *But poor sleep affects the entire body and can complicate or cause many conditions…*

•**Diabetes.** Poor sleep imbalances blood sugar levels, putting you at higher risk of type 2 diabetes, which kills more than 100,000 Americans yearly. Sleep is such an important regulator of blood sugar that poor sleep by itself, with no other factor involved, can cause prediabetes.

•**Obesity.** The risk of obesity is worsened by poor sleep, which imbalances the satiety hormones that tell you when you're hungry and when you're full.

•**Immunity.** The immune system is weakened by poor sleep, making infection-fighting T cells less able to identify and kill invaders.

•**Psychiatric disorders.** Every major psychiatric condition is worsened by poor sleep, including clinical depression, bipolar disorder, anxiety disorders, post-traumatic stress disorder, psychotic disorders, and eating disorders.

•**Mental health.** Everyday emotions are also affected by poor sleep, which makes you less able to handle social and psychological stress.

An estimated 50 to 70 million Americans suffer from poor sleep—in many cases, because of stress and worry. All of us live in a nonstop world of constant information, pressure, and deadlines, with little or no downtime. Relentless stress generates high levels of the stress hormone cortisol, which raises core body temperature and heart rate, making restful sleep more difficult.

Are You Sleeping Poorly?

People often don't know the exact amount of time they sleep each night. Take this quiz to see if it's likely you need more sleep.

•**When you wake up in the morning, could you fall back asleep by 10 or 11 a.m.?** (*Yes = poor sleep*)

•**Can you function optimally without caffeine before noon?** (*No = poor sleep*)

•**If you didn't set an alarm, how much longer would you sleep?** (*1 hour or more = poor sleep*)

•**Do you frequently read the same passage over and over again without assimilating it?** (*Yes = poor sleep*)

If you had a "poor sleep" answer to two or more questions, it's likely a lack of sleep is hurting your health.

If you find yourself awake in the middle of the night, practice what sleep experts call the 20-20 rule. Get out of bed after 20 minutes of wakefulness and spend 20 minutes in a side chair or couch before getting back into bed. This ensures that you won't associate your bed with wakefulness.

Finally, keep your bedroom dark and quiet, the ideal conditions for sleep. Again, the most important factor in sleeping well is consistency. For consistent levels of darkness, wear an eye mask. For consistent levels of quiet, wear earplugs.

BLUE LIGHT

The "blue light" wavelength from screens such as smartphones, computers, and TVs suppresses the production of melatonin, the hormone that helps control the sleep-wake cycle. If you use your phone before bedtime (but not in bed!), turn on the blue light filter. If you use your computer or watch TV in the hours before bedtime, consider wearing a pair of glasses that block blue light.

SLEEPING PILLS

Sleeping pills are problematic for several reasons. They sedate the brain so that you can get to sleep, but the sleep you get isn't natural: It's disrupted, with less restorative deep sleep and dreaming (REM) sleep.

There's also the issue of psychological dependence: If you take a sleeping pill every night, you start to believe that you can't sleep without it—whether that belief is true or not.

ALCOHOL AND CAFFEINE

Alcohol helps you fall asleep, but it doesn't help you stay asleep or achieve deep, high-quality, restorative sleep. That's because once the alcohol is metabolized, you wake up and can find yourself tossing and turning all night, unable to get to the deeper, restorative layers of sleep. It takes three to four hours to metabolize alcohol, so stop drinking alcoholic beverages four hours before bedtime.

Caffeine works, in part, by blocking adenosine, the neurotransmitter that induces sleepiness. That's great for earlier in the day, but problematic in the evening. Like napping, don't ingest caffeine after 2 p.m. If a 2 p.m. cup of coffee interferes with sleep, stop even earlier.

EXERCISE

Exercising any time during the day helps you get to sleep at bedtime. But because exercise raises body temperature, it can be problematic for sleep if you exercise two to three hours before bedtime. Exercise earlier in the day—ideally, the same time every day.

MEDICAL CARE

Many medical conditions can interfere with sleep, such as sleep apnea, restless legs syndrome, hyperthyroidism, prostate problems, and chronic pain. If you suspect that a medical problem is causing your insomnia, talk to your doctor.

GET MORNING LIGHT

If you get a good dose of sunlight in the morning, you'll suppress melatonin—which will build up later in the day, helping you sleep. There are many ways to get morning sunlight. Exercise outside. Sit on your patio and sip a cup of tea. And don't wear your sunglasses—unfiltered sunlight has to go in through your eyeball to suppress melatonin.

Conquer Insomnia Now

Aric A. Prather, Ph.D., professor of psychiatry and behavioral sciences and practicing psychologist at the Neuro/Psych Sleep Clinic at University of California, San Francisco. He is author of *The Sleep Prescription: Seven Days to Unlocking Your Best Rest*. UCSFHealth. org/providers/aric-prather

Tossing, turning, thoughts racing—insomnia has become widespread since the pandemic. In fact, more than 60 percent of people report an increase in trouble falling and staying asleep, according to the *Journal of Sleep Research.*

If you are among them, you likely have tried all the popular methods for better sleep, including going to bed at the same time every night and/or taking an over-the-counter supplement or even a prescription medication. Some people even try monitoring their sleep patterns with a phone app.

Renowned sleep scientist Aric A. Prather, Ph.D., says these tips and tricks don't address the real culprit—*you*. Your stress and anxiety over sleep—or actually, *not* sleeping—may be what's interfering with your ability to get your shut-eye. What's more, your angst often leads you to do things that make sense in the short term but end up undermining how your sleep naturally works.

Dr. Prather, a practicing clinician who has helped hundreds of sleep-clinic patients, spoke to us about the cognitive behavioral therapy techniques he uses, as well as some unconventional strategies that you should be trying...

YOU ARE BUILT FOR SLEEP

Sleep isn't something you do as much as it is something that *happens* to you. *Two powerful biological mechanisms that guide the process of falling and staying asleep are at work in your body...*

•**Homeostatic sleep pressure** is a buildup of neurochemicals such as *adenosine* that are byproducts of the brain's activity and that increase the longer you are awake.

•**Circadian rhythms** are more nuanced. They are a "master clock" reliant on environmental cues such as natural light. Through the buildup and release of hormones and proteins, circadian rhythms track cellular functions and allow your body to anticipate and respond to physiological needs such as sleep.

These two biological cycles are influenced by all kinds of external factors, including stimulants (think sugar and caffeine), exercise, temperature, social interactions...and rumination. Not surprisingly, ruminating in bed at night—when your mind starts racing with anxious thoughts—can profoundly disrupt your internal cycles and compromise your ability to sleep.

But there are things you can do to influence your homeostatic sleep pressure and circadian rhythms in positive ways and to avoid rumination.

DURING THE DAY

Get up at the same time every day. Most people with insomnia think the key is going to bed at the same time each night, but this scenario involves forcing yourself to fall asleep, which just creates more anxiety.

Better: It is much easier to control when you wake up, and it helps regulate and stabilize your ability to grow tired and sleep at the end of the day. You don't have to suddenly become an early bird—choose a wake-up time that you can consistently maintain both on workdays and weekends. It should realistically suit your life and allow an ideal amount of sleep time for you each night (most adults should plan for seven hours).

•**Load-manage your stress.** Many people go full tilt all day and into the evening, then try to unwind just before heading to bed. It's challenging to work off that pent-up stress, and that is why you are so restless when you turn off the lights.

Better: Keep your overall stress levels manageable by taking five five-to-10-minute microbreaks throughout the day. Each break should be screen-free and phone-free. You can use the time to meditate, take a walk, talk to a friend, listen to a podcast, and/or garden.

•**Worry early.** Days can be so busy that it's easy to distract yourself from worrying and save it all up for when you climb into bed.

Better: Set aside 15 minutes during the mid- to late afternoon for "emotional worry" time. Set a timer, and give yourself the freedom to fret about whatever is bothering you most. Don't try to come up with solutions to your problems. The goal is to give your pesky thoughts free rein. Jot them down on a piece of paper. When the timer goes off, discharge your thoughts by crumpling up the paper and throwing it in the trash before you go on with your day. Then if you do start to ruminate in bed, tell yourself, *I'll save this stuff for tomorrow and obsess over it in my next emotional worry session.*

•**Stick your head in the freezer.** We often hit a valley of low energy in midafternoon—that is a preprogrammed part of our circadian rhythms. And we commonly turn to coffee or napping, but these fixes can compromise sleep later on that night.

Better: Give yourself a mild physical shock. Cold jump-starts the nervous system, raises your heart rate, and makes you more alert. If you can't easily put your head in the freezer, fill a sink with cold water and immerse your face or forearms for 15 seconds.

DURING THE EVENING

Set an alarm to go off two hours before you go to sleep. By mid-evening—when the retinal cells in your eyes start to process the dimming of natural light in your environment—your body's pineal gland starts producing the hormone *melatonin.* That's when you should move into wind-down mode. Wrap up your work, e-mail, and to-do lists. Keep artificial lights low. Try especially hard to avoid the stimulus-reward loop of social media and phone apps—they seem relaxing but actually are designed to stoke your attention and can cause a rise in the stress hormone *cortisol,* which provides an energy boost and keeps you up. *Instead…*

•**Focus on wind-down activities that are relaxing and tranquil.**

Suggestions: Reading…knitting…bathing or showering, which promotes sleep by cooling your core body temperature as the water evaporates from your skin afterward…and watching TV, but skip the nail-biter dramas and stick with reruns of TV sitcoms you've enjoyed watching before.

•**Make your bed a haven.** Avoid doing wind-down activities there. Don't climb into bed until your eyelids are heavy and you want to sleep. The idea is to break the association between your bed and your wakefulness and angst. Think about it—you wouldn't sit at the dinner table for hours waiting to get hungry.

WHEN YOU ARE LYING IN BED

•**If your mind starts to race, slow it with measured breathing.** Focusing on and controlling your breath is a basic way to influence how you feel and think.

Resource: Through its app and online content offerings, Headspace.com offers meditation and relaxation instructions that are geared to helping you sleep.

Cost: 14-day free trial…then about $12.99 a month.

•**Stand on the platform, and watch the trains go by.** This meditative technique can be used to disengage from rumination. If you experience intrusive, troublesome thoughts, envision them as train cars rumbling by while you observe them from the safety of the platform. Don't get on the train because it will take you to places you don't want to go. Instead, watch the cars with curiosity as they move past and down the track out of sight.

•**If you don't fall asleep after 20 minutes, get out of bed.** Transition back to your wind-down activities until you feel sleepy again. The idea is to let your homeostatic sleep pressure continue to build. Some people worry that getting up will be stimulating, but if you can't sleep, you are already awake and mentally aroused. Continuing to lie there and struggle just reinforces the wrong associations with your bed.

•**If you wake up in the middle of the night, the same "rules of bed" apply.** If you can't return to sleep quickly, get up and resume wind-down activities.

Caution: If you are older and/or have chronic pain, it may not be easy or safe to move around your home in the middle of the night. In that case, at least sit all the way up in bed to make it clear to your body that you are no longer in sleep mode. Or try what I used to do as a kid—turn yourself around so your head is at the bottom of the bed and your feet near your pillow. I used to read like that until I got sleepy, then I returned to my normal sleep position.

If you have a spouse or partner: Accommodating your partner can make it hard to implement the above strategies.

Example: Getting up whenever you can't sleep might disturb the other person.

Suggestion: Sleep apart for a few weeks if you are suffering from insomnia. Do your reconditioning in a guest room if you have one. If that's too disruptive, try more creative solutions.

Example: One patient set up a comfy space in the living room with his wife that became their "before bed" nook. They shared quality time there, then each partner went off to the bedroom to sleep when he/she grew tired.

What You Eat Can Help or Hurt Your Sleep

Carrie Ali, editor, *Bottom Line Health*.

If you're struggling to sleep, it could be time to change your diet. Researchers at Columbia University Vagelos College of Physicians and Surgeons reported in the *American Journal of Clinical Nutrition* that there's a link between high-glycemic foods and the risk of developing insomnia.

The glycemic index (GI) assigns values to foods based on how rapidly they increase blood sugar. Foods are categorized as low (≤55), intermediate (56–69), or high (≥70) on a 100-point scale. When we eat low- or intermediate-glycemic foods, blood sugar rises gradually and the body releases insulin to balance the glucose. High-glycemic foods, however, set off a roller-coaster reaction. Blood sugar soars to a high level in what's called *postprandial* (after a meal) *hyperglycemia* (high blood sugar). To compensate, the body releases a large burst of insulin that can lower blood sugar too much too quickly. If blood sugar drops below about 70 milligrams per deciliter, the brain doesn't

have enough glucose, its primary fuel, so the body releases adrenaline and the stress hormone cortisol. Release of those counterregulatory hormones can cause heart palpitations, tremors, cold sweats, anxiety, irritability, and hunger. If that's not enough to disrupt sleep, high-GI diets can also cause an inflammatory immune response that inhibits sleep, as well as intestinal dysbiosis.

While high-GI foods appeared to increase insomnia risk in this study, foods such as whole grains, vegetables, and whole fruits—but not juices—lowered it. Although fruit is full of natural sugar, its fiber helps prevent blood sugar spikes.

While this study focused on postmenopausal women, the authors speculated that the findings are likely universal. For anyone struggling with insomnia, replacing high-GI foods with minimally processed, whole ones—including carbohydrates like whole grains and sweet fruit—could provide some relief.

Get the Restorative Benefits of Sleep While You're Awake

Sara C. Mednick, Ph.D., cognitive neuroscientist and professor of psychology in the department of cognitive sciences at University of California, Irvine, and author of *The Power of the Downstate: Recharge Your Life Using Your Body's Own Restorative Systems* and *Take a Nap! Change Your Life.* Dr. Mednick is director of the UC Irvine Sleep and Cognition (SaC) Lab. SaraMednick.com

As a neuroscientist and director of the Sleep and Cognition Lab at the University of California, Irvine, Sara C. Mednick, Ph.D., would never tell you to skimp on sleep. The seven to eight hours you spend in bed every night are the ultimate restorative journey, as your brain leaves conscious thought behind and begins sorting through the day's clutter. Memories are consolidated…energy stores replenished…hormone levels regulated…and much of the cellular wear and tear that naturally occurs during 16 or so hours of living is repaired.

But what if Dr. Mednick told you that you could reap those benefits during the day while you're awake? That in addition to sleep, you can rejuvenate your brain, heart, muscles, and more by exercising a certain way…eating a certain way…breathing a certain way? You can do that by tapping into the power of your body's restorative systems using the *downstate*.

INTRODUCING YOUR DOWNSTATE

Healthy brains are surprisingly active during sleep, switching on and off in one-second periods called *upstates*, when brain activity is high… and *downstates* when it's low. Sleep researchers believe that sleep's restorative benefits emerge from these lightning-fast downstates.

Dr. Mednick has taken the sleep research concept of restorative sleep that takes place during deep, non-rapid eye movement (NREM) sleep and flipped it on its head to describe any time deep rejuvenation takes place. The average person's upstate is when life activities require energy, focus, action, and mobilization of mental and physical energy…and so the downstate is when our metaphorical tanks are refilled. That recharging takes place during meditation, while spending time in nature, while engaging in heart-pumping exercise, and while spending quality time with loved ones. These healthy activities trigger hormonal and chemical cascades similar to the ones that occur during deep sleep.

Downstate-boosting activities promote *autonomic balance*—a healthy balance between the sympathetic nervous system (the fight-or-flight response that kicks in not just during moments of stress but whenever we think or act)…and the parasympathetic nervous system (the rest-and-digest system that calms us, decreases inflammation, and supports mental and emotional processing). Modern-day life—full of work pressures, family responsibilities, and general stress—has most people tipped into autonomic imbalance. Their sympathetic branch revs all day long and even at night, with little time spent in rejuvenation mode. This imbalance is responsible for the lion's share of premature aging, including deteriorating memory and immunity, heart disease, obesity, and more.

Anytime you engage in an activity that balances your autonomic nervous system, you are harnessing the power of the downstate. *Examples…*

•**Exercise.** During a challenging workout, your sympathetic nervous system revs up, increasing heart rate, powering muscles and more. After the workout, the parasympathetic system takes over to reverse those processes and bring you back to baseline—your heart rate slows, temperature drops, and muscles relax. This parasympathetic recovery floods cells with restorative nutrients…lowers levels of the stress hormone *cortisol*…and triggers production of *brain-derived neurotrophic factor* (BDNF) and other neuroprotective hormones that stimulate the growth of new brain cells.

•**Deep breathing.** You've likely heard that deep breathing helps relieve stress, but breathing in a specific way—about 10 to 12 seconds per breath, five to six breaths per minute—not only is relaxing, it also promotes autonomic balance by stimulating the *vagus nerve*, the conductor of the orchestra that is our parasympathetic nervous system.

SECRET WEAPON FOR HEALTHY AGING

Regular exercise and slow, deep breathing also balance the autonomic nervous system by improving *heart-rate variability* (HRV), the amount of variation between heartbeats. Most people think the heart beats like a metronome, with the exact same amount of milliseconds between beats. But there's variation, and that's a good thing. People who have high HRV, which is desirable, have *more* variation when it comes to the timing between heartbeats, although the variation is subtle. This sign of autonomic balance is linked with everything from enhanced memory and stress management to reduced rates of heart disease, diabetes, and obesity. Unfortunately, HRV diminishes as we age. The timing between heartbeats becomes more uniform. That is indicative of the body becoming less tolerant of stress and is linked with many chronic health conditions. *It happens for several reasons…*

•**The 50-and-older set is significantly less likely to dedicate time to downstate-regulating activities.** In a 2021 study by researchers at Florida Atlantic University, 55 percent of adults over age 60 said that they were less physically active than they had been two to three years prior. And 40 percent of Americans over age 75 are entirely inactive.

•**Older adults spend less time in nature.** Most US adults spend five or fewer hours a week in nature.

•**And they spend more time alone.** Nearly one-quarter of adults ages 65 and up are considered socially isolated.

Statistics like these are the main reason that aging seems to come with dramatic dips in physical, mental and cognitive functioning—people stop taking proactive steps to stimulate their downstate.

Not only do older adults tend to stop engaging in these daytime downstate activities, but their sleep quality suffers with every passing year. Once people hit their 40s, the time spent in *slow wave sleep* (SWS) naturally reduces. This is unfortunate because all the vital processes occur during SWS. Stress hormones pause while growth hormone and other hormones critical for muscle, organ and tissue repair, immune and metabolic function, and inflammation control are released. The parasympathetic nervous system is never as strong as it is during SWS, which is why so much restoration happens here in our 20s and 30s… only to peter out as we get older.

Good news: Engaging in downstate activities during the day can help make up for the natural loss in SWS.

Recent study: Young people and seniors were hooked up to electrodes to measure their brain activity and HRV as they move through the stages of sleep. In healthy young adults, there are giant increases in parasympathetic activity as they move from lighter to deeper sleep, and their HRV skyrockets. But in participants age 60 and up, there's basically a flatline between their waking HRV and sleeping HRV. Simply by virtue of age, they fail to have any meaningful downstate recovery while they sleep.

FIVE WAYS TO BOOST YOUR HRV

Sleep is the ultimate downstate supporter. *But here are other ways to improve your HRV and show your downstate some love during waking hours…*

•**Exercise for 30 minutes at least three times a week.** Make your workouts challenging—an easy walk won't boost sympathetic activity enough to initiate a significant parasympathetic rebound. Schedule these workouts for the mornings—that gives your nervous system the time it needs (about a day) to fully recover, leading to HRV benefits.

•**Stop eating by 8 p.m.** Our digestive organs prefer to be in rest-and-digest mode overnight. Snacking at 10 p.m kickstarts your sympathetic nervous system. This is why eating late at night makes it tricky to fall asleep—you are asking your energy-production centers to power on, even though you want your brain to power off.

•**Limit eating to 12, 10, or even eight hours a day.** When you shorten your eating window to 12 hours or less (for example, 7 a.m. to 6 p.m. or 9:30 a.m. to 7:30 p.m.), you expand that recovery time, improving HRV and restoring autonomic balance. Twelve hours of eating a day is attainable. Try it, and, after a week, reduce the window by one hour until you reach eight hours of eating a day. This way of eating is called *intermittent fasting* or *time-restricted eating.*

•**Connect with nature several times a week.** Over the past several hundred years, people have gradually shifted from working outside on farms and in fields toward a more sedentary life in offices and homes. Today, the average American spends more than 90 percent of his/her time indoors. Yet, study after study shows that more time spent in Mother Nature's company leads to improvements in HRV. It also lowers stress levels (by flooding the body with calming, feel-good hormones) and improves immune function by increasing intake of *phytoncides*, aromatic plant compounds released by trees and other plants that trigger production of immune-supportive white blood cells.

•**Partner up.** Intimacy promotes autonomic balance by making you feel cared for, safe and part of a community, all of which are known to tip autonomic balance in the right direction. Romantic or sexual intimacy works (anything from holding hands to having sex), as does platonic friendship, spending time with loved ones, and even caring for a pet.

Sound Sleep Isn't What You Think

Mouse study by researchers at the University of Copenhagen, Denmark, published in *Nature Neuroscience*.

Many people believe that a night's sleep should be uninterrupted, but sleep is not a constant state.

Recent finding: The neurotransmitter *noradrenaline*, a stress hormone, causes the brain to wake up more than 100 times a night. But the awakenings—called micro-arousals—are so brief that sleepers don't notice them. These awakenings reset the brain so it can store memory during sleep. That means these micro interruptions to sleep are a sign of sleeping well.

Drinks That Keep You Up... Or Help You Sleep

Drinks that keep you up: Alcohol may cause you to fall asleep faster but interferes with sleep in the second half of the night. An after-dinner espresso, hot cocoa, and green tea may sound relaxing, but they contain the stimulant caffeine. Sugary drinks such as soda, fruit drinks, especially with added sugar, and sports drinks tend to stimulate the body and may contain caffeine.

Sleep-inducing drinks: Herbal teas such as holy basil, valerian, passionflower, and chamomile...a turmeric latte made with warm milk, which contains the sleep-promoting amino acid *tryptophan*, and spiced with nutmeg, clove and/or cinnamon for an anti-inflammatory boost...fruit-infused water...unsweetened tart cherry juice...beverages containing ashwagandha, an herb that has been shown to reduce levels of the stress hormone cortisol.

Health.com

When Sleep Isn't Refreshing

Chris Iliades, M.D., retired ear, nose, throat, head, and neck surgeon who now dedicates his time to educating patients through writing.

Insomnia is the most common sleep disorder, affecting about 10 percent of Americans, the American Sleep Association reports. Another 30 percent of Americans complain of excessive daytime sleepiness (EDS)—a condition that is so common that it is considered to be a major public health problem. EDS causes one out of five motor vehicle accidents, decreased work production, and many work-related injuries.

For most people with EDS, sleepiness is caused by not getting enough sleep. But for about 5 percent of us, it strikes even after a good night's sleep. This condition is called *hypersomnia*, and it can be a major quality-of-life issue. Hypersomnia can be a symptom of another disease, or it can be a condition on its own.

PRIMARY HYPERSOMNIA

When it is not caused by another condition, it is called primary hypersomnia. It is usually diagnosed between the ages of 17 and 24 and remains a long-term condition after diagnosis. There are three known types of primary hypersomnia: narcolepsy, idiopathic hypersomnia, and Kleine-Levin syndrome. The best known and most common cause is narcolepsy.

•**Narcolepsy** is a brain disease caused by not having enough of a brain messenger (neurotransmitter) called *hypocretin*. This messenger helps control sleeping and waking cycles. About 75 percent of people with narcolepsy have a symptom not seen in other types of hypersomnia called *cataplexy*. Cataplexy is a complete and sudden loss of muscle tone that causes a person to collapse. It can be triggered by strong emotions. Another symptom of narcolepsy is vivid dreams or hallucinations and an inability to move just before falling asleep.

The most common treatment for narcolepsy is *modafinil* (Provigil). A drug called sodium oxybate is added to treat people with cataplexy.

Idiopathic primary hypersomnia is less common. The word *idiopathic* means unknown cause. When it was first diagnosed in the 1950s, it was called sleep drunkenness. People with this type of primary hypersomnia have normal brain hypocretin levels. Part of the cause may be abnormal genes passed down through families, since about 40 percent of people with this condition have a family history.

Idiopathic hypersomnia may also respond to stimulant drugs. The FDA recently approved another medication for this condition called Xywav, which includes the minerals calcium and magnesium along with the cataplexy drug sodium oxybate.

•**Kleine-Levin syndrome is very rare.** The cause is unknown. People with this syndrome have periods of prolonged sleep lasting up to 20 hours. They only wake up to eat. When they wake up, they may be very hungry and may have strange personality changes. This condition has also been called hibernation or sleeping-beauty syndrome. Prolonged sleep periods usually last about 10 days and recur about every three months. Between attacks, these people return to normal sleep and behavior. Attacks may be triggered by drinking alcohol or by an infection, and they tend to become less frequent with older age.

Kleine-Levin syndrome does not have any approved drug treatment. Since the condition comes and goes, affected people may just have a doctor's note allowing them to miss work or school during periods of prolonged sleep. The medication lithium may decrease the frequency of sleeping episodes for some people, and steroids may shorten the episodes.

SECONDARY HYPERSOMNIA

When hypersomnia is caused by another disease, such as sleep apnea, drug or alcohol abuse, hypothyroidism, Parkinson's disease, a brain tumor, brain trauma, or depression, it's called secondary hypersomnia. In these cases, hypersomnia can occur at any age and usually goes away when the underlying disease is treated. Until the cause can be controlled, people may be treated with modafinil.

Symptoms of Hypersomnia

•**Excessive daytime sleepiness** despite getting at least seven hours of sleep

•**Falling asleep several times every day** or sleeping more than nine hours at night and having sleep drunkenness during the day

•**Slowed thinking and poor memory**

•**Anxiety, restlessness, or irritability**

•**Depression**

•**Frequent headaches**

•**Lack of energy**

For a hypersomnia diagnosis, these symptoms must occur at least three times per week for at least three months and interfere with a person's quality of life, causing problems at work, school, or home.

All people with hypersomnia can benefit from mental health support, exercise, planned naps, and avoiding stimulants such as nicotine, caffeine, and alcohol. Sleep hygiene is also important. Sleep hygiene means setting regular hours for sleeping and waking, relaxing before sleeping, and keeping the bedroom dark and quiet.

Hypersomnia is a common problem that can be difficult to live with. It can even be dangerous if you have a sleep attack or cataplexy while driving or going down a staircase. It can interfere with your ability to function normally. Talk to your doctor if you have EDS or other symptoms of hypersomnia. Diagnosing the type of hypersomnia and getting on the best treatment can help control this condition and improve your quality of life.

Media Use Before Bed Can Be Good for Sleep

Study by researchers in College of Arts and Sciences, University at Buffalo, New York, published in *Journal of Sleep Research*.

Most reports say using media just before bed—such as watching TV or playing video games—can make it harder to fall asleep.

Recent finding: Watching a streaming service or listening to a podcast before bed can be a passive, calming activity that makes sleep better.

Also: Use just before bed of traditional media—TV, radio, video games, and books—is associated with more total sleep time, as long as the media use lasts a relatively short time (no more than an hour) and you are not multitasking.

Short Sleepers May Be Shielded from Sleep-Related Cognitive Problems

University of California, San Francisco.

People with familial natural short sleep (FNSS), the preference to sleep for just four to six hours per night, may be immune to the neurodegenerative effects of sleep loss. Researchers note that in people with FNSS, the brain efficiently accomplishes its needed sleep tasks in a shorter time. FNSS runs in families and is associated with five known genes.

A New Type of Vacation for Wellness

Susie Ellis, leading authority on wellness trends. She is chair and CEO of the nonprofit Global Wellness Institute, the industry's leading global research and educational resource, and cofounder, chair and CEO of the Global Wellness Summit, an organization that facilitates collaboration amongst industry thought leaders. GlobalWellnessInstitute.org

Is it time for a wellness vacation—one where you spend time destressing and focusing on your mental and physical well-being? According to recent research from the Global Wellness Institute, wellness travel is an estimated $816 billion market and is expected to explode to $1.1 trillion by 2025.

During the decade before the pandemic, people had already started rethinking what they wanted from travel, questioning the century-old model of indulging in excessive food and alcohol and getting too little sleep at tourist-crushed destinations. Today, these manic getaways are being replaced by slower, more mindful experiences, with health and safety front and center.

ENTER THE WELLNESS VACATION

Today's wellness resorts offer healthy food, ultra-comfortable bedding, soft lighting, and well-filtered air and water. These properties have wellness built into their DNA, including fitness activities such as yoga, tai chi, hiking and biking…relaxation and meditation practices…spa treatments…and culinary classes and nutrition counseling. Some even offer medical testing and counseling. And many are situated on large pieces of land that allow for social distancing and vigorous outdoor activities.

Many wellness resorts are all-inclusive and have a variety of activities scheduled for every hour of the day. But that doesn't mean you have to engage in strenuous physical activity if you don't want to. You can take relaxation classes, lounge by the pool and book spa services to boost your health.

Benefits: A Cedars-Sinai Hospital study revealed that a 45-minute massage significantly reduces levels of stress hormones and strengthens immunity. Other research has found that massage therapy, mudpacks, and mineral-water baths can lower blood pressure, and heart rate, as well as relieve head, back, and neck pain.

WHERE TO GO

Wellness resorts (also called "destination spas") are found throughout the U.S. and the world. You can go for a day, a few days, a week or more. Many can be booked for extended stays (so-called wellness sabbaticals), and there is a trend toward residences and second homes attached to wellness resorts.

What about price? A wellness vacation can be expensive, given the luxury accommodations, fitness and stress-reducing programs, farm-to-table cuisine, and spa services. But the cost can be comparable to visiting Disney World with the family or a trip to Europe.

Some notable properties in the US…

• **Canyon Ranch—Lenox, Massachusetts …Tucson, Arizona…Las Vegas…and Woodside, California.** One of the original spa resorts, Canyon Ranch was created with wellness in mind. Guests can select from 14 pathways that include personalized services based on wellness intentions.

Examples: Optimize your health and habits…age well and live longer…reach a healthy weight. You also can book a medical-based immersive experience called "Pathways Plus," that revolves around a battery of diagnostic services to zero in on targeted health improvements. CanyonRanch.com

• **Miraval Resorts—Lenox, Massachusetts …Tucson, Arizona…Austin, Texas.** Another pioneering spa resort, now owned by Hyatt Hotels, Miraval Resorts helps guests create a balanced life. Each property reflects its location. The Massachusetts resort is situated amidst the Berkshire Mountains and offers hiking and biking alongside wooded and lakeside trails, kayaking and paddleboarding, and cross-country skiing. Miraval is well-known for its equine therapy, a mindfulness experience involving horses. MiravalResorts.com

• **The Lodge at Woodloch, Hawley, Pennsylvania.** A luxurious spa resort, The Lodge at Woodloch is in the Pocono Mountains, just over two hours from New York City. Activities include hiking…kayaking or paddleboarding on a small pond…biking…relaxing under a hydromassage waterfall…doing a hot-cold room circuit to boost circulation…creating art…or taking a cooking class. TheLodgeAt Woodloch.com

• **Chateau Elan Winery and Resort, Braselton, Georgia.** This unique North Georgia resort, also a winery, features a chateau-style inn that overlooks 3,500 acres of vineyards, hills, and forests. You can play golf or tennis… take holistic wellness classes such as meditation and yoga…hike and bike. Afternoon tea, picnics, and fireside s'mores are always on the menu, and there are several restaurants on the property. ChateauElan.com

• **Destination Kohler, Kohler, Wisconsin.** The Kohler plumbing company is well-known for its Kohler Waters Spas, featuring hydrotherapy treatments such as water-based massages, Vichy rod showers (vertical bars that pour warm water over your body as you lay on a massage table), and therapeutic bathing pools. Accommodations available at the main property in Wisconsin range from three- to five-star hotels. Golf, yoga, indoor cycling, and fitness classes are signature offerings. Kohler Waters Spas also are located in Lincoln Park and Burr Ridge, Illinois…Green Bay, Wisconsin…and St. Andrews, Scotland. DestinationKohler.com

• **Lake Austin Spa Resort, Texas.** This secluded resort—just 40 rooms—is in the Texas Hill Country 30 minutes from Austin. The focus is on lake activities, including boating, kayaking and paddleboarding…and floating yoga, stretching, and meditation classes. All of the traditionally styled rooms have views of the lake. Pets are allowed. LakeAustin.com

• **The Ranch Malibu, California.** This West Coast 200-acre resort was voted *Travel & Leisure*'s #1 destination spa in the U.S. for 2022. The strict group-oriented program includes daily four-hour hikes, guided low-impact exercise classes, massages, and plant-based meals. The Ranch Private program can be tailored to meet your fitness levels. The resort limits the number of guests to just 25 per stay…a minimum seven-day stay is required running from Sunday to Saturday. There is no cell phone service, nor are there TVs in rooms and Wi-Fi access is limited. The Ranch Italy (which offers four-day stays) takes place at the medical-wellness retreat Palazzo Fiuggi, a historic property less than 50 minutes from Rome. TheRanchMalibu.com

MODERATELY PRICED RESORTS

• **Le Monastère des Augustines, Québec City, Québec, Canada.** A monastery hidden in the middle of Old Québec that is now a wellness center, Le Monastère welcomes people of all faiths, cultures and beliefs. Wellness activities include silent, meditative walks through the Old City, gentle yoga classes, and holistic wellness assessments. Meals focus on healthy, mindful eating. Breakfast is silent. Monastere. ca/en

•**Kripalu Center for Yoga and Health, Stockbridge, Massachusetts.** This iconic yoga center is the place for yoga and meditation classes—numerous styles of each practice are offered daily—hiking and vegetarian/vegan dining (all meals are served buffet-style, and breakfast is silent). Some poultry and fish are included. Accommodations range from bunk beds in a communal room with a bathroom down the hall to private rooms in the new Annex building. The astoundingly beautiful property is just up the road from the famed Tanglewood concert center. Kripalu.org

•**Red Mountain Resort, Ivins, Utah.** This desert canyon resort, within an hour's drive of Zion National Park, offers the ultimate back-to-nature vacation. Hiking and e-biking are top activities, along with yoga and stretching classes. Guest rooms and villas are available with views of the Utah mountains. You can book an all-inclusive package or opt for accommodation-only rates. RedMountainResort.com

Sleep Medications, Dementia, and Race

Journal of Alzheimer's Disease.

A new study showed that white people who take sleep medications have a higher risk of dementia. In the study, approximately 3,000 older adults without dementia were followed over an average duration of nine years. White participants who "often" or "almost always" took sleep medications had a 79 percent higher chance of developing dementia compared to those who "never" or "rarely" used them. Among Black participants, whose consumption of sleep aids was markedly lower, frequent users had a similar likelihood of developing dementia than those who abstained or rarely used the medications. The researchers found that whites were three times as likely as Blacks to take sleep medications. They were twice as likely to use benzodiazepines, 10 times as likely to take trazodone (Desyrel and Oleptro), and more than seven times as likely to take "Z-drugs," such as Ambien.

CHAPTER 19

Women's Health

How to Find Cancer in Dense Breasts

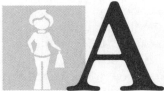About four out of 10 women have dense breasts. Density has nothing to do with size—it just means that dense breasts have more connective tissue than fatty tissue. Women with dense breasts are five times more likely to develop breast cancer than other women.

Denser breasts also make breast cancer harder to find because both cancers and dense connective tissue areas look the same on a mammogram. They both appear as thick white globs. Fatty tissue appears dark and transparent, so tumors show up more easily. In fact, dense breasts reduce the ability of mammograms to find cancer by about 50 percent.

HIGHER RISK AND HARD TO FIND

To learn more about why dense breasts develop more cancers and how to find these cancers on an imaging study, researchers from the Linköping University in Sweden used two technologies. One is an MRI imaging study with a contrast dye that can measure the movement (diffusion) of water molecules through breast tissue. The other is called *microdialysis*. This technology measures the fluid between breast cells, called the microenvironment.

The results of the study are published in the *British Journal of Cancer*. Forty-four women with healthy breasts had their breast density measured by a mammography exam called the Breast Imaging Reporting and Data System (BI-RADS). Breast density in the study

Study titled "Breast Density Is Strongly Associated with Multiparametric Magnetic Resonance Imaging Biomarkers and Pro-Tumorigenic Proteins in Situ," by researchers at Linköping University, Sweden, published in the *British Journal of Cancer*.

group ranged from non-dense to dense. All the women were postmenopausal.

Microdialysis was done by placing a small tube (catheter) into breast tissue to withdraw a fluid sample. The study found that women with dense breasts had higher levels of 124 proteins. These proteins are linked to faster cell growth, more blood vessel growth, and inflammation. All of these factors are associated with cancerous tumor growth. The imaging studies found that breast perfusion (or passage of blood volume) was delayed in dense breasts.

A NEW KIND OF MRI

An MRI picks up more growths (or lesions) in dense breasts than a mammogram, but it cannot determine the difference between a cancerous and noncancerous lesion. The researchers propose that the new imaging technique of an MRI along with perfusion measurement could be a way to identify tumors in dense breasts. This combo type of imaging may also reduce unnecessary biopsies.

A WAY TO LOWER CANCER RISK?

The study also suggests that altering the microenvironment in dense breasts could reduce cancer risk. This could be done by reducing or blocking these proteins. About one-third of women between the ages of 40 and 50 have cells in their breasts that have the potential to become cancerous, but only about one percent of these women develop cancer. This study suggests that density of breast tissue and the microenvironment may be a key to identifying women at risk. Altering the microenvironment may offer new ways to prevent or reduce the risk of breast cancer in dense breasts. The next study for the research team is to find out if anti-inflammatory treatment can change the cancer risk in dense breasts.

What Causes Cognitive Problems in Breast Cancer Survivors?

Study titled "Elevated C-Reactive Protein and Subsequent Patient-Reported Cognitive Problems in Older Breast Cancer Survivors: The Thinking and Living with Cancer Study," by researchers at UCLA's Cousins Center for Psycho-neuroimmunology and Jonsson Comprehensive Cancer Center, Los Angeles, published in *Journal of Clinical Oncology*.

If you're a breast cancer survivor, your memory might not be as sharp as it used to be. Cognitive problems (not just memory loss, but depleted concentration and problem solving) often occur even after the treatment and cancer has ended. Researchers at UCLA have been conducting a long-term study to find out why that happens.

One possible explanation for the brain fade is long-term inflammation that occurs along with cancer survival. To learn more about the link between inflammation and cognitive problems in breast cancer survivors, a team of researchers from UCLA followed 400 breast cancer survivors for up to five years to see if higher levels of inflammation were associated with these cognitive problems. This type of long-term study is called a longitudinal study, and the researchers named it *Thinking and Living with Cancer* (TLC) Study.

Four hundred women age 60 or older participated. The average age was between 67 and 68. All the women were diagnosed with stage 0 to stage 3 breast cancer. These women were compared to a control group of 329 women enrolled and matched for age without breast cancer. Women with a prior diagnosis of cancer, neurologic disease, or dementia were excluded from the study. Results of the TLC study are published in the *Journal of Clinical Oncology*.

To measure their cognitive problems, the women were given a common questionnaire that featured questions about cognitive abilities such as memory and task completion. The test was called the Functional Assessment of Cancer Therapy–Cognitive Function scale.

HOW TO MEASURE INFLAMMATION

To measure inflammation, the women had blood tests for C-reactive protein (CRP). CRP is a protein your liver releases during times of inflammation, such as when your immune system is fighting an infection, injury, or cancer. CRP is also used to diagnose inflammation caused by heart disease. Normally CRP should be low, less than 2 milligrams per liter (mg/L). For example, a higher risk for heart attack starts at 2 mg/L.

All the women had their CRP measured at the start of the study, which was conducted from 2010 through 2020. Women diagnosed with breast cancer had the blood test before they started treatment. Blood tests and cognitive questionnaires were repeated up to six times over five years. *These were the key findings…*

- **Compared to women in the control group,** women with breast cancer had higher CRP levels at the beginning of the study and at 12, 24, and 60 months.

- **Higher CRP results predicted lower cognition marks** on the cognition questionnaire in the breast cancer group.

- **Breast cancer survivors scored 9.5 points lower in the cognition assessment** than the control group when their CRP levels were 3 mg/L and 14.2 points lower when their CRP levels were 10 mg/L.

- **CRP levels were not associated with cognition in the control group.**

- **The strongest evidence of cognitive loss was less ability to complete tasks,** concentrate, and remember things during everyday activities.

CURBING INFLAMMATION AND COGNITIVE DECLINE

The research team concludes that their study supports the role of chronic inflammation in the development of cognitive problems for older women surviving breast cancer. They suggest CRP testing as one way to find or predict cognitive problems at an early stage. Early interventions may then be effective for reducing inflammation and cognitive decline. These interventions might include physical activity, better sleep, and anti-inflammatory medications.

Women Have Gotten Off Track with Cancer Screenings

Compared to 2018, 2.1 million fewer women were screened for breast cancer in 2020, a drop of 6 percent…and 4.5 million fewer women were screened for cervical cancer, an 11 percent drop. Many of those who dropped out of screening still have not resumed. The ripple effects of this gap may take years to manifest fully.

Study by researchers at the American Cancer Society, Atlanta, published in *JAMA Network Open*.

Ultra-Processed Foods Linked to Female Cancers

Study titled "Ultra-Processed Food Consumption, Cancer Risk and Cancer Mortality: A Large-Scale Prospective Analysis Within the U.K. Biobank," led by researchers at Imperial College London, U.K., published in *eClinicalMedicine*.

You've probably heard more than once that whole foods are the way to go for a healthy diet. And science continues to show that this is good advice. There's a growing body of research linking ultra-processed foods (UPFs) to an increased risk for obesity, type 2 diabetes, and heart disease. Now, what has been described as the most comprehensive assessment to date finds an association between ultra-processed foods and the risk for developing cancers, especially breast and ovarian. The review is published in the British medical journal *eClinicalMedicine*. The new study finds a significant link between UPFs and the risk of being diagnosed and dying from cancer.

UPFs are the opposite of whole foods. They are made mostly from the extracted fats, starches, and sugars of foods and may have additives like artificial colors, preservatives, and flavorings. Examples include frozen meals, soft drinks, hot dogs and cold cuts, fast food, packaged cakes or cookies, and salty snacks.

This new study comes from a collaboration of international researchers led by the School of Public Health at Imperial College London. In this observational study, the research team reviewed records of close to 200,000 British adults ages 40 to 69 from the United Kingdom Biobank.

UPFS INCREASE RISK FOR FEMALE CANCERS

Between 2009 and 2012, people in the biobank provided detailed information about their daily diet. They were followed over the next 10 years to compare their intake of UPFs as a percent of their total diet to their risk of being diagnosed or dying from 34 types of cancer.

These were some of the key findings…

•**People in the study reported about 23 percent of their diet was UPFs.**

•**During the follow-up period there were about 16,000 cancers diagnosed and 4,000 cancer deaths.**

•**For every 10 percent increase in UPFs,** the research team found a 2 percent increase in all cancers, including a 19 percent increase in ovarian cancers.

•**They found a 6 percent increase in death from all cancers,** including a 16 percent risk of death from breast cancer, and a 30 percent risk of death from ovarian cancer.

Although this type of observational study does not prove a link between ultra-processed foods and cancer, it is strongly suggestive. The risk of cancer was found after adjusting for other cancer risk factors such as smoking, physical activity, and obesity. *These are some of the ways that UPFs may increase cancer risk…*

•**They are high in salt, fat, and sugar.**

•**They may contain cancer-causing additives or contaminants.**

•**Processing reduces fiber and the availability of important nutrients from whole foods.**

•**Packaging material of these foods may contain cancer causing chemicals that get into processed foods.**

•**Processed foods are dense in calories leading to weight gain and the obesity increased cancer risk.**

UPF INTAKE DANGEROUSLY HIGH IN LOWER-INCOME POPULATIONS

This study found that their participants, which included primarily white and middle-class individuals, consumed about a 23 percent level of ultra-processed foods. In other studies that include minorities and lower-income populations suggest more than 50 percent of the American and U.K. diet is made up of ultra-processed foods.

The global cancer rate has been steadily increasing. Diets high in UPFs are becoming recognized as an important risk factor for cancer, obesity, type 2 diabetes, and heart disease. But these foods are hard to avoid since they're heavily advertised, inexpensive, and convenient. The World Health Organization and the United Nations recommend limiting UPFs as part of a healthy, sustainable diet. The research teams concludes that their study supports a growing body of evidence for the limiting of UPF consumption.

New Hope for Advanced Ovarian Cancer

Study of 76 patients by researchers at Yale Cancer Center, New Haven, Connecticut, and University of Maryland School of Medicine, Baltimore, published in *British Journal of Cancer.*

Ovarian cancer is the most lethal gynecological cancer, and current treatments, such as *ixabepilone* (IXA), have been only limited in effectiveness.

Recent finding: Combining IXA with *bevacizumab* (BEV), an antibody that prevents new blood vessels from forming, improves patient survival and slows further spread of the cancer… and the combined drugs are as well-tolerated as IXA alone.

Vitamin D Could Halt Ovarian Cancer

Kazuhisa Kitami, M.D., Ph.D., researcher of obstetrics and gynecology at Nagoya University School of Medicine, Nagoya, Japan, and lead author of a study published in *Matrix Biology*.

Injections of vitamin D helped prevent ovarian cancer in mice and stopped metastasized cancer from spreading. Vitamin D restores a layer of cells in the peritoneal cavity to their cancer-protective state. While not yet tested in humans, supplementing with up to 2,000 international units (IU) of vitamin D and getting 30 minutes of sunlight daily are considered safe.

Uterine Cancer Deaths Are Up

Victoria Bae-Jump, M.D., Ph.D., director of Lineberger Comprehensive Cancer Center at UNC-Chapel Hill, North Carolina, commenting on a National Cancer Institute study published in *JAMA Oncology*. UNCLineberger.org

Overall rates increased 1.8 percent per year over eight years, while rates from aggressive uterine cancer have risen 2.7 percent per year. Up to 65 percent of women who develop any form of uterine cancer are obese.

Self-defense: Maintain a healthy weight. Postmenopausal women who experience vaginal bleeding and premenopausal women who experience menstrual disruptions should talk to their doctors.

Phthalates Are Linked to Uterine Fibroids

Northwestern University.

Women with a high exposure to certain phthalates—toxic pollutants that are found in food packaging, hair and makeup products, shower curtains, and more—have an elevated risk of symptomatic uterine fibroids. Symptoms can include excessive and uncontrolled uterine bleeding, anemia, miscarriages, infertility, and large abdominal tumors. DEHP, the most widely used phthalate, settles on floors and other surfaces and can accumulate in dust and air.

Women: Watch Antibiotic Intake

Antibiotics for Recurring UTIs Might Backfire

Taking antibiotics for recurring urinary tract infections may predispose women to developing more infections. Repeated cycles of antibiotics only partially clear UTI-causing bacteria from the gut and can cause repeat infections by disrupting the gut microbiome. Those surviving bacteria can then multiply and spread back to the bladder. Women with recurrent UTIs in a clinical trial had less diversity of healthy gut microbial species, which could provide more opportunities for bacteria to gain a foothold and multiply. The microbiomes of women with recurrent UTIs were particularly scarce in bacteria that produce butyrate, a short-chain fatty acid with anti-inflammatory effects.

Washington University School of Medicine.

Antibiotics Linked to Memory Loss in Women

Taking antibiotics for a cumulative total of more than two months during middle age was associated with cognition and memory changes that are typical in women three to four years older.

Best: Take antibiotics only when your doctor thinks them necessary.

Raaj Mehta, M.D., gastroenterologist at Massachusetts General Hospital, Boston, and coleader of a study of 14,542 older women published in *PLOS One*.

Women Have Higher Risk of A-fib

Cedars-Sinai Medical Center.

Science has long shown that men are at greater risk for developing atrial fibrillation (A-fib) than women, but new research shows the opposite. Height is associated with a higher risk of A-fib. Most women are shorter than men, which may explain the perception that their risk is lower. But this study showed that if a man and a woman have the same height, the woman would be 50 percent more likely to develop A-fib. Further, once a woman is diagnosed, she is more likely to experience stroke or heart failure than a man, making prevention exceedingly important. The most effective prevention strategies against A-fib include maintaining a healthy weight, controlling blood pressure, limiting alcohol use, and exercising moderately. Patients diagnosed with the condition can be treated with blood thinners, outpatient procedures such as cardioversion or ablation, or heart surgery.

Blurry Vision? You Might Have Thyroid Eye Disease

Madhura A. Tamhankar, M.D., associate professor of ophthalmology and neurology at the Hospital of the University of Pennsylvania. She is part of a team of physicians who see patients with thyroid eye disease and other complex eye conditions at the Scheie Eye Institute, at Penn Presbyterian Medical Center, Philadelphia. Dr. Tamhankar has worked as a consultant with Horizon Therapeutics, the maker of *Teprotumumab-trbw* (Tepezza).

If you have blurry vision and eyes that are red, dry, or watery, you might suspect anything from allergies to dry eyes. Many eye-care providers might treat your eye problem with antihistamines, artificial tears, or a round of antibiotics. But if your real ailment is a condition called thyroid eye disease (TED)—which has additional signs and symptoms that set it apart from other conditions—such remedies will not get to the root of your problems and, in fact, may exacerbate your symptoms.

Knowing more about this uncommon but potentially devastating eye condition could mean getting the help you need faster. And that could make a lifelong difference in your vision, appearance, and quality of life.

WHAT IS TED?

TED is an autoimmune disease, meaning it's caused by your own immune system attacking tissues in your eyes. About 90 percent of people with TED have harmfully high levels of thyroid hormones, a condition known as hyperthyroidism or Graves' disease, which is caused by an immune attack on the thyroid gland. The immune proteins that target the thyroid gland can also target muscles and fatty tissues surrounding the eyes. TED can develop before or after thyroid hormone levels rise, and rarely some people with TED may have normal thyroid levels. It's even possible to have TED with low thyroid levels.

Thyroid eye disease progresses during an active, initial stage that typically lasts for six months to two years. Some people recover fully after this stage, but others have lingering effects.

SYMPTOMS OF TED

The hallmark of TED is a distinctive change in appearance. The eyes bulge or seem to constantly stare and can get inflamed, and swelling in the back of the eye can push the eyeballs forward. At first, the changes may be subtle, but a doctor who knows what to look for will see a telltale sign: the upper lid will sit higher than the colored part of the eye—like a window shade opened a little too widely. Affected individuals may have a staring, wide-eyed look.

Many people become anxious or depressed about the change in their appearance. They say they don't look or feel like themselves. But TED isn't just a cosmetic issue. *Other signs and symptoms can include...*

•**Dryness or a feeling of grittiness in the eyes.** This results, in part, from the front of the eye being more exposed to air and dust as the eye pushes forward and the eyelids retract.

•**Redness in the eyes** and red, swollen eyelids.

•**Bags around the eyes,** caused by swollen tissues.

•**Pain in or around the eyes,** especially when looking up, down, or sideways.

•**A low tolerance for bright lights.**

•**Difficulty or pain with moving the eyes,** which can result in blurred or double vision. These vision changes can make it hard to drive, read, and do other everyday tasks.

•**Visual loss.** This can happen if the corneas, the clear front windows of the eyes, are severely damaged by extreme dryness or if swelling tissues compress and damage the optic nerve, the cable at the back of each eye that sends visual signals to the brain. These complications happen in a small number of patients.

DIAGNOSIS

If a doctor suspects you have TED, the first step will be to take blood samples to test for thyroid levels and levels of certain antibodies involved in the disease. You might also get some imaging tests, such as an ultrasound, a CT scan, or MRI, so your doctor can look for any changes in the tissues around your eyes.

TREATMENT

Since most people with TED have high thyroid levels, which can cause symptoms such as anxiety, tremors, weight loss, and excess sweating, it's a good idea to see an endocrinologist, a doctor who specializes in hormone disorders. The specialist or a primary care doctor will prescribe treatments to normalize thyroid levels. These can include medications and surgery. Keeping thyroid levels stable and normal is very important and can greatly help the eye symptoms.

One treatment for high thyroid levels, radioactive iodine, has been shown to worsen eye disease in some patients. But doctors can adjust the ways they administer the drug to minimize those effects.

An ophthalmologist, a medical doctor specializing in eye health, can offer additional treatments to address the eye problems associated with TED. Early treatment, during the

---

Risk Factors

Women are much more likely than men to get TED. About half of cases are in people younger than age 43, and half are in older people.

Smoking is a major risk factor: The more cigarettes you smoke, the higher your risk. Quitting lowers the risk.

---

active stage of the disease, can often reverse or limit progression.

If you have mild symptoms, you may get relief with a few simple remedies and lifestyle changes…

•**Artificial tears are available without a prescription.** These can help lubricate the eyes and ease dryness. Some people with more severe dryness may need lubricating ointments or gels.

•**Quitting smoking.** Smoking worsens inflammation, and people who quit after their diagnosis are less likely to progress to more severe symptoms.

•**Dietary changes.** A diet that lowers inflammation throughout the body can make a difference. That means limiting sugar, highly processed foods, and alcohol and loading up on leafy greens, other vegetables, fruits, and whole foods. Foods rich in omega-3 fatty acids, such as fish, and/or nutritional supplements may also help. It's also important to get enough vitamin D.

•**Selenium supplements.** Studies show that taking 200 micrograms of the mineral selenium each day can help reduce TED symptoms. You can get selenium in most multivitamins. (But don't rely on vitamins to make up for a poor diet.)

•**Prism eyeglasses.** These glasses with special lenses can help correct double vision. Sunglasses also can help with light sensitivity.

People with more severe symptoms may need to see an ophthalmology team that specializes in TED and can offer more aggressive treatments…

•**Infusions with a recently approved medication called *teprotumumab-trbw* (Tepezza).** This drug can reduce eye bulging and double vision and may allow many patients who would otherwise need surgery to avoid it. It is given intravenously as eight infusions, spaced three weeks apart. Side effects can include nausea, diarrhea, and muscle spasms. Some people with diabetes see increases in blood sugar, and some patients report hearing loss.

•**Steroid pills or injections.** Drugs such as prednisone can be used temporarily to reduce inflammation and swelling. These drugs can cause mood swings, fluid retention, and other side effects.

•**Radiation.** In some cases, orbital radiation may be used to reduce eye swelling. This therapy is used less commonly today.

•**Surgery.** If the optic nerve is at risk, a procedure to relieve pressure on the nerve, called decompression surgery, may be done while the disease is still in the active stage. In the rehabilitative phase of the disease, decompression surgery can be done to relieve the bulging of the eyes. Eye muscle surgery is performed for double vision and eyelid surgery to improve appearance and function.

Cluster Headaches Are More Severe in Women

Study titled "Sex Differences in Clinical Features, Treatment, and Lifestyle Factors in Patients with Cluster Headache," by researchers at the Karolinska Institute, Stockholm, Sweden, published in *Neurology*.

A cluster headache is as bad as it sounds. It's a rare but very severe type of headache, even worse than migraine pain. Although migraine headaches occur more often in women, cluster headaches are more common in men. In the past, it was thought that these headaches were more frequent in men, but recent research suggests that women experience them more than previously thought. An earlier study by the Karolinska Institute in Sweden suggested that women may get a more severe type of cluster headache, but other research has been mixed when it comes to the differences between the sexes and cluster headaches.

CLUSTER HEADACHES DEFINED

Cluster headaches get their name from their frequency pattern. They come in clusters lasting weeks or months. There may be up to eight attacks per day lasting from 30 to 45 minutes. The headaches eventually stop for months or years. For some people, the attacks can return within a few months. This is called a chronic cluster headache. A new study from Karolinska Institute, in Stockholm, Sweden, is the largest survey of data on sex differences in cluster headaches to date. The findings are published in the journal *Neurology.*

The main symptom of a cluster headache is severe one-sided head pain that comes on quickly. The pain is centered around one eye. Other symptoms include one-sided nasal congestion, pain radiating to one side of the face and head, a drooping eyelid, and restlessness. The new study looked at the differences between men and women in 874 patients diagnosed with cluster headache from 2014 to 2020.

WOMEN EXPERIENCE SEVERE CLUSTER HEADACHE SYMPTOMS

Patients answered a detailed questionnaire about their symptoms, triggers, treatment, and lifestyle. Sixty-six percent of the patients were men. *These were the key results…*

•**Women were more likely to have chronic type cluster headaches than men** (18 percent for women vs. 9 percent for men).

•**Women had longer bouts of headaches and were more likely to use treatment to prevent headaches** (60 percent to 48 percent).

•**Women were more likely to have drooping eyelids, called ptosis** (61 percent to 47 percent).

•**Women were more likely to experience restlessness** (54 percent to 46 percent).

•**Women were more likely to have a family history of cluster headaches** (15 percent to 7 percent).

•**Women were more likely to have a daily pattern of attacks** (74 percent to 63 percent).

Other differences included women being less likely to have attacks triggered by drinking alcohol and more likely to have headaches triggered by loss of sleep. The researchers conclude that these significant differences between men and women can help doctors diagnose and choose treatment for women as well as predict the prognosis of their cluster headaches. They plan to do future studies using a biobank of 900 DNA samples to learn more about the cause and treatment of these debilitating headaches.

Cluster headaches occur in about one out of 500 people. Men experience them at roughly a three-to-one ratio. The average age at which these headaches start is 20 to 40 years. In addition to alcohol and sleep deprivation, other triggers include smoking and sleep apnea. The cause is unknown but thought to be linked to the biologic (circadian) clock controlled by an area of the brain called the hypothalamus. There is no cure for cluster headaches, but medications can help stop an attack and reduce the number of episodes.

Vegetarian Diets Increase Hip Fracture Risk in Women

Study titled "Risk of Hip Fracture in Meat-Eaters, Pescatarians, and Vegetarians: Results from the U.K. Women's Cohort Study," by researchers at the University of Leeds, Woodhouse, England, published in *BMC Medicine*.

Both vegetarian diets and hip fractures are becoming more common with women. In the U.S., about 5 percent of the population practices meat-free eating. Unfortunately, it might not be the right dietary choice for women who need to protect their bones, according to a recent study.

DIET AFFECTS HIP HEALTH

Hip fractures are the most common type of fracture in older women, and these injuries have a huge impact on long-term health and quality of life. Recognizing this fact, researchers from the School of Food Science and Nutrition at University of Leeds in the U.K. compared the risk of hip fracture in women during a specific age span. The women were divided into groups based on their diets. The groups included vegetarians (vegans were combined with vegetarians due to the small number of participants), occasional meat-eaters, regular meat-eaters, and women who did not eat meat, but did eat fish (pescatarians). The only diet associated with a higher risk of hip fracture was the vegetarian diet. The results of the study are published in *BMC Medicine*.

The study included more than 26,000 women living in the U.K. between ages 35 and 69. Their diet groups were based on a 217-item food frequency questionnaire that the women began between 1995 and 1998. Women who ate meat five or more times per week were in the regular meat-eater group. Women who ate meat less than five times per week were placed in the occasional meat-eater group. Using hospital records, the researchers identified 822 hip fractures over about 20 years in these women. Hip fractures occurred in 3 percent of the women.

The key finding of the study was that after adjusting for other hip fracture risks such as smoking and age, women on a vegetarian diet had a 33 percent higher risk of hip fracture than women who were regular meat eaters. None of the other diets had any association with an increased or decreased risk of hip fracture.

WHY BECOME A VEGETARIAN?

Many people switch to a vegetarian diet because they believe it to be healthier than an omnivorous plan. And several studies support this view—people on vegetarian diets show a reduced risk of chronic diseases such as diabetes, heart disease and cancer. Another benefit is environmental. Vegetarians produce a lower carbon footprint that will hopefully reduce global warming.

WHY STRICTLY PLANT BASED MIGHT HURT OUR BONES

In the U.K, about 6 percent of the population follows a vegetarian diet. Although healthier in some ways, studies also show that a diet without animal protein from fish or meat is associated with lower bone mineral density. This may result in weaker bones that can break easily. Loss of mineral density may be due to a lack of proteins and nutrients such as calcium, vitamin D, vitamin B_{12}, and omega-3 fatty acids that are more abundant in animal products than in plants.

Another factor that may contribute to fractures in vegetarians is body mass index (BMI). BMI is a measure of body fat based on height and weight. Vegetarians tend to have a lower BMI than meat eaters and low BMI has been associated with a higher risk for hip fractures. A nutrient that may also be deficient in vegetarian diets and add to the risk of hip fracture is insulin-like growth factor (IGF-1).

The research team concludes that vegetarians are at a higher risk for hip fracture than regular meat eaters. This does not mean that they encourage women to abandon vegetarian diets. They call for further research to confirm their findings and to find out if vegetarian diets in men also increase hip fractures. They would like to see further research into the role of BMI and how specific nutrients in animal-based foods

that reduce fracture risks could be replaced in a vegetarian diet. These studies could lead to effective interventions to reduce hip fractures in people on vegetarian diets.

Unpaid Labor Affects Women's Mental Health

Study of 70,000 people by researchers at the University of Melbourne, Australia, published in *The Lancet Public Health*.

Women are more often diagnosed with depression and anxiety, and new research suggests one reason why.

Recent finding: The burden of housework, child rearing, and elder care falls more heavily on women than men even when women are holding down a paying job...and the more of this unpaid work women do, the worse their mental (and sometimes physical) health.

Women Make More Inflation-Driven Adjustments to Their Lifestyles Than Men Do

BMO Real Financial Progress Index by Bank of Montreal. BMO.com

Forty-seven percent of women say they adjust or will adjust how they shop for groceries, compared with 36 percent of men...49 percent of women say they will dine out less, versus 43 percent of men...25 percent of women say they will cancel subscriptions, versus 20 percent of men. In all, 80 percent of Americans are changing their actions to offset the impact of inflation—including 31 percent who are driving less because of the cost of fuel and 23 percent who are spending less on vacations or forgoing them completely. One-quarter of Americans say they will need to delay retirement...36 percent have reduced their savings...and 21 percent have reduced retirement savings.

Dietary Changes May Reduce the Risk of Hip Fracture in Women

An observational study of 26,000 women found that eating 25 grams of additional protein each day cut the risk of hip fracture by 14 percent. Further, every cup of tea or coffee reduced risk by 4 percent. Both drinks contain biologically active compounds called *polyphenols* and *phytoestrogens* that may help to maintain bone health. In a separate study, researchers found that women who ate more than 100 daily micrograms (mcg) of vitamin K_1 were 31 percent less likely to have any fracture, compared with participants who consumed less than 60 mcg per day. One to two servings of vegetables such as spinach, kale, broccoli, and cabbage provide ample vitamin K_1.

University of Leeds, Edith Cowan University.

Index